Prevention Effectiveness

Prevention Effectiveness

A Guide to Decision Analysis and Economic Evaluation

SECOND EDITION

Edited by

ANNE C. HADDIX, Ph.D.

STEVEN M. TEUTSCH, M.D., M.P.H.

PHAEDRA S. CORSO, Ph.D.

OXFORD
UNIVERSITY PRESS
2003

OXFORD

UNIVERSITY PRESS

Oxford   New York
Auckland   Bangkok   Buenos Aires   Cape Town   Chennai
Dar es Salaam   Delhi   Hong Kong   Istanbul   Karachi   Kolkata
Kuala Lumpur   Madrid   Melbourne   Mexico City   Mumbai   Nairobi
São Paulo   Shanghai   Singapore   Taipei   Tokyo   Toronto

Copyright © 2003 by Oxford Univesity Press, Inc.

Published by Oxford University Press, Inc.
198 Madison Avenue, New York, New York, 10016

http://www.oup-usa.org

Oxford is a registered trademark of Oxford University Press

Library of Congress Cataloging-in-Publication data
Prevention effectiveness : a guide to decision analysis and economic evaluation /
edited by Anne C. Haddix, Steven M. Teutsch, Phaedra S. Corso.—2nd ed.
p. cm.
Includes bibliographical references and index.
ISBN 0-19-514897-5
1. Medicine, Preventive—Evaluation. 2. Medicine, Preventive—Decision making.
3. Medicine, Preventive—Cost effectiveness—Evaluation.
4. Medicine, Preventive—Economic aspects.
I. Haddix, Anne C. II. Teutsch, Steven M. III. Corso, Phaedra S.
RA427 .M385   2002
614.4—dc21   2002022446

9 8 7 6 5 4 3 2 1

Printed in the United States of America
on acid-free paper

This book is dedicated to the employees of
the Centers for Disease Control and Prevention,
who work tirelessly to protect
and improve the quality
of human life

Foreword

Two questions above all must be addressed by those who favor more preventive interventions to improve the health of our population. The first is "What works?" The second and tougher question is "What works *best* to solve a defined problem?" This slim volume gives an essential road map for answering these two bedeviling though deceptively simple queries.

Prevention approaches for ameliorating a specific health problem range widely. Consider, for example, the growing toll of type 2 (adult onset) diabetes mellitus. It ranks high as a cause of premature mortality, disability, and excess health-care costs.[1] Are there preventive approaches available that can reduce the health and economic consequences? If so, how are they partitioned among primary prevention (health promotion), secondary prevention (screening, diagnosis, and prevention-oriented therapies), and tertiary prevention (treatment to prevent or postpone complications)? Potentially effective approaches might be found in federal, state, or local policy; in community health-improvement programs; or in computer-based programs to help patients improve health habits in areas like nutrition and physical activity.

In one aspect of this complex puzzle of causality and prevention effectiveness, there is strong evidence that increased physical activity in adults can reduce the risk of developing diabetes. This is true whether applied to the overall population or to the subset at higher risk due to family history and overweight/obesity.[2,3] However, getting people to increase their physical activity is not a simple matter. We are left to ponder what are the best strategies, ranging from worksite fitness programs to getting parents to turn off the TV, computers, and video games that their children are overusing. How to identify reasonable alternatives and select the best approach, through systematic searches for evidence using standard methods, is the road map this volume provides. Its distinguished authors offer an excellent primer on how to think about this common but complex problem, to analyze the available data, and to draw reasonable inferences. Analysis of this type is essential if decision makers in health-care organizations and public health, education, and other governmental agencies, including Congress and state and local elected officials, are to make better decisions about where to invest time, money, and political capital.

Knowing what can work is often not sufficient to guide decisions because choices need to be made among the set of effective interventions. If you cannot do everything, where do you start? Answering this question requires marrying analysis of effectiveness with economic analysis, as the authors have admirably shown in the second part of this volume. What are the relative costs and returns, in dollars or health, of alternative investments to achieve the same goal? Precise answers to these questions are not easy to acquire. Yet the research and discovery process often reveals differences in likely returns on investment using common-sense assumptions for missing variables. Moreover, the analytic process uncovers gaps in knowledge that additional research can remedy.

The practical benefit of using the recommended approaches to determine prevention effectiveness and return on investment is large. If decision makers take heed and utilize the results of the best analyses of which we are capable today, significant reductions in the toll of major diseases and other health conditions are achievable, as are improvements in the cost effectiveness of our health-care and public health systems.

Nonetheless, we should heed the authors' admonitions not to oversell the value of these techniques, and we need to continue to refine both methods and the data on which they are based for all types of preventive maneuver. Efforts are growing to distill the data on effectiveness and cost effectiveness and to develop actionable recommendations for clinicians and public health decision makers. For example, Partnership for Prevention has used these approaches to prioritize clinical preventive services,[4] and the British Medical Journal Publishing Group has published five issues of the eminently useful *Clinical Evidence*, a compilation of effectiveness literature relevant to clinical practice.[5]

However, even consistent findings from randomized control trials do not prove that clinical interventions are the most effective or the most cost–effective real-world strategies to address a clinical problem. We need more of those still rare analyses that cut across clinical and population-based interventions and combine economic with effectiveness analysis.

As evidence-based decision making becomes the mantra for those charged with the responsibility for population and clinical prevention, so does the necessity of frequent updates. A review of the current validity of 17 clinical practice guidelines published by the U.S. Agency for Healthcare Research and Quality found that for seven new evidence and expert judgment indicated that a major update was required and that six needed at least a minor update.[6]

A particularly valuable piece of advice in this book is to think hard about the question one wants to ask and consider alternatives. This is the first item on the checklist for evaluating a decision analysis. In our diabetes example, an increase in physical activity was identified as a high-priority intervention to reduce the health and economic toll of the disease. This was a correct answer to our question, but did we ask the right question? Did we fall prey to the common mistake of partitioning the world of effectiveness research into various disease states? A more important public policy question may be the overall health effectiveness of a particular investment in physical activity improvement versus a comparable investment in enhanced clinical control of diabetes. Analysis of physical activity promotion solely as an effective prevention strategy for diabetes ignores the effectiveness of more exercise in improving other health outcomes, depreciating its true health impact. Increased physical activity also reduces blood pressure and coronary artery disease, permits better function for many arthritics, and enhances cognitive ability in older adults.

Even if we limit our focus to what is effective at reducing the toll of diabetes, we could benefit from a broad view of its determinants in populations, from physiological factors and individual lifestyle influences to broader environmental factors such as occupation and geographic locale as well as overarching social structures that are likely to be affected only by macro policy decisions.[7] What we ask is at least as important as how we find the answer. The thoughtful approaches in this book help with both questions.

Jonathan E. Fielding

REFERENCES

1. Centers for Disease Control and Prevention. *Diabetes: A Serious Public Health Problem, 2001.* Atlanta: CDC, 2001. Available from http://www.cdc.gov/diabetes/pubs/pdf/diabete.pdf.
2. Tuomilehto J, Lindstrom J, Eriksson JG, et al. Prevention of type 2 diabetes mellitus by changes in lifestyle among subjects with impaired glucose tolerance. *N Engl J Med 2001;* 344:1343–50.
3. Task Force on Community Preventive Services. Strategies for reducing morbidity and mortality from diabetes through health-care system interventions and diabetes self-management education in community settings. A report on recommendations of the Task Force on Community Preventive Services. *MMWR Morb Mortal Wkly Rep 2001;* 50:1–15.
4. Coffield AB, Maciosek MV, McGinnis JM, et al. Priorities among recommended clinical preventive services. *Am J Prev Med 2001;* 21:1–9.
5. Barton, S. *Clinical Evidence.* London: British Medical Publishing Group, 2001.
6. Shekelle PG, Ortiz E, Rhodes S, et al. Validity of the Agency for Healthcare Research and Quality clinical practice guidelines. *JAMA 2001;* 286:1461–7.
7. McKinlay J, Marceau L. US public health and the 21st century: diabetes mellitus. *Lancet 2000;* 356:757–61.

Preface

As public accountability has increased and resources have become scarcer, public health, like clinical medicine, has been forced to reexamine the benefits and costs of its activities to assure that it implements effective interventions and allocates resources efficiently. Decision and economic analyses are basic tools in carrying out that mission. These methods have become standard practice in clinical medicine and health-services research. This book was written in an effort to apply and adapt that experience to public health situations.

The book was originally written to introduce Centers for Disease Control and Prevention staff to the concepts of decision and economic analyses, to provide guidance on methods to maximize comparability of studies, and to provide access to frequently used reference information. It has been adapted to meet the needs of scientists and managers in state and local health departments and managed-care organizations as well as students in schools of public health and clinicians for an introductory text, a text that shows how these methods can be applied in population-based practice; to facilitate better comparability of studies; and to solidify understanding of the scientific basis for use of these tools in decision making. Decision makers will learn how these studies are conducted so they can be critical consumers—understanding the strengths and limitations—and apply findings to policy and practice.

The second edition updates and expands the standard methodology for conducting prevention-effectiveness analyses. The book has been reorganized. Following the introduction, Chapters 2 through 6 provide the individual components of a prevention study, Chapters 7 through 9 integrate those components into decision analysis and economic evaluations, and Chapter 10 addresses the critical issue of how to make the information actionable by decision makers. The appendices provide valuable reference resources for conducting studies. Each chapter has been revised or rewritten. In particular, the chapters on measuring effectiveness (Chapter 3), decision analysis (Chapter 7), and making information useful for decision makers (Chapter 10) as well as several appendices are entirely new. The chapters on cost, time preference, cost–benefit analysis, and appendices have had substantial revision and updates. The recommendations throughout the book are now consistent with those made by the Panel on Cost Effectiveness in Health and Medicine.[1]

Prevention-effectiveness studies have three essential steps: (1) framing the study, (2) structuring the decision model, and (3) analyzing the model and interpreting the results. The steps must be completed in order, and it is especially important that the first two steps are done thoroughly and carefully.

Each chapter provides an introduction to the methods and options for conducting a prevention-effectiveness study and the basic concepts, underlying principles, and rationales for choosing among alternative approaches. The recommendations presented in each chapter are especially important. Use of the recommendations will increase the credibility of prevention-effectiveness studies and enhance the comparability of results across studies.

Prevention effectiveness is the systematic assessment of the impact of public health policies, programs, and practices on health outcomes. Chapter 1 gives an overview of the application of prevention effectiveness to public health problems and introduces readers to the methodology.

The first step in any prevention-effectiveness study, whether a decision analysis or an economic evaluation, is the framing of the study. This step is critical to the entire process of prevention-effectiveness research. Chapter 2 identifies key issues that must be addressed before structuring and analyzing a problem. Each issue is discussed and recommendations are made where appropriate. The chapter concludes by providing a useful checklist for evaluating a prevention-effectiveness study, protocol, or scope of work.

Chapter 3 examines the measures of effectiveness that can be used in prevention-effectiveness studies. These are the probabilities that link an intervention to a health outcome. Many of the variables common to prevention-effectiveness models are identified, including characteristics of the population, screening, preventability, and risk. The chapter concludes with a catalog of sources for obtaining estimates of variable values. This chapter also presents the concepts of study design and quality-of-evidence methods that will be of particular value for readers less familiar with these concepts.

Chapter 4 defines costs, describes methods for measuring the cost of prevention interventions, and discusses cost-of-illness methods for assessing the value of health outcomes. A method for estimating intervention costs is presented that includes a set of worksheets for cost inventory and analysis.

Chapter 5 discusses why and how quality-adjusted life years (QALYs) are measured, identifies sources of data for measuring quality adjustments, and provides an example of using QALYs in a cost–utility analysis. The usefulness, limitations, and alternatives to the QALY model are also discussed.

Chapter 6 addresses time preference and the adjusting of costs and benefits in a multiperiod model. The methods for discounting, inflating, and annuitizing costs and benefits are presented. Discounting of both monetary and nonmonetary costs and benefits is discussed.

Chapter 7 presents the theoretical basis for decision analysis, explains when and how to do a decision analysis, and discusses how to evaluate the results. Addressing uncertainty with sensitivity analysis is also explained and illustrated. Some benefits of using decision analysis in public health are also addressed.

Cost–benefit analysis (CBA) attempts to weigh all of the impacts of a prevention intervention, valued in monetary terms, for the purpose of assessing whether the benefits exceed the costs. Chapter 8 discusses the theoretical basis for CBA, describes the method for conducting a CBA within the decision-analytic framework described in the book, and discusses the two most common summary measures derived from a CBA. Two approaches to estimating the cost of health outcomes are compared: willingness to pay and cost of illness. Alternative techniques to measure willingness to pay are explored. The chapter concludes with a discussion of the usefulness and limitations of CBA in evaluating public health programs.

Cost–effectiveness analysis (CEA) looks at the cost per unit of health outcome for all intervention options available. It is the most frequently used technique to compare alternative treatment courses or interventions. Chapter 9 addresses data requirements for conducting CEAs, provides guidelines for identifying interventions and health outcomes, and discusses the interpretation of CEA results. The cost-of-illness approach for estimating health-outcome costs is presented, including estimation of medical and nonmedical costs and productivity losses. The limitations of CEA are discussed. Cost–utility analysis is a special kind of CEA in which the health outcome is measured in standardized quality adjusted units, such as QALYs.

Chapter 10, new to this edition, examines the use of prevention-effectiveness studies in public health decision making. This chapter focuses on some of the common issues that underlie reluctance to use economic evaluations and decision analyses, efforts to address these problems, and recommendations for analysts to facilitate the use of prevention-effectiveness studies by public health decision makers.

A set of appendices follows the main body of the book. These appendices are meant to provide practical information for undertaking a prevention-effectiveness study. Included in the appendices are a glossary; a compilation of the recommendations interspersed throughout the book; a catalog of software for decision and economic analyses; a cost–effectiveness case study; a list of sources for cost-of-illness data; a table with 2000 statewide average operating cost-to-charge ratios for urban and rural hospitals; discount and annuity factor tables; the Consumer Price Index (1960–2000), including the Medical Care and Medical Care Services components; and updated productivity loss tables. Based on the 2000 U.S. census data and shown by age and gender, these tables are included so that estimation of productivity losses can be standardized in prevention-effectiveness studies.

As prevention-effectiveness methods are applied with increasing frequency, our understanding of how they can be used most effectively will continue to be refined. We invited our readers to comment on the book's content, user friendliness, and orientation of the first edition. We have incorporated many of those suggestions in this edition. We extend the invitation for feedback again.

Atlanta, Georgia   A. C. H.
West Point, Pennsylvania   S. M. T.
Atlanta, Georgia   P. S. C.

REFERENCES

1. Gold et al. *Cost–Effectiveness in Health and Medicine.* New York: Oxford University Press, 1996.

Acknowledgments

The editors express their appreciation to William L. Roper, MD, MPH, former Director of CDC, who provided the initial leadership for prevention-effectiveness research at CDC.

We thank the federal and nonfederal experts who reviewed the first edition of *Prevention Effectiveness: A Guide to Decision Analysis and Economic Evaluation*. The workshop held in Atlanta, Georgia, in 1993 served as a forum for establishing the methodological foundation for this book.

We also thank Vilma Carande-Kulis, PhD, and Bill Lawrence, MD, MPH, for their comments on various chapters in the second edition and Lexie Walker for preparing many of the tables and figures.

While reviewers' comments and suggestions were of tremendous assistance, the authors and editors are responsible for the final content.

Contents

Contributors, xix

1. Introduction, 1
   Steven M. Teutsch, Jeffrey R. Harris

2. Study Design, 11
   Paul G. Farnham, Anne C. Haddix

3. Measuring Effectiveness, 28
   K. Robin Yabroff, Jeanne Mandelblatt

4. Costs, 53
   Anne C. Haddix, Phaedra S. Corso, Robin D. Gorsky

5. Quality of Life, 77
   Erik J. Dasbach, Steven M. Teutsch

6. Time Effects, 92
   Phaedra S. Corso, Anne C. Haddix

7. Decision Analysis, 103
   Sue J. Goldie, Phaedra S. Corso

8. Cost–Benefit Analysis, 127
   Mark Messonnier, Martin Meltzer

9. Cost–Effectiveness Analysis, 156
   Thomas L. Gift, Anne C. Haddix, Phaedra S. Corso

10. Using Economic Evaluations in Decision Making, 178
    Joanna E. Siegel, Carolyn M. Clancy

Appendices

A. Glossary, 199

B. Recommendations, 211

C. Software, 214
   Richard D. Rheingans

D. Worked Example: Cost–Effectiveness of Postexposure Prophylaxis Following
   Sexual Exposure to Human Immunodeficiency Virus, 217
   Harrell W. Chesson, Steven D. Pinkerton

E. Sources for Collecting Cost-of-Illness Data, 232
   Laurie A. Ferrell

F. Cost-to-Charge Ratios, 239

G. Discount and Annuitization Tables, 241

H. Consumer Price Index, 244

I. Productivity Loss Tables, 245
   Scott D. Grosse

   Index, 259

Contributors

HARRELL W. CHESSON, PhD
Economist
Division of STD Prevention
National Center for HIV, STD, and TB
Prevention
CDC

CAROLYN M. CLANCY, MD
Acting Director
Agency for Healthcare Research and
Quality

PHAEDRA S. CORSO, PhD, MPA
Health Economist
Prevention Effectiveness Branch
Epidemiology Program Office
CDC

ERIK J. DASBACH, PhD
Director
Health Economic Statistics
Biostatistics and Research Decision Sciences
Merck Research Laboratories

PAUL G. FARNHAM, PhD
Associate Professor
Department of Economics
Andrew Young School of Policy Studies
Georgia State University

LAURIE A. FERRELL, MPH
Senior Financial Analyst
Rollins School of Public Health
Emory University

JONATHAN FIELDING, MD, MPH,
MBA
Professor of Health Services and Pediatrics
School of Public Health
University of California
Director of Public Health and Health Officer
Department of Health Services
County of Los Angeles

THOMAS L. GIFT, PhD
Health Economist
Division of STD Prevention
National Center for HIV, STD, and TB
Prevention
CDC

SUE J. GOLDIE, MD, MPH
Assistant Professor of Health Policy and
Decision Science
Center for Risk Analysis
Department of Health Policy and
Management
Harvard School of Public Health

ROBIN D. GORSKY, PhD†
Associate Professor
University of New Hampshire

SCOTT D. GROSSE, PhD
Economist
Office of the Director
National Center on Birth Defects and
Developmental Disabilities
CDC

†Deceased

ANNE C. HADDIX, PhD
Associate Professor of Health Economics
Department of International Health
Rollins School of Public Health
Emory University

JEFFREY R. HARRIS, MD, MPH
Senior Lecturer
Health Promotion Research Center
Department of Health Services
University of Washington School of
  Community Medicine and Public Health

JEANNE MANDELBLATT, MD, MPH
Professor
Department of Oncology and
  Medicine
Georgetown University Medical Center
Director
Cancer Control Program
Lombardi Cancer Center
Georgetown University

MARTIN MELTZER, PhD
Economist
Office of Surveillance
National Center for Infectious Diseases
CDC

MARK MESSONNIER, PhD
Economist

STEVEN D. PINKERTON, PhD
Associate Professor of Psychiatry and
  Behavioral Medicine
Center for AIDS Intervention Research
Department of Psychiatry and Behavioral
  Medicine
Medical College of Wisconsin

RICHARD D. RHEINGANS, DFES
Assistant Professor of Health and
  Environmental Economics
Department of International Health
Rollins School of Public Health
Emory University

JOANNA E. SIEGEL, ScD
Director
Research Initiative in Clinical Economics
  Center
Center for Outcomes and Effectiveness Research
Agency for Healthcare Research and Quality

STEVEN M. TEUTSCH, MD MPH
Senior Director
Outcomes Research and Management
Merck & Co., Inc.

K. ROBIN YABROFF, PhD, MBA
Research Assistant Professor
Cancer Control Program
Lombardi Cancer Center
Georgetown University

Prevention Effectiveness

1

Introduction

STEVEN M. TEUTSCH
JEFFREY R. HARRIS

Prevention effectiveness studies assess the impact of public health policies, pro grams, and practices on health outcomes[1] by determining their effectiveness, safety, and cost. The roots of prevention effectiveness lie in the assessment of medical technology and in research on health services and outcomes and build on operations research, epidemiology, statistics, economics, psychology, and other decision sciences. The results of prevention-effectiveness studies provide a basis for recommendations regarding public health programs, guidelines for prevention and control, and decision making about resource allocations; they are at the core of evidence-based public health. Sound decisions require timely, high-quality, comparable, and appropriately directed information. Prevention-effectiveness studies can provide this information.

For many years, particularly in the arena of medical care, it was sufficient to show that the benefits of a technology exceed its harms before using it. Now, in a world of limited resources for public health, officials must use resources as efficiently as possible and must demonstrate that a technology delivers value for the resources expended. By the same token, policies and programs should also be scrutinized for the value they deliver.

Prevention-effectiveness studies help meet these goals. They provide a systematic approach to organizing the available information about prevention strategies so that policy makers can have a scientific framework for making decisions. The concept pulls together information from epidemiology and public health surveillance, intervention studies, and economic analyses, using direct evidence when available and indirect evidence when necessary. It addresses basic questions, such as the following:

- What is the magnitude of the problem addressed by the prevention strategy (burden of illness and injury, descriptive epidemiology, and public health surveillance)?
- Can the intervention work (efficacy)?
- Does the intervention work (effectiveness)?

- What are the benefits and harms of the intervention (net benefits)?
- What does the intervention cost (cost analysis)?
- How do the benefits compare with the costs (cost–effectiveness, cost–benefit, and cost–utility analyses)?
- What additional benefit could be obtained with additional resources (marginal and incremental analyses)?

CONCEPTUAL MODEL FOR THE DEVELOPMENT OF PREVENTION STRATEGIES

Public health strategies evolve from basic science and applied research through community demonstrations into widespread use (Fig. 1.1). The information available at each stage and the methods for analyzing and synthesizing that information differ.

Information on biological risk factors is derived from basic research. Bench and epidemiologic research identify risk factors and the magnitude of their impact, as well as the biological and social underpinnings of disease and injury. Understanding these risk factors focuses attention on initial targets for potential intervention programs. Once major risk factors are identified (e.g., hypercholesterolemia for myocardial infarction, use of seat belts for automobile-crash injuries, or social isolation for mental health), potential interventions can be developed. Applied research, such as randomized controlled trials, can be conducted to provide information on the efficacy of these interventions. Research on efficacy shows the degree to which intervention strategies can work under idealized conditions with carefully selected populations and, in many cases, optimal resources.

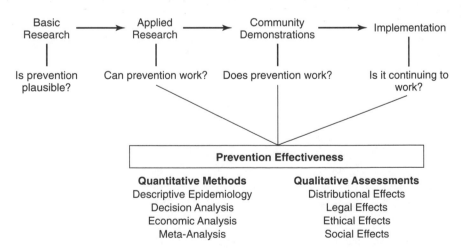

Figure 1.1   Development and implementation of prevention strategies and the role of prevention effectiveness. *Source*: Teutsch, SM. A framework for assessing the effectiveness of disease and injury prevention. MMWR 1992: 41 (No. RR-3).

After determining which strategies are efficacious, the next step is to determine how well these strategies actually work in community settings. Such community-based demonstrations are used to assess the real-world effectiveness of the prevention strategy. We define *effectiveness* as the impact that an intervention achieves in the real world under practical resource constraints in an entire unselected population or in specified subgroups of a population. It is axiomatic that effectiveness so defined will almost certainly be lower than efficacy because of resource constraints, individual adherence, and coverage of an intervention strategy, although there are some exceptions, such as herd immunity from immunizations.

Effectiveness research is outcome-oriented. Rather than focusing on the process of disease prevention and control (e.g., measuring how many people receive an intervention), prevention-effectiveness research seeks to directly link the intervention with the health outcome of interest (e.g., mortality, quality of life, or functional status). In this respect, the focus of prevention-effectiveness research differs from that of program evaluation. A prevention-effectiveness study would show, for example, how mortality is decreased by a particular intervention rather than how an intervention was administered.

As prevention strategies are implemented more widely, there is a growing need to maximize the intended impact with the resources available or to obtain a particular impact with as little expenditure of resources as possible. Thus, the efficiency of various approaches needs to be examined. There are always competing uses for resources, so the opportunity costs for each of our choices must be considered.

We enter the domain of prevention effectiveness as the results of applied research begin to demonstrate the efficacy of intervention strategies, including technologies, policies, and programs. The process continues throughout the development of the intervention into practical public health tools and their application in real settings (Fig. 1.1). Various methods are available for use at each stage of development and implementation.

TRADITIONAL APPROACHES

Attributable Risk and Prevented Fraction

In assessing an intervention strategy, one must know what it can realistically accomplish in terms of health outcomes. The first evidence usually comes from research on cause-and-effect relationships associated with health problems, in which the link between a risk factor and an outcome is identified, for example, the relationship between hypertension and coronary artery disease. The *relative risk* associated with the risk factor provides a traditional epidemiological measure of the potential impact. However, the overall public health impact is based not only on the relative risk but also on the frequency at which the condition occurs in the population. The impact is measured in terms of *attributable risk*, a measure of the amount of disease or injury that could be eliminated if the risk factor never occurred in a given population. It is the maximal limit of disease or injury that could be averted by avoiding a particular risk factor. In that sense, it is analogous to efficacy (i.e., what could be achieved under ideal circumstances). In contrast, the *prevented fraction* is a measure of the amount of a health problem that has actually been avoided by a prevention strategy and reflects what can be achieved in a real-world setting (i.e., it is analogous to effectiveness).

Program Evaluation and Prevention Effectiveness

Program evaluation supports prevention-effectiveness research. *Program evaluation* assesses the structure, processes, and outcomes of intervention programs, with particular attention paid to the purposes and expectations of stakeholders.[2] Research on evaluation includes a complex array of experimental and quasi-experimental designs. These methods form the basis for determining the effectiveness and efficiency of prevention strategies by providing data on how programs are implemented and consumed.

ADDITIONAL METHODS FOR PREVENTION EFFECTIVENESS

Decision Models

Models are useful in conducting prevention-effectiveness studies, especially when evidence of effectiveness is indirect or uncertain. In some instances, a prevention strategy demonstrably improves a health outcome, and direct evidence of this is available. For example, mammography screening and follow-up for women over 50 years of age have been confirmed to reduce mortality from breast cancer. In many instances, however, such direct effects cannot be measured. When they cannot, we must rely on indirect evidence of the effectiveness of an intervention. For example, former smokers have lowered their risk of lung cancer, yet no studies have been conducted to show that a specific smoking-cessation strategy prevents lung cancer. A model would rely on indirect evidence that the smoking-cessation strategy decreases smoking and on the knowledge that cessation decreases the risk of developing lung cancer. Such indirect evidence can be used with confidence because each link in the chain of causality can be clearly documented.

Models can be very helpful in making assumptions explicit and in forcing examination of the logic, coherence, and evidence for each step in the process. The evidence for each step should be assessed using systematic methods and rules of evidence, such as systematic evidence reviews and, where needed, meta-analyses (see Chapters 3 and 10). Although assessments can also include literature reviews or the consensus of experts, such approaches may be subject to bias unless the rules of evidence are followed uniformly.

In addition to structuring effectiveness studies, models are useful in structuring other types of analysis. A basic decision analysis uses a decision-tree model to compare alternate strategies (see Chapter 7). Decision trees include information about the likelihood of each outcome (probabilities) and can incorporate preferences (utilities) or costs or both for different outcomes. Other approaches model more complex situations, such as infectious disease transmission. Markov models define sets of probabilities for transitions among health states for each intervention to assess how outcomes are affected, Monte Carlo simulations provide a probabilistic approach, mathematical models incorporate complex mathematical relationships, and microsimulation attempts to replicate details of clinical processes.

In decision trees and other models, sensitivity analyses permit assessment of values for which there is uncertainty. Sensitivity analyses can identify critical steps that are likely to make a substantial difference in choosing one strategy over another.

Modeling may help to identify the important issues for which data are needed and thereby help to formulate a research agenda; it may also pinpoint issues for which more precise estimates will not affect a decision. Economic analyses are often based on such models. The use of models makes the decision process explicit and can help to clarify the criteria upon which decisions are based.

Economic Models

Resources are always constrained. Economics provides a range of tools to understand how resources are allocated as well as to help make choices about future allocation. The methods discussed in this volume are cost–benefit, cost–effectiveness, and cost–utility analyses. Each method allows comparison of different intervention strategies based on the resources they consume and the outputs they generate. Each requires a careful cost analysis (i.e., identification of costs associated with a prevention activity) and assessment of outcomes, both harms and benefits. The scope of an analysis usually determines the appropriate analytical method and range of consequences to consider. Cost–benefit analysis includes all costs, benefits, and harms and values them in dollars or another monetary unit. It includes costs of programs, costs to patients and others such as medical costs, direct out-of-pocket expenses, productivity and leisure losses, and intangible costs (e.g., grief, pain, suffering). It requires that the health outcomes be valued in monetary terms. Cost–benefit analysis is particularly suited to comparisons with interventions that include cross-sectoral considerations, for example, housing, education, or transportation interventions. Cost–effectiveness usually examines direct medical, nonmedical, and productivity costs. It compares those costs with outcomes in standard health units, such as cost per case averted. It is most suitable when comparing interventions that have similar health outcomes. Cost–utility analysis compares direct medical and nonmedical costs with health outcomes converted to a standard health unit, often a quality-adjusted life year, which combines both morbidity and mortality. Because it provides a general health measure, cost–utility analysis is often used to compare health interventions which have different types of health outcome. Each of these types of analysis is covered in more detail in later chapters. Users should recognize that these analyses provide a great deal of information about interventions, how they can be targeted, modified, or made more efficient. Using them for this purpose can be particularly valuable in modifying program strategies. Our choices have opportunity costs: one choice inevitably means that we forego another. These techniques help us to understand the costs and consequences of our choices when allocating resources.

USES AND LIMITATIONS

Prevention-effectiveness studies are only tools in the decision-making process. They certainly do not make the decisions themselves. Decision processes should be based on solid technical information, such as that obtained from prevention-effectiveness studies; but quantitative information must be combined with an understanding of preferences and values of the stakeholders that are not intrinsically technical in nature. Judgments about those preferences, including acceptability, feasibility, and consistency with strategy, are central to effective decision-making processes. The information generated by these techniques can help to focus discussions among stakeholders and decision makers, allowing them to discern the trade-offs and consequences among alternative strategies, potentially redirecting energy toward a better understanding of the nature of the problem and identifying acceptable solutions.

The application of economic analysis in public health is still a relatively new and dynamic area. Although there is general agreement on many of the principles of economic analysis, controversy about their application in public health persists. Thus, issues such as choice of discount rates, valuation of life, and discounting of future benefits have not been fully resolved. Because public health economics is an evolving field, researchers are urged to consult economists or decision analysts when they begin to design a study. This collaboration can assure that acceptable methods and current and appropriate data sources are used.

Many of the basic decision techniques described in this book can be used at an individual level or a population level. A clinically relevant decision analysis can use individual patient preferences to help guide prevention and therapeutic choices. Similar types of analysis can inform policy choices as well.

SOCIAL, LEGAL, AND EQUITY ASPECTS

Although the decision-making aids described in this book can assist in the process of making policy decisions, they are still just aids. Other considerations must also be included in the decision-making process. Many prevention strategies have much broader effects than those directly related to the health outcomes at which they are aimed. This scope of effect is often not included explicitly in the decision-making process. The social impact of an intervention strategy is well illustrated by the many ramifications associated with human immunodeficiency virus/acquired immunodeficiency syndrome (HIV/AIDS). Intervention strategies implemented for AIDS have raised issues about civil rights among high-risk groups. Sex education and the distribution of condoms in public schools have raised a panoply of concerns reflecting conflicting social values involving students, parents, educators, and public health officials.

It is apparent that prevention strategies must be compatible with the law, but they do raise issues regarding regulations and have an influence on the legal system and precedents. Counseling and testing for HIV/AIDS, for instance, have raised important issues relating to the right to privacy (confidentiality). Many important advances in public health have required changes in regulations (e.g., limitations on smoking in public places, the worksite, or commercial air travel).

Equity and distributional aspects must also be considered. In the context of limited resources, prevention programs can be focused in different ways. They can be directed intensively toward high-risk populations or, less intensively, toward an entire population. These alternate strategies may have very similar costs and benefits, yet the groups that benefit may differ substantially. Similarly, the group that benefits and the group that is harmed may be different, thus raising issues of equity. For example, fortification of flour with folic acid to prevent neural tube defects is accompanied by the risk of permanent neurological disease because diagnosis of vitamin B_{12} deficiency may be delayed. The benefits accrue to infants and their families and the harms to a generally older population. Prevention-effectiveness studies can identify, but cannot resolve, these concerns.

TYPES OF PREVENTION STRATEGIES

Traditional biomedical studies on prevention focus on such clinical strategies to prevent disease and injury as surgical intervention and screening. Prevention-effectiveness studies, however, focus on prevention strategies that encompass the entire domain of public health practice. As a result, many elements of the outcomes and costs are measured differently in prevention-effectiveness studies compared to clinical prevention studies. In preventing lead poisoning, for example, costs related to a prevention strategy might include the nonmedical costs of removing lead paint from older buildings and replacing plumbing that contains lead, in addition to the medical costs of screening and treating persons with elevated blood-lead levels.

Prevention strategies often embody a variety of intervention approaches. In general, however, strategies can be classified as clinical, behavioral, environmental, or systemic. *Clinical* prevention strategies are those conveyed by a health-care provider to a patient, often within a clinical setting (e.g., vaccinations, screening and treatment for diabetic eye disease, and monitoring treatment for tuberculosis). *Behavioral* interventions require individual action, such as eating a healthful diet, exercising, stopping smoking, or wearing a bicycle helmet. They may employ a clinical or a population-based implementation strategy. *Environmental* strategies are those that society can impose and that may require little effort on the part of an individual. Examples of such strategies are laws that limit smoking in public places, dictate the removal of lead from gasoline, prescribe the addition of fluoride to public water supplies, and require the use of seat belts in motor vehicles. *Systemic* changes involve changing the fundamental community processes. For example, improved access to care may require basic changes in the health-care system and financing.

These four approaches should be distinguished from the traditional medical model of prevention based on three stages in disease and injury processes. *Primary prevention* targets risk factors to prevent occurrence of disease or injury. *Secondary prevention* targets subclinical disease through early identification and treatment.

Tertiary prevention is aimed at an established disease or injury to ameliorate progression and maximize function for the person affected.

In keeping with expectations for an introductory text, this book is not intended to be exhaustive, nor does it provide an in-depth theoretical basis for analytic methods. Similarly, this book does not provide an in-depth discussion of systematic literature reviews and synthesis. Such information is available elsewhere (see the bibliography at the end of each chapter). A guide to computer software is also included in Appendix C.

Although program evaluation supports prevention-effectiveness research, program-evaluation methods are not specifically addressed in this book, nor do we discuss in depth many social, legal, and distributional issues that are important parts of many policy decisions.

REFERENCES

1. Teutsch SM. A framework for assessing the effectiveness of disease and injury prevention. *MMWR Morb Mortal Wkly Rep 1992;* 41:i–iv, 1–12.
2. Milstein RL, Wetterhall SF. CDC. Framework for program evaluation in public health. *MMWR Morb Mortal Wkly Rep 1999;* 48.

BIBLIOGRAPHY

Prevention Effectiveness

Bierman H Jr, Bonini CP, Hausman WH. *Quantitative Analysis for Business Decisions*, 8th ed. Homewood, IL: Irwin, 1991.

Bunker JP, Barnes BA, Mosteller F, eds. *Costs, Risks, and Benefits of Surgery*. New York: Oxford University Press, 1977.

Drummond MF, O'Brien B, Stoddart GL, Torrance GW. *Methods for the Economic Evaluation of Health Care Programmes*, 2d ed. Oxford: Oxford Medical Publications, 1997.

Eddy DM, Hasselblad V, Shachter R. *Meta-analysis by the Confidence Profile Method*. Boston: Academic Press, 1992.

Halperin W, Baker EL, Monson RR. *Public Health Surveillance*. Boston: Little, Brown, 1992.

Hedges LV, Olkin I. *Statistical Methods for Meta-analysis*. Boston: Academic Press, 1985.

National Research Council. *Valuing Health Risks, Costs, and Benefits for Environmental Decision Making: Report of a Conference*. Washington DC: National Academy Press, 1990.

National Research Council Institute of Medicine. *Toward a National Health Care Survey: A Data System for the 21st Century*. Washington DC: National Academy Press, 1992.

Petitti DB. *Meta-analysis, Decision Analysis, and Cost–Effectiveness Analysis: Methods for Quantitative Synthesis in Medicine*, 2d ed. New York: Oxford University Press, 2000.

Russell LB. *Is Prevention Better than Cure?* Washington DC: Brookings Institution, 1986.

Russell LB. *Evaluating Preventive Care: Report on a Workshop*. Washington DC: Brookings Institution, 1987.

Scriven M. *Evaluation Thesaurus*, 4th ed. Newbury Park, CA: Sage, 1991.

Sox H, Blatt M, Higgins M, Marton K. *Medical Decision Making.* Stoneham, MA: Butterworth-Heinemann, 1988.

Stokey E, Zeckhauser R. *A Primer for Policy Analysis.* New York: Norton, 1978.

Teutsch SM. A framework for assessing the effectiveness of disease and injury prevention. *MMWR Morb Mortal Wkly Rep 1992;* 41:i–iv, 1–12.

Teutsch SM, Churchill RE. *Principles and Practice of Public Health Surveillance*, 2d ed. New York: Oxford University Press, 2000.

Weinstein MC, Fineberg HV. *Clinical Decision Analysis.* Philadelphia: Saunders, 1980.

Winterfeldt D, Edwards W. *Decision Analysis and Behavioral Research.* Cambridge: Cambridge University Press, 1986.

Economic Analysis

Borus MEJ, Buntz CG, Tash WR. *Evaluating the Impact of Health Programs: Primer.* Cambridge: Cambridge University Press, 1982.

Cohen DR, Henderson JB. *Health, Prevention and Economics.* Oxford: Oxford University Press, 1982.

Drummond MF. Survey of cost–effectiveness and cost–benefit analyses in industrialized countries. *World Health Stat Q 1985;* 38:383–401.

Drummond MF, Davies L. Economic analyses along side clinical trials. *Int J Technol Assess Health Care 1991;* 7:561–73.

Drummond MF, O'Brien B, Stoddart GL, Torrance GW. *Methods for the Economic Evaluation of Health Care Programmes*, 2d ed. Oxford: Oxford Medical Publications, 1997.

Eisenberg JM. Clinical economics: a guide to the economic analysis of clinical practices. *JAMA 1989;* 262:2879–86.

Eisenberg JM, Koffer H, Finkler SA. Economic analysis of a new drug: potential savings in hospital operating costs from the use of a once-daily regimen of a parenteral cephalosporin. *Rev Infect Dis 1984;* 6:S909–23.

Feldstein P. *Health Care Economics*, 3rd ed. New York: John Wiley and Sons, 1988.

Gold MR, Siegel JE, Russell LB, Weinstein MC. *Cost–Effectiveness in Health and Medicine.* New York: Oxford University Press, 1996.

Gramlich EM. *A Guide to Benefit–Cost Analysis*, 2d ed. Englewood Cliffs, NJ: Prentice-Hall, 1990.

Harrington W, Krupnick AJ, Spofford WO. *Economics and Episodic Disease: The Benefits of Preventing a Giardiasis Outbreak.* Washington DC: Resources for the Future, 1991.

Hartunian NS. The incidence and economic costs of cancer, motor vehicle injuries, coronary heart disease and stroke: a comparative analysis. *Am J Public Health 1980;* 70:1249–60.

Luce BR, Elixhauser A. *Standards for Socioeconomic Evaluation of Health Care Products and Services.* New York: Springer-Verlag, 1990.

Manning WG, et al. The taxes of sin: do smokers and drinkers pay their way? *JAMA 1989;* 261:1604–9.

Mills A. Survey and examples of economic evaluation of health programmes in developing countries. *World Health Stat Q 1985;* 39:402–31.

Mohr LB. *Impact Analysis for Program Evaluation.* Pacific Grove, CA: Dorsey, 1988.

Petitti DB. *Meta-analysis, Decision Analysis, and Cost–Effectiveness Analysis: Methods for Quantitative Synthesis in Medicine*, 2d ed. New York: Oxford University Press, 2000.

Rice DP, Hodgson TA, Kopgtein AN. The economic costs of illness: a replication and update. *Health Care Financ Rev 1985;* 7:61–80.

Richardson AW, Gafni A. Treatment of capital costs in evaluating health-care programs. *Cost Manage 1983;* 26–30.

Robinson JC. Philosophical origins of the economic valuation of life. *Milbank Q 1986;* 64:133–55.

Scitovsky A, Rice D. Estimates of the direct and indirect costs of acquired immunodeficiency syndrome in the U.S. 1985, 1986, 1987. *Public Health Rep 1987;* 102:5–17.

Scitovsky AA. Estimating the direct costs of illness. *Milbank Memorial Fund Q 1982;* 60:463–91.

Shepard DS, Thompson MS. First principles of cost–effectiveness analysis. *Public Health Rep 1979;* 94:535–43.

Warner KE, Luce BR. *Cost–Benefit and Cost–Effectiveness Analysis in Health Care.* Ann Arbor, MI: Health Administration Press, 1982.

Weinstein MC, Stason WB. Foundations of cost–effectiveness analysis for health and medical practices. *N Engl J Med 1977;* 236:716–21.

2

Study Design

PAUL G. FARNHAM
ANNE C. HADDIX

Before beginning a prevention-effectiveness analysis, researchers must address a number of issues. The perspective of the study, the analytic methods, and other key issues affect not only the nature of the analysis but also the interpretation and usefulness of the results. This process is referred to as *framing* the study. Its successful completion is one of the most important steps in designing a study.

This chapter identifies the key points that must be addressed before the analytic process begins, discusses each point, and provides a set of questions that can be used to evaluate a prevention-effectiveness study or protocol for quality or adherence to guidelines. After reading this chapter, the reader should be able to identify answers for each of these key questions as they pertain to a study. Examples are drawn from a variety of prevention-effectiveness studies to show how issues might be addressed.

The key points highlighted in this chapter are not always addressed in the order presented. Their order depends on the type of analysis under consideration. For example, in a decision analysis examining strategies to maximize quality of life, the health outcome may be selected first. Other, points may be considered simultaneously. Often, it is difficult to describe the problem or study question without also considering the audience. Therefore, the list below is meant to serve as a guide, not a strict road map.

Throughout this and subsequent chapters, recommendations for study design, structure, analysis, and interpretation are embedded in the text. These recommendations are meant to assist in standardizing prevention-effectiveness methodology and to increase the credibility and comparability of studies.

FRAMING THE QUESTION: A LIST OF KEY POINTS

1. Define the audience for the evaluation. Identify the users of the results of the analysis, and indicate how the results will be used. Determine the information needs of the target audience in reference to the program or intervention.
2. Define operationally the *problem* or *question* to be analyzed. This process

will influence the types of effects and costs to be included and will help to determine which analytic method is most appropriate.

3. Indicate clearly the *prevention strategies* being evaluated, including the baseline *comparator* (the strategy that best represents current practice or the best alternative) for the evaluation.

4. Specify the *perspective* of the analysis. The perspective taken will determine which costs and benefits are included. Limit perspectives to those relevant to the study question.

5. Define the relevant *time frame* and *analytic horizon* for the analysis. Determine the time period (time frame) in which the interventions will be evaluated. Determine how far into the future (analytic horizon) costs and effects that accrue from the intervention will be considered.

6. Determine the *analytic method* or methods. The methods described in this book are decision analysis, cost–benefit analysis, cost–effectiveness analysis, and cost–utility analysis. The choice of analytic method will depend on the policy question, the outcomes of interest, and the availability of data.

7. Determine whether the analysis is to be a *marginal* or an *incremental* one. A marginal analysis examines the effect of expanding or contracting an intervention. An incremental analysis compares the effects of alternative programs.

8. Identify the relevant *costs*. For economic evaluations, identify the program costs and determine whether the health outcomes will be evaluated using the cost-of-illness or the willingness-to-pay approach. If the cost-of-illness approach is used, determine whether productivity losses will be included. Identify other relevant costs or monetary benefits.

9. Identify the *health outcome* or outcomes of interest. Determine whether the outcomes of interest are final health outcomes. The number and nature of outcomes will also help to identify the appropriate analytic method.

10. Specify the *discount rate* or time preference for monetary and nonmonetary costs and outcomes that would occur in the future.

11. Identify the *sources of uncertainty* and plan *sensitivity analyses*. There may be uncertainty about the effectiveness of a program option at achieving specified health outcomes or the values of parameters in the model.

12. Determine the *summary measures* that will be reported.

13. Evaluate if the distribution of the costs and benefits in the population will differ for the alternative prevention-intervention options, including the baseline comparator. Determine the feasibility of analyzing the *distributional effects* of alternate strategies.

The following sections deal with each of these points in greater detail, including examples and recommendations relevant to various types of prevention programs.

AUDIENCE

One of the first steps in designing a prevention-effectiveness study is to identify the audience. The audience can be defined as the consumers of the study results.

Studies must be framed so that the results will provide information useful for the kinds of decision that need to be made. Generally, two types of consumers can be identified: policy decision makers and program decision makers.

Policy decision makers include elected officials, agency heads, and state and local public health officials. Examples of studies that provide economic data for policy decisions include determining the cost–effectiveness of requiring folic acid fortification of cereal grains to prevent neural tube defects and determining the costs and benefits associated with gasoline additives to reduce carbon monoxide emissions (as mandated by the Clean Air Act).

Program decision makers may use the results of prevention-effectiveness studies to make decisions about different approaches to a prevention program. For instance, an economic analysis for program decision making might determine the most cost–effective smoke alarm distribution program to reduce mortality from house fires. It might study whether to implement universal or selected screening for *Chlamydia trachomatis* in public sexually transmitted disease (STD) clinics.

In addition to policy makers and program decision makers, other interested parties may use the results of economic analyses for decision making. These may include managed-care organizations, insurance companies, other researchers, patients, health-care workers, the general public, and the press. For example, managed-care organizations and insurance companies may be interested in the costs and effects of various cancer-screening strategies to determine their coverage of these strategies. Identifying the target audience for a study before framing the study question will help to ensure that the analyses conducted will provide the information needed by a particular audience in a form useful for that audience.

STUDY QUESTION

Developing a well-constructed and clearly articulated study question is also one of the first steps in designing a prevention-effectiveness study. The study question must address the policy or program issues that drive the analysis and identify the target audience. The study should be framed to reflect the needs of the users of the evaluation results. For example, when evaluating the cost–effectiveness of an expanded vaccination program, it may be more useful to ask "What is the cost–effectiveness of an expanded program versus the current program?" rather than "What is the cost–effectiveness of the current program versus no program?" In the case of cervical cancer screening, the issue may be how often to recommend screening: every 5 years, 3 years, or annually?

A carefully and clearly stated study question provides the basis for determining other key elements in an economic analysis. Decisions about the perspective of the analysis, the time frame, the analytic method, the costs to be included, and the benefits or health outcomes of interest are often made on the basis of the study question.

INTERVENTION STRATEGIES

Once the study question is clearly defined, the alternate strategies to be analyzed are selected. These strategies may be apparent from the study question. A sound strategy clearly defines three components: (*1*) the intervention, (*2*) the target population for the intervention, and (*3*) the delivery system. However, strategies must be operationally feasible. The availability of data that link the intervention to the health outcome of interest may also determine whether a particular strategy should be included. Lack of evidence of effectiveness may eliminate some strategies from consideration. The analyst must also be careful to select only a limited number of options to prevent the analysis from being too cumbersome. However, the analyst must still include all appropriate options so that the study provides the information needed for decision making.

In addition to new strategies to be considered, a baseline comparator must be selected. The baseline comparator may be the existing-program/strategy option or the option "no program" if no program exists at the time of the evaluation. In clinical prevention–effectiveness studies, the baseline comparator is often the current standard of care or the best alternative therapy. The results of the analysis may show that the baseline comparator is the most cost-effective strategy, but this cannot be demonstrated unless it is explicitly included. For example, when the Centers For Disease Control (CDC) issued guidelines for the voluntary human immunodeficiency virus (HIV) counseling and testing of pregnant women and the use of zidovudine (ZDV) to prevent HIV transmission from mother to child, the first prevention-effectiveness studies compared this policy to a policy of no program, the situation that existed before the effectiveness of the ZDV intervention was known and the guidelines were established. Subsequent analyses examined the universal testing of women, the testing of newborns, and the use of additional HIV tests during pregnancy. In these cases, the guidelines for voluntary counseling and testing of pregnant women became the alternative against which the other policies were compared.

Screening strategies can be compared on both the intensive and extensive margins. Studies that compare strategies on the *intensive margin* are those that examine the effects of changes in the periodicity of screening on the same group of individuals. Studies that compare screening strategies on the *extensive margin* are those that examine the effects of the same intervention on different groups of individuals. For example, when the costs and effects of screening a group of women more frequently for cervical cancer are analyzed, this is a question of additional screening on the intensive margin. For mammography screening for breast cancer, protocols typically focus on women over 50 years old, where the incidence of the disease is the greatest. The costs and outcomes of extending this screening to women between the ages of 40 and 50 or between 30 and 40 years old could then be considered. Applying this procedure to different groups would be additional screening on the extensive margin.

In all of these studies, analysts need to consider what may happen under the different policy alternatives regarding such issues as the behavior of the participants, the quality of screening procedures used, and the prevalence of the health condition in various populations. Each of these factors will influence the costs and outcomes of the alternatives. The question is always what would happen with a given policy compared to what would happen without the policy or with a specific alternative. The prevention-effectiveness analysis involves a "with and without" comparison, not a "before and after" one. Since there are often no empirical data on what might have happened if the policy had not been in place or what could happen under some hypothetical alternative, the policy analyst must often use a modeling technique, such as decision analysis, to compare alternative policy options.

Recommendation 2.1: The list of alternative strategies in prevention-effectiveness studies should include all reasonable options and a baseline comparator.

PERSPECTIVE

Once the study question has been crafted, the next step is to identify the appropriate perspective or perspectives the analysis will take. The *perspective* is the viewpoint from which the analysis is conducted and refers to which costs and benefits are included. Prevention-effectiveness analyses typically take the societal perspective, analyzing all benefits of a program (no matter who receives them) and all costs of a program (no matter who pays them). For most public health studies, the societal perspective is appropriate because the goal of the research is to analyze the allocation of societal resources among competing activities. Studies from the perspective of a health-care provider or some other vantage point may be appropriate in such specific instances as those described below.

When an analysis is done from the societal perspective, the costs of a prevention strategy must reflect what members of society give up now and in the future to implement the prevention intervention. This is called the *opportunity cost.* Opportunity costs include all monetary and nonmonetary costs of a strategy regardless of whether they are incurred by an agency, a provider, or a consumer. Thus, cost figures may need to be collected for a clinic, a participant, and a public health agency to develop a complete measure of program costs. Opportunity costs include more than just the dollar costs associated with providing or receiving health-care services. They also include the resources not available to society because of an illness or injury. If an individual is unable to work, society loses the benefit of that person's contribution in the work force. That loss is described as an opportunity cost. Another opportunity cost would be the value assigned to a person's healthy time that has been forfeited. Because opportunity costs may not appear as a monetary figure in anyone's budget, they may have to be imputed. The opportunity cost of lost work from an illness or injury, also referred to as *productivity losses,* may be reported separately in the study. In some types of cost utility analyses, the productivity losses associated with the health outcome may have been incorporated into the outcome measure and, therefore, should not be included as a cost. See Chapter 4 for a more complete discussion.

In the context of preventing HIV infection, for example, counseling and testing activities at STD clinics may be supported by both federal and state funds. When program costs are estimated from the societal perspective, data from both the counseling and testing activities of the program must be collected. Focusing only on the costs incurred by one component may produce a misleading picture of opportunity costs.

Prevention programs that involve outreach into the community may involve volunteers or may have the salaries of some employees subsidized from other sources. Implicit or shadow prices must be developed for the volunteers' time, and budgetary figures may have to be adjusted to reflect the external subsidies in order to measure these costs accurately from the societal perspective. For example, the implicit costs of volunteer time were very important for HIV prevention and treatment programs in the early years of the acquired immunodeficiency syndrome (AIDS) epidemic. Since the use of volunteers was much more widespread in San Francisco than in other parts of the country, these implicit costs could have accounted for geographic differences in the explicit money costs of treating HIV/AIDS. In addition to time, factors such as transportation, space, materials, telephone, and postage must be included in total costs. An analysis done from the societal perspective should incorporate all of these costs.

Other Perspectives

The costs and outcomes of prevention programs can also be measured from the perspective of various individuals or groups. Societal costs and benefits, which are relevant for overall resource-allocation decisions, may not be relevant to individuals or organizations that are making a decision about providing or paying for a specific prevention program. For example, hospital administrators may be more concerned about who is paying the cost of a screening intervention than about its societal cost since the hospital does not want to provide excessive amounts of services that may turn into uncompensated care.

Other perspectives include those of (1) federal, state, and local governments (the impact on the budgets of specific agencies undertaking a prevention program or on programs such as Medicaid or Medicare, which fund the purchase of health services); (2) health-care providers (the costs imposed on various types of hospitals, managed-care organizations, or other providers because of the adoption of particular prevention programs); (3) businesses (the impact of illnesses or prevention activities on health-related employee benefits and productivity); and (4) individuals (the costs of undertaking a current prevention activity with uncertain future benefits or the costs of illness paid out-of-pocket). For example, to answer questions from the business community about the impact of HIV in the workplace and to engage the business community in HIV prevention, the CDC requested a study of the costs to business of an HIV-infected worker.[1] This study focused on the impact of HIV on employee health and life insurance, company retraining costs, and employee pension plans, costs that are accounted for differently when estimating the cost of illness from a societal perspective.

Recommendation 2.2: For decisions that impact public health, prevention-effectiveness studies should take the societal perspective. Additional perspectives may also be studied when relevant to the study question. The perspectives of the analysis should be clearly stated.

Recommendation 2.3: All measurable opportunity costs, representing all groups that are affected by a program or intervention, should be included in the societal perspective.

TIME FRAME AND ANALYTIC HORIZON

The *time frame* of an analysis is the specified period in which the intervention strategies are actually applied. The *analytic horizon* is the period over which the costs and benefits of health outcomes that occur as a result of the intervention are considered. Thus, the analytic horizon is often longer than the time frame because the benefits of an intervention may continue after an intervention is completed. Figure 2.1 illustrates the distinction between these two concepts. The figure is based on an example of an intervention delivered over a 1-year period that has a lifetime effect on the individuals who receive it. The lifetime (analytic horizon) effect of chronic heart disease prevented in persons who participate in a cholesterol-screening and education program during a 1-year period (time frame) is one such example. Time frame and analytic horizon together are often referred to as the *time horizon* for the study. Regardless, it is important to specify the duration of each of the two components.

The time pattern of benefits and costs plays an especially important role in the economic evaluation of prevention activities. Prevention interventions often occur in the absence of acute health events. Indeed, many years may elapse between the adoption of a prevention behavior and the expected development of a health problem that the prevention behavior was designed to prevent. The gain in life expectancy or quality of life from a prevention activity may occur far in the future.

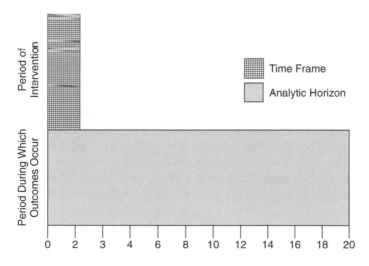

Figure 2.1   The distinction between time frame and analytic horizon.

It is important to specify a time frame that is long enough to account for several factors: (*1*) seasonal variations in costs or health outcomes, (*2*) start-up and ongoing maintenance costs, and (*3*) the achievement of a steady-state health outcome. As an example, a community bicycle helmet program may initially achieve a sharp increase in the rates at which bicycle helmets are used. As publicity about the program decreases, rates of helmet use may taper off. The time frame for the bicycle helmet program should be long enough to temper the effects of the initial publicity about the program and allow an examination of the lasting results of the program. These same factors also affect the evaluation of HIV-prevention programs. In addition, there is the possibility of relapse to risky behavior that can occur in future years with these interventions.

Although it is important that the time frame of the analysis be of an appropriate length, it should not be overextended. Changes in technology may lead to the obsolescence of a current prevention method within a few years. The choice of time frame should reflect reasonable assumptions about what technology will be used during the time period considered. For example, in evaluating a current screening program, such as mammography, if a major new therapy is expected to be available within a few years, a short time frame (perhaps 3–7 years) might be chosen. This short time frame should reflect a reasonable assumption about how long the current therapy will still be in use.

Because the time frame for each study must be carefully matched to the intervention being studied, no particular time frame can be generally recommended. However, the time frame of the analysis should always be clearly stated at the beginning of the study.

Recommendation 2.4: The time frame for a prevention-effectiveness study must be long enough to cover the implementation of the program being evaluated.

The analytic horizon is the period of time for which costs and benefits related to a particular intervention are measured. Costs may be incurred before an intervention is implemented (e.g., setting up a clinic, training counselors). Costs may also continue after an intervention is implemented (e.g., costs of staff to report statistics). In the case of prevention interventions, benefits are expected to continue after the intervention is completed (e.g., long-term benefits in the form of reduction in high-risk behavior as a result of a specific health-education program).

In prevention-effectiveness analyses of public health interventions, the ideal analytic horizon is the portion of the lifetime of the persons affected by a prevention intervention, during which time the costs of the intervention are incurred and the benefits received. An analytic horizon that does not encompass this period may not capture all of the benefits associated with the intervention. If a shorter analytic horizon is selected and some benefits are not captured, the study's comparability with other evaluations of prevention effectiveness is limited. However, horizons that capture multigenerational benefits, although relevant, may be overly complex and computationally difficult. In some cases, intergeneration effects are crucial. One such case is the evaluation of genetic screening programs for potential parents. For these reasons, the following recommendation is made.

Recommendation 2.5: The analytic horizon of a prevention-effectiveness study should extend over the time period during which the costs, harms, and benefits of the intervention are incurred.

ANALYTIC METHOD

The purpose of a prevention-effectiveness analysis is to identify, measure, value, and compare the costs and consequences of alternate prevention strategies. In addition to a decision analysis, which may only include health outcomes, three methods are commonly used for economic evaluations: cost–benefit analysis, cost–effectiveness analysis, and cost–utility analysis. Selection of the appropriate method or methods depends on the target audience for the study, the study question, and the availability of data. In some instances, more than one method may be employed in one study to answer specific policy questions.

Cost–Benefit Analysis

Cost–benefit analysis (CBA) is often considered the gold standard for economic evaluations. Because it is the one method in which the costs and benefits are reported using a common metric (generally dollars), results from CBAs can be compared with results from studies of a wide range of public programs. The CBA compares society's total willingness to pay for the outcomes of a program or policy (the benefits) with the opportunity costs of the program. The opportunity costs reflect what is sacrificed to produce those outcomes. A program makes the best use of society's limited resources and is termed "efficient" if the benefits exceed the costs because the valuation people place on the program outcomes is greater than the cost of producing them. Benefits and costs are calculated without regard to who receives the benefits and who pays the costs. The CBA is often used when comparing programs with significant nonhealth benefits (e.g., environmental programs that may improve property values) and may be used to make decisions on program funding.

With CBA, program outcomes or benefits are assigned a monetary value. Results of a CBA are expressed as net benefits (program benefits minus program costs). The net benefits can then be used in comparing a range of activities with dissimilar measures of health outcome. Results of CBAs indicate whether a specific strategy leads to a net gain or net loss. This information can help decision makers select among various programs or strategies within a program. Less desirably, results reported in the literature have been expressed as benefit–cost ratios (net benefits divided by net costs). However, because benefit-cost ratios can be distorted, they should not be used. See Chapter 8 for a more complete discussion.

Because all costs and benefits are converted into dollar values, CBA raises some controversial questions. What is the exact value of saving one life? More precisely, what is society willing to pay to reduce the probability of death by a certain amount? Is the life of an older person worth as much as the life of a younger person? Should different values be placed on an outcome that leads to a life with a physical disability and an outcome that leads to a life without disability? If so, does society value persons with disabilities more or less than those who have none? The issues involved with calculating society's willingness to pay to save a life and the use of proxies such as future earnings are discussed in detail in Chapter 8.

In summary, the primary advantage of CBA is the comparability of health-related results with those from other types of programs or policies. The primary disadvantage of CBA for prevention-effectiveness studies is that all benefits are converted into monetary values. Assigning a monetary value to health outcomes, especially a human life, is a difficult and controversial task. The value of averting pain and suffering (classified as an intangible cost) presents a similar problem. Because of the difficulty in measuring and valuing qualitative benefits, prevention-effectiveness practitioners more commonly use cost–effectiveness and cost–utility analyses. However, as our ability to quantify intangibles improves, CBA is becoming a more comprehensive and a more complete measure of changes in societal welfare.

Cost–Effectiveness Analysis

In cost–effectiveness analysis (CEA), no attempt is made to assign a monetary value to health outcomes. Instead of dollars, outcomes are measured in the most appropriate natural effects or physical units. For example, in comparing programs to promote the use of bicycle helmets, the unit of measure for the CEA might be "head injuries averted." Other units of measures for CEA might include disease prevented or number of lives saved. The unit of measure selected is the outcome most relevant for the analysis. Cost–utility analyses (CUAs) use a measure of health-related quality of life to capture the effects of an intervention and are a special type of CEA. In this book, if the outcome measure of a CEA is health-related quality of life, a study is referred to as a CUA. All other CEAs in which the outcomes are other than health-related quality of life are referred to as CEAs.

The most commonly performed economic analyses in the health arena are CEAs. Effectiveness data on outcomes are more generally available and more easily understood than outcome measures for either CBA or CUA. Although CEA uses a unit of measure related to health outcome, it still considers the costs of a program and the costs saved by the program (the net cost). Operationally, it is defined as the net cost divided by the net effectiveness (see Chapter 9 for more details).

In CEA, the net cost of implementing an intervention is combined with the effectiveness of the intervention. Results are expressed in various ways depending on the health outcome selected (e.g., CEA results might be stated as "cost per life saved" or "cost per injury averted").

When the goal is to identify the most cost-effective prevention strategy from a set of alternate interventions that produce a common effect, CEA is most useful. The disadvantage of CEA is that the comparability of cost–effectiveness studies for different health conditions is limited because there is no single outcome measure. Also, judgments about the value and quality of lives must be made implicitly by the user of the study results because the value to society of a life and the quality of life in excess of a person's economic contribution is not included in a CEA.

Cost–Utility Analysis

The CUA allows prevention strategies for more than one disease or health problem to be compared. In CUA, as in CEA, a common measure is used to compare alternative program outcomes. In CUA, outcomes are expressed as number of life years saved, with a quality-of-life adjustment. Thus, the common measure for CUA is quality-adjusted life years (QALYs). The QALY measure has an intuitive appeal to decision makers. Rather than relying on implicit judgments about the value and quality of life, CUA makes these values explicit in the calculation. In some international studies, the disability-adjusted life year (DALY) may be used. However, QALYs and DALYs can be subjective determinations that are difficult to measure and may not be universally accepted.

The CBA, CEA, and CUA methods are appropriate in different circumstances. The availability of data, the way a study question is framed, and the information needs of the audience influence the selection of the type of analytic method. In addition, the selection of an analytic method or methods is also linked to the selection of outcome measures, as discussed below.

All three types, CBA, CEA, and CUA, utilize data and methods described in subsequent chapters. The CBA is described in more detail in Chapter 8 and CEA and CUA in Chapter 9. Specific recommendations regarding the use of these methods are found in these chapters as well.

MARGINAL AND INCREMENTAL ANALYSES

Prevention-effectiveness studies, in general, examine the effects of alternative strategies at their margins. In other words, the objective is to examine the *additional* effects (additional costs and outcomes) produced by one strategy when compared to another strategy. Studies may examine the additional effects produced by either expanding or contracting an intervention or when comparing two or more different interventions.

Marginal analysis examines the effect on health outcomes of making an additional investment in an intervention. For example, determining the cost-effectiveness of spending an additional $2 million in a cereal grain fortification program to double the folic acid level to prevent neural tube defects requires a marginal analysis because the policy question addresses the effect of adding resources to an existing intervention. In contrast, incremental analysis examines the relationship between making an investment in a different intervention and the health outcomes expected to be produced by that strategy. Determining whether fortification of cereal grains is a more cost–effective strategy to prevent neural tube defects than a vitamin-supplementation program requires an incremental analysis.

Marginal and incremental analyses are fundamental to prevention-effectiveness studies. They are the basic foundation of the comparative measures used to decide among strategies. Average costs are typically a poor substitute for marginal and incremental costs. Average costs provide information about only a particular strategy. Marginal and incremental costs allow for comparison among strategies and ranking them by their marginal returns.

Recommendation 2.6: Marginal or incremental analysis should always be performed in a prevention-effectiveness study for comparing programs or interventions. Average analyses are acceptable for independent programs or interventions.

COSTS

It is useful to identify all relevant costs in the evaluation before constructing the model. The availability of data on cost may affect decisions about the perspective of the analysis and the analytic method. Sources of data on cost should also be identified. Chapter 4 contains a complete discussion of intervention costs and costs of illness. The willingness-to-pay approach to estimating the monetary value of health outcomes and other benefits is included in Chapter 8. A list of data sources for costs is provided in Appendix E.

OUTCOMES

In prevention-effectiveness studies, outcomes are the results of implementing a prevention strategy. Outcomes are usually expressed as health conditions (e.g., QALYs or cases prevented). The first is an outcome measure that would be used in a CUA. The second outcome measure would be more frequently used in a CEA. The value of either, expressed in monetary terms, as well as the value of other outcomes not related to health would be used in a CBA.

Outcomes in prevention-effectiveness studies include both benefits and harms resulting from an intervention. Regardless, all outcomes that result from the intervention should be included. For example, one intervention designed to reduce the long-term health impacts associated with obesity may be a program to promote physical activity. However, increased physical activity may result in exercise-related injuries. The impact of these injuries should be included as an outcome in the analysis along with such benefits as the reduction in cardiovascular disease and diabetes.

Selection of the outcome measure is guided not only by the analytic method used but also by the policy question to be answered and the kind of data that can reasonably be collected. Lack of data to conduct a particular type of analysis may make it necessary to select another analytic method and another, perhaps less preferable, outcome measure. For example, in a recent study of the cost–effectiveness of programs to promote the use of bicycle helmets among children, it was determined that the use of QALYs saved would best answer the policy question because this would allow both fatal and nonfatal head injuries to be included in one measure. However, data did not exist on the severity of the head injuries; only data regarding the number of head injuries were available. Thus, it was not possible to use a quality-adjusted measure. Because of this, two outcome measures were selected: head injuries prevented and fatalities prevented. Therefore, cost–effectiveness ratios were calculated for each.

For many public health prevention strategies implemented outside the clinical arena, benefits other than health outcomes may also be of interest. For example, in a study of the impact on health after the installation of municipal water and sewer systems in *colonias* on the United States–Mexico border, one of the primary benefits was an increase in property values. Without taking this benefit into account as one of the outcomes, the study would fail to convey the full measure of benefits of the program. Therefore, it was decided that a CBA would best capture both economic and health benefits in a single summary measure.

A more complete discussion on selection and measurement of outcomes is included in Chapters 3, 5, 8, and 9.

Recommendation 2.7: Prevention-effectiveness studies should include all benefits and harms that have a meaningful impact on the results of the analysis.

DISCOUNT RATE

Time affects both monetary and nonmonetary valuations of program outcomes and costs because individuals generally weigh benefits and costs in the near future more heavily than those in the distant future. A dollar that an individual receives this year is worth more than a dollar that will be received 10 years from now. This is because this year's dollar can be invested so that in 10 years' time it will be worth more than a dollar. This argument applies to the valuation of capital and investments and to health outcomes. A dollar may also be worth more now because the individual prefers to make purchases today rather than to postpone consumption until the future. A health outcome that is achieved today may be worth more than the same health outcome produced 10 years from now. This concept is referred to as *time preference*. As a rule, the societal preference is for health benefits received today versus health benefits received in the future (see Chapter 6 for a more complete discussion).

The discount rate used in prevention-effectiveness studies is not related to inflation. Even in a world of zero inflation, the value of a dollar received today would be greater than the value of a dollar received in the future (see Chapter 6). Using a discount rate in an economic analysis provides a method of adjusting the value of receiving benefits today versus receiving benefits in the future or of incurring costs in the present versus incurring costs in the future.

Since most public health projects involve benefits and costs that continue into the future, it is necessary to calculate the present value of these benefits and costs to make them comparable in terms of the time dimension. This calculation of present value involves the choice of a discount rate. The choice of a discount rate can have a significant impact on the results of the analysis. This issue is explored in greater depth and recommendations about specific discount rates and discounting of health outcomes are given in Chapter 6.

UNCERTAINTY

In prevention-effectiveness studies, precise estimates often are not available for certain variables. This may reflect limitations of previous studies or the fact that studies in different population settings have yielded a range of estimates. The initial assumptions made about a study definitely influence its results. Therefore, it is important to list all of the assumptions upon which the values of variables are based and to perform sensitivity analyses on key variables to determine if different values of these variables would impact the overall study results. For example, in a study of HIV counseling and testing of pregnant women and the administration of ZDV to reduce HIV transmission from mothers to infants, researchers performed sensitivity analyses on four key variables: maternal HIV seroprevalence, the proportion of women accepting HIV counseling and testing, the proportion of women receiving ZDV treatment, and the lifetime cost of medical treatment for an HIV-infected infant.[2]

Sensitivity-analysis techniques and interpretation are covered in more detail in Chapter 7.

Recommendation 2.8: Univariate and multivariable sensitivity analyses should be performed and the results reported for a prevention-effectiveness study.

SUMMARY MEASURES

A number of summary ratios can be reported in a prevention-effectiveness study. As noted earlier, it is important to identify the outcome measures that most accurately address the study questions before beginning an analysis. Once the outcome measures have been identified, the decision analysis can be structured with the desired output in mind. However, regardless of the analytic method used, a marginal or incremental analysis should be performed, as described above. The marginal or incremental measure should then be used as a primary summary measure for the study.

Examples of summary measures include the incremental net present value of benefits (CBA), the incremental cost–effectiveness ratio (CEA), and the incremental cost-utility ratio (CUA). Average summary measures may also be reported but should not be used to compare prevention strategies. Summary measures and their calculations are discussed in detail in Chapters 7–9.

DISTRIBUTIONAL EFFECTS

As discussed above, the way a prevention intervention is implemented may affect the distribution of costs and benefits. "Who pays the most?" and "Who receives the greatest benefit?" are questions with legal, ethical, political, and practical implications. Policy makers should consider distributional effects when making decisions about prevention programs. For example, targeting an effective intervention to a specific population will benefit that population rather than another.

In economic analyses, identification of the potential shifts in distribution of costs is useful for ensuring the collection of appropriate data and classifying costs and benefits. Examination of subpopulations or selection of an additional perspective for the analysis may be based on potential distributional effects.

Recommendation 2.9: When possible, the distributional and ethical implications of a prevention–effectiveness study should be examined and discussed.

COMPARABILITY OF STUDY RESULTS

It is extremely important for persons who conduct prevention–effectiveness studies to clearly state all assumptions about the factors discussed in this chapter. Study results should be reported with all assumptions explicitly identified, including audience perspective, outcome and cost measures, use of discounting, and discount rate.

Unfortunately, this policy has not always been followed in the studies reported in the literature. A review of 228 CUAs in the medical literature indicated that only 52% explicitly stated what perspective the analysis used, with the rest leaving the determination of the perspective to the readers.[3] The lack of clear definition of assumptions seriously compromises the scientific integrity of a study and makes the results virtually useless for comparison purposes. In the HIV-prevention literature, researchers have advocated the standardization of cost-of-illness and quality-of-life estimates to increase the comparability of the evaluation of different prevention interventions.[4]

Analyses of prevention programs should also indicate the robustness of their results through the use of sensitivity analysis or other techniques. Because studies incorporate a wide variety of assumptions and data of inconsistent quality, users of the study need to know which assumptions and data are most important to the overall results. Users can then incorporate their own estimates of these factors if they are not satisfied with the decisions made or the assumptions used in the analysis.

Recommendation 2.10: All assumptions should be explicitly stated, including assumptions about the study structure, probabilities, outcome measures, and costs.

CONCLUSION

The key points discussed above are essential for conducting and evaluating prevention–effectiveness studies. Each of the key points may have a substantial impact on the results of an analysis. Not only should they be addressed when conducting a study, they should also be clearly reported. A checklist of key points follows.

CHECKLIST FOR EVALUATING THE PROTOCOL OR SCOPE OF WORK FOR A PREVENTION-EFFECTIVENESS STUDY

1. Was the audience for the study clearly identified?
2. Was the study question clearly defined? Did the question follow a clear description of the public health problem?
3. Were the alternate prevention strategies clearly identified and described? Were the target populations and mechanisms identified and described? Was an appropriate baseline comparator included as a strategy?
4. Was the perspective of the analysis stated? Will the analysis take a societal perspective? Will another perspective also be taken?
5. Were the time frame and the analytic horizon defined? What is the time period over which the alternate strategies will be evaluated? Over what period of time will the costs and benefits of health outcomes be measured?
6. Were the analytic method or methods specified? Is the study a decision analysis, CBA, CEA, or CUA? Will a marginal or incremental analysis be conducted?
7. Were the costs clearly identified? Were the costs of the alternate strategies included? Will the study take the cost-of-illness or willingness-to-pay approach to measure the value of health outcomes or adverse health effects? If the cost-of-illness approach is chosen, will productivity losses be included? Were other relevant costs included (e.g., cost to government, business)?
8. Was the health outcome clearly identified? Are there multiple outcomes? Are the outcomes final?
9. Was the discount rate specified? Will sensitivity analysis be conducted on the discount rate?
10. Were the sources of uncertainty in the model identified? Will appropriate sensitivity and threshold analyses be conducted? Have the assumptions of the study been clearly identified?
11. Were the summary measures identified?
12. Will the distributional effects of the alternate strategies be examined?

REFERENCES

1. Farnham PG, Gorsky RD. Cost to business for an HIV-infected worker. *Inquiry 1994;* 31: 76–88.
2. Gorsky RD, Farnham PG, Straus W, et al. Preventing perinatal transmission of HIV—costs and effectiveness of a recommended intervention. *Public Health Rep 1996;* 111:335–40.
3. Neumann PJ, Stone PW, Chapman RH, et al. The quality of reporting in published cost–utility analyses, 1976–1997. *Ann Intern Med 2000;* 132:964–72.
4. Holtgrave DR, Pinkerton SD. Updates of cost of illness and quality of life estimates for use in economic evaluations of HIV prevention programs. *J AIDS 1997;* 16:54–62.

BIBLIOGRAPHY

Barry PZ, DeFriese GF. Cost–benefit and cost–effectiveness analysis for health promotion programs. *Am J Health Promot 1990;* 4:448–52.

Drummond MF, O'Brien B, Stoddart GL, Torrance, GW. *Methods for the Economic Evaluation of Health Care Programmes*, 2d ed. New York: Oxford University Press, 1997.

Gold ME, Siegel JE, Russell LB, Weinstein MC. *Cost–Effectiveness in Health and Medicine.* New York: Oxford University Press, 1996.

Lave JR, Lave LB. Cost–benefit concepts in health: examination of some prevention efforts. *Prev Med 1978;* 7:414–23.

Murphy RJ, Gasparotto G, Opatz JP. Methodological challenges to program evaluation. *Am J Health Promot 1987;* 1:33–40.

O'Donnell MP, Ainsworth TH. *Health Promotion in the Workplace.* New York: John Wiley and Sons, 1984.

Patrick DL, Erickson, P. *Health Status and Health Policy. Allocating Resources to Health Care.* New York: Oxford University Press, 1993.

Russell LB. *Is Prevention Better than Cure?* Washington DC: Brookings Institution, 1986.

Russell LB. *Evaluating Preventive Care.* Washington DC: Brookings Institution, 1987.

Russell LB. *Educated Guesses: Making Policy about Medical Screening Tests.* Berkeley: University of California Press, 1994.

Sloan FA. *Valuing Health Care Costs, Benefits, and Effectiveness of Pharmaceuticals and Other Medical Technologies.* New York: Cambridge University Press, 1995.

Tolley G, Kenkel D, Fabian R. *Valuing Health for Policy.* Chicago: University of Chicago Press, 1994.

Udvarhelyi IS, Colditz GA, Rai A, Epstein AM. Cost–effectiveness and cost–benefit analyses in the medical literature. *Ann Intern Med 1992;* 116:238–44.

US Preventive Services Task Force. *Guide to Clinical Preventive Services*, 2d ed. Baltimore: Williams and Wilkins, 1996.

Warner KE. The economic evaluation of preventive health care. *Soc Sci Med 1979;* 13C: 227–37.

Warner KE, Luce, BR. *Cost–Benefit and Cost–Effectiveness Analysis in Health Care.* Ann Arbor, MI: Health Administration Press, 1982.

3

Measuring Effectiveness

K. ROBIN YABROFF
JEANNE MANDELBLATT

Decision models and cost–effectiveness analyses are most commonly developed to provide timely information to clinicians or health policy makers about the most likely impact of disease-prevention strategies in the absence of definitive studies. These models summarize the benefits and harms (and costs) of a prevention strategy in a single measure. They can be used to assess the impact of prevention strategies in reducing the development of disease, detecting disease earlier in its natural history when treatment may be more effective, or reducing morbidity through effective treatment.

Developing a decision model requires specifying the study question and study population, mapping out the underlying process of disease and the intervention strategy, identifying an appropriate baseline or comparison strategy, and identifying all possible downstream effects of the intervention. This chapter focuses on estimating the many different types of parameters used in decision models. It begins with basic concepts and then reviews population measures and risk estimates, study design, and sources of data. Finally, issues for special consideration in modeling prevention effectiveness are identified and discussed.

PUBLIC HEALTH ISSUES IN THE DEVELOPMENT OF DECISION MODELS

This section reviews issues in the development of decision models, including the types of interventions to be assessed, the appropriate population for the models, and measures of population effects.

Prevention interventions can range from very specific clinical strategies, such as increasing the rate of immunizations in well-child visits with provider reminders, to the use of mass media to increase knowledge, such as for human immunodeficiency virus (HIV)–prevention behaviors, to broader environmental interventions, such as housing regulations to limit exposures to lead-based paint.

Broader system changes, such as changing eligibility criteria for national or state-based insurance programs or mandating insurance coverage for specific procedures or services, are also examples of prevention interventions that can be assessed with decision analysis. These different intervention strategies will vary in the composition of the intervention and expected change in behavior or risk factor, mechanism of intervention delivery, target population for the intervention, and expected penetrance of the intervention in target populations. Provider reminders, for example, may consist of a checklist placed on a patient's chart, whereas implementing broad health-care system changes, such as changes in insurance coverage for screening tests, may be significantly more complex. Even with interventions that focus on behavioral change, there may be variability in content and intensity. Some may require a single behavioral change (e.g., immunization), while others will require ongoing participation or modification of long-term attitudes or habits. Exercise or diet modification, smoking-cessation, use of bike helmets, and safe sex practices are all examples of prevention behaviors that may require intensive interventions, multiple reinforcements, and multiple time periods for assessment. For example, smoking-cessation programs utilizing counseling, nicotine replacement, or other medications may lead to short-term (3-month) quit rates up to approximately 40%.[1–4] When measured for longer periods of time, however, many program participants will start smoking again and quit rates can drop even lower.[1,5] Assessment of the intervention at 3 months would overestimate intervention effectiveness.

Given the breadth of these public health interventions, specifying the target population is a critical component of parameter estimation. The content of the intervention may also change based on the target population. For example, mass media strategies used to increase knowledge of HIV prevention and related behaviors (and their potential impact) will vary dramatically if developed for the general population or for a high-risk population, such as injection drug users. Additionally, the mass media intervention may be delivered in a specific geographic area; nationally through radio, television, newspapers, or an organization-specific newsletter; or in a closed-circuit setting within a health-care facility. The population reached by these means will vary based on where they live; their radio listening, television viewing, or newspaper reading habits; or their organizational membership and use of health care. Like any other intervention strategy, mass media interventions will affect only the individuals who see or hear the message, understand and internalize the content of the message, and as a result change their behavior. The extent to which an intervention reaches its intended target is the intervention *penetrance* and should be considered when outlining and estimating intervention effects.

The examples listed previously have different target populations of individuals with different characteristics and risks of disease. Thus, detailing the intervention and defining the target population based on age distribution, gender, race, or any other factors that might impact disease risk are critical to model development since all parameters must be specific to the target population. The measurement of population effects and their use in decision models are reviewed in the next section.

POPULATION EFFECTS

Models to assess prevention strategies utilize many different measures of disease within a specified population. For example, a model of the cost effectiveness of interventions to increase mammography use in women aged 50 and older would require information about the frequency of new cases of breast cancer, current use of mammography, differences in stage of disease at diagnosis for women receiving mammography, impact of diagnosis with breast cancer on a patient's mental and physical well-being, and ultimately mortality. As illustrated by this example, common measures of population effects used in decision models of prevention interventions include disease incidence, prevalence, morbidity, and mortality. All of these measures would be specific to a general population of women aged 50 and older; assessing the impact of interventions to increase mammography use in a population with a genetic predisposition to developing breast cancer (high risk) would require estimates of incidence, prevalence, morbidity, and mortality from a similar high-risk population. Additionally, since women with a genetic predisposition to breast cancer may be more likely to develop disease at a younger age, all estimates should be based on a high-risk, age-appropriate population.[6] Definitions of these population effects and examples of their use in decision models are described below.

The *penetrance* of an intervention reflects the degree to which an intervention reaches the intended population. Interventions may be delivered only to a subset of a population because of targeting, resource limitations, or feasibility, thus influencing penetrance.

Incidence is the number of new cases of disease in a defined population initially free of disease but at risk for developing disease within a specified time period. Incidence can also refer to health events such as hospitalizations within a defined population over a specified period of time. Estimation of new cases is an important natural history component of disease models as well as prevention strategies that reduce the incidence of disease or increase the incidence of preventive behaviors. For example, a decision model might be used to assess the impact of a prevention strategy in reducing new cases of disease by increasing the utilization of influenza vaccination among the elderly,[7,8] increasing rubella vaccination among children,[9] or reducing dental caries by fluoridating drinking water. Chemopreventive agents for breast cancer, such as tamoxifen or raloxifene, are evaluated for their effectiveness at reducing the number of new breast cancer cases among women at risk.[10]

The total number of cases in a defined population at risk for developing disease within a specified time period is the disease *prevalence*. Prevalence can be used to describe the baseline risk in a population in the absence of any intervention and includes both new and existing cases of disease. In the example of an intervention to increase mammography use, previously unscreened women with subclinical disease detected at a single screening would be defined as prevalent cases. As with incidence, health events, such as cause-specific hospitalizations or symptoms of disease, can be reported by their prevalence. Prevention strategies can impact the prevalence of disease by reducing the length of time an individual might suffer from disease or by affecting the development of new cases or both. The Papanicolaou smear, which is used to identify pre-invasive and invasive cervical cancer, is an example of an intervention that can reduce cervical cancer prevalence by both mechanisms. Diagnosis and treatment of pre-invasive disease can prevent the development of new cases of cervical cancer (incidence). Additionally, the diagnosis and treatment of invasive cervical cancer early in its natural history are associated with shorter duration of disease and higher rates of cure.[11]

Mortality is typically expressed as a rate and is the number of individuals within a defined population who die during a specific period. Mortality rates can be expressed as all-cause mortality or cause-specific mortality. *Cause-specific mortality* is the number of deaths from a particular disease among individuals at risk for developing or dying from disease. For example, prostate cancer mortality rates are reported only for men. Higher rates of cause specific mortality are usually found in populations with higher rates of underlying disease incidence. Cause-specific mortality is not deaths among individuals or cases with disease; this is *case fatality*. Another closely related concept is *survival*, which is the period from assessment of health characteristics and diagnosis with a disease or condition until death or the end of an observation period. Survival can be reported as median time from the beginning of assessment or as a time-specific rate depending on the typical duration of survival. Acute events where short-term survival is low (e.g., head injury) might be reported as a 30-day rate, whereas more chronic diseases, such as cancer, where patients live longer, are routinely reported as a 5-year survival rate. As with other parameters, mortality, case fatality, and survival rates should be estimated for the underlying population in the decision model. In the model of interventions to increase mammography screening, separate mortality or survival estimates would be made for women never diagnosed with breast cancer and for women diagnosed with breast cancer by stage of disease at diagnosis and specific treatment.

Morbidity is broadly defined as the absence of health or physical or psychological well-being. Strictly speaking, the incidence or development of disease may be associated with some morbidity, although for many diseases, this process may be asymptomatic and patients are unaware of their disease. Morbidity measures are especially important where prevention strategies are equally effective at reducing incidence, prevalence, or mortality; but improvements in these outcomes are associated with a temporary or permanent decrement in physical or mental health. Morbidity involves a broad group of measures used to express the burden of disease, including disability, injury, quality of life, and utility. Service utilization, such as hospitalizations and emergency room visits, are also measures of morbidity. *Disability* is usually defined as the temporary or long-term reduction in an individual's functional capacity. Prevention or minimization of disability is commonly used as an outcome in decision analysis. For example, cochlear implants may minimize the disability and costs associated with profound deafness in children.[12]

Injuries are unintentional or intentional events that cause physical or mental harm and may lead to disability or death. Examples of intentional injuries include homicide, abuse, and suicide, whereas unintentional injuries are most commonly the result of motor vehicle collisions and falls. In 1996, unintentional injuries were the fifth leading cause of death in the United States,[13] leading to interest in injury-prevention counseling and other interventions that promote the use of automobile seat belts, smoke detectors, as well as motorcycle and bicycle helmets.

Quality of life is a multidimensional measure of the physical, emotional, and social effects of disease, treatment, or sequela of injury and disability and is usually measured using standardized, validated instruments. Many of the first measures of quality of life were based on objective assessments completed by physicians (e.g., Karnofsky Performance Scale),[14] but patients currently complete most measures. Measures of quality of life include general or generic ones, which can be used by all individuals, as well as disease-specific ones, which provide additional detail on symptoms of disease and side effects of treatment. Generic measures are comparable across studies and diseases but may not fully measure disease-specific burdens.

The morbidity measures described above are most commonly used as outcomes of decision models; however, a related concept, utility, is the only measure used to "quality-adjust" survival time in the denominator of decision models. *Utility* represents the value an individual places on a specific outcome. Quality of life and utility are described in greater detail in Chapter 5.

Each of these measures can be used to describe the burden of disease or health outcome in a specific population. However, because the development of most diseases is associated with multiple risk factors and health behaviors, yet individuals without risk factors or behaviors can still develop disease, estimates of association between risk factors or health characteristics and disease are usually quantified as relative. In the following section, the most commonly used relative estimates of risk are reviewed.

MEASURES OF OVERALL IMPACT OF RISK FACTORS AND INTERVENTIONS

This section reviews measures of association between interventions, health behaviors, or risk factors and the health outcomes described above. Commonly used measures of association include attributable risks, relative risks, and odds ratios. These measures reflect the risk of disease in a population with the risk factor or treatment compared to the risk of disease in a population without the risk factor or treatment.

Attributable risk is the rate of disease or other outcomes in individuals with the risk factor or health behavior that can be attributed to that risk factor or behavior. Attributable risk is usually calculated only from studies where measures of the risk factor or behavior are made before disease or health outcome. It is calculated by subtracting the rate of the outcome among individuals without the risk factor from the rate of the outcome among individuals with the risk factor. An important assumption in the calculation of attributable risk is that risk factors other than the one under investigation have had equal effects on individuals who develop disease and on those who do not. Similar concepts include the *population attributable risk*, which is used to calculate attributable risk for the entire population. For example, in the United States, smoking attributable mortality is estimated to be approximately 400,000 deaths per year.[15,16] Thus, eliminating cigarette smoking and any risk former smokers have after quitting could reduce mortality rates by 400,000 per year. This measure is the maximum benefit in an ideal setting where the behavior or risk factor and associated risk could be completely eliminated.

The prevented fraction is related to the attributable risk but reflects the maximum benefit of an intervention in a real-world or typical setting. The *prevented fraction* is a measure of the proportion of disease or other outcome in individuals exposed to a protective factor or health behavior that can be attributed to that risk factor or behavior. It is calculated by subtracting incidence in the exposed population (I_e) from the incidence in the unexposed population (I_u) and dividing by the incidence in the unexposed population [$(I_u - I_e)/I_u$].

Relative risk is the ratio of the risk of developing disease (incidence) or death (mortality) in the group with the risk factor or health behavior of interest (I_e) to the risk of disease or death in the group without the risk factor or health behavior of interest (I_u). The relative risk is I_e/I_u. As with attributable risk, relative risk can be calculated only directly from studies where the measurement of the risk factor or health behavior precedes the occurrence of the outcome (i.e., cohort studies, randomized controlled trials). An analogous relative measure of risk in studies of survival or time-to-event is the *relative hazard*, the ratio of the survival time in the group with the risk factor divided by the survival time in the group without the risk factor.

The *odds ratio* is a commonly used measure of association that relies on a ratio of odds rather than probabilities. The odds of an event are the probability of an event happening (p) divided by the probability of an event not happening ($1 - p$) [$p/(1 - p)$]. For example, in a population of 100 individuals with a risk factor where 25 develop the disease, the odds of developing disease are 25/(100–25), or 33%, whereas the probability of developing disease is 25/100, or 25%. The odds ratio can be calculated for study designs where measurement of exposure precedes disease where measurement of exposure occurs simultaneously or where measurement of disease precedes measurement of exposure, although its conceptualization is slightly different. In studies where measurement of exposure precedes disease, the odds ratio is the ratio of the odds of disease in a population with the health characteristic or risk factor to the odds of disease in a population without the health characteristic or risk factor. In case-control studies, where disease is measured prior to measurement of the health characteristic, the odds ratio is also the odds of having a health characteristic or risk factor among a population with disease to the odds of having a health characteristic or risk factor among a population without disease.

Relative measures of risk, such as relative risk and odds ratio, are commonly used in models of prevention strategies that interrupt an underlying natural history of disease. For example, natural history models of cervical cancer in women with HIV disease[17] or fracture among women on hormone replacement therapy[18] are based, in part, on estimates of relative risk. In observational studies, the relative risk and odds ratio are usually risk–outcome associations, rather than intervention–outcome associations. Although associations between interventions or specific treatments and disease outcomes may be estimated in cohort studies where this information is collected, these estimates may be limited by patient selection.

Once an intervention is mapped out and the appropriate population defined, measures of intervention effectiveness and other parameters must be estimated. In the next sections, the distinctions between efficacy and effectiveness are discussed, with attention to issues related to adherence, and study design is reviewed to highlight issues concerned with the selection of different types of parameters.

Effectiveness and Efficacy

A health service or intervention is considered to be effective if it improves health outcomes in a typical community or health-care setting. Effectiveness is distinguished from efficacy in that *efficacy* is the extent to which a health service or intervention results in improved health under ideal conditions. Since the interpretation of a decision analysis of a prevention strategy is usually for a typical community, *effectiveness* is the measure of intervention impact desired. However, results from randomized controlled trials (RCTs) conducted in well-defined and carefully monitored populations represent the efficacy, not the effectiveness, of an intervention in improving health outcomes (see Study Design, below). As a result of differences between ideal and typical settings, characteristics of provider and patient populations, as well as patient and provider adherence, estimates of intervention effectiveness are almost always lower than estimates of intervention efficacy. Model structure should incorporate these issues; they are discussed in greater detail below.

Efficacy estimates from RCTs may not translate directly into effectiveness in general practice, where both providers and patients may differ from those that participate in trials. RCTs are usually conducted in carefully selected settings, such as academic centers, and may differ from community-based settings, where resources may be more limited, adherence or follow-up may be less complete, or patients and providers may be less carefully selected.[19] Additionally, interventions conducted in an RCT setting may include more extensive monitoring, with more direct provider involvement than may occur in a typical practice or community.

Additionally, many RCTs are typically conducted in younger, healthier, nonminority populations with higher socioeconomic status and better preventive health behaviors and overall health than the general population with disease.[20–22] Although these healthier populations are represented in intervention and control arms, use of select populations in randomized trials may limit the generalizability of findings to the general population. For instance, a review of cancer patients in New Mexico between 1969 and 1982 noted that only 2% of cases in the tumor registry participated in Southwestern Oncology Group RCT protocols. Cancer patients over the age of 65 were underrepresented in trials without age restrictions and excluded from trials with age restrictions.[21] This lack of representation is of particular concern since this population is at highest risk of developing the most common cancers[11] and may have higher rates of disease complication or side effect,[23, 24] which may in turn lower the anticipated effectiveness of new therapies. Thus, extrapolation of efficacy estimates from RCTs should be carefully reviewed for the target population since a lack of generalizability may affect policy recommendations. In the example described here, decisions about Medicare coverage for specific treatments of cancer in an elderly population may be limited by the representativeness of the underlying studies for the elderly.

In real-world settings, as opposed to most RCT settings, patients or providers may not fully adhere to specific treatment regimens or medical advice, potentially reducing the impact of the intervention on health outcomes when applied to the general population. Some RCTs utilize eligibility criteria that include predictors of treatment or program adherence and exclude potentially nonadherent subjects. This is particularly relevant since, in several randomized trials, adherence to treatment, including placebo, is associated with improved outcomes over subjects who are nonadherent.[25] This may further reduce the generalizability of RCT findings.

In clinical settings, providers may not adhere to recommended guidelines and services, provide prevention-oriented advice, or provide sufficient monitoring of complex regimens.[26] This may be because they are not aware of guidelines, are forgetful, or face time constraints.[27] However, if the effectiveness of an intervention is estimated from guideline-based performance, lower than expected levels of adherence will overestimate actual effectiveness. Even when providers do adhere to guidelines, however, patients may not adhere to recommended prevention-oriented changes in diet, physical activity, cancer screening tests, or safe sexual practices.[28,29] In the case of cervical cancer screening, 20%–57% of women with abnormal test results do not complete timely follow-up.[22,30,31] Such women may be less likely to return to regular screening or to seek care if symptoms develop in the future. Lack of patient adherence to recommended follow-up will reduce the effectiveness of interventions at improving breast and cervical cancer outcomes and may increase the costs associated with multiple reminders or other strategies to improve follow-up. An extreme example of patient nonadherence is related to the resurgence of drug-resistant tuberculosis, which is associated with incomplete treatment.[32] Directly observed therapy programs, which exert more control over patient adherence, are associated with lower rates of drug resistance and relapse[33] as well as further transmission.[34] Thus, an important component for modeling the effectiveness of prevention strategies includes estimation of the multiple types of adherence, from the perspectives of the provider and the patient, and the distinct consequences for adherent and nonadherent individuals.

In the next sections, study design is reviewed in greater detail and selection among studies for specific types of parameter estimate are discussed.

STUDY DESIGN

Understanding the strengths and weaknesses of study design is critical for selecting the most appropriate data from the best available study for estimating parameters. A single model may use data from multiple types of study, including RCTs, observational studies, syntheses of estimates from other studies, and expert opinion or consensus panel estimates.

Several features of all study designs are key to the underlying quality and, potentially, the suitability of the study for use in a decision model. The setting and process of selection of eligible subjects provide information about generalizability and appropriateness of the sample as well as potential biases that may affect the interpretation of study findings. Specification of explicit inclusion and exclusion criteria and high participation rates are critical components of selection for all studies. The unbiased and standardized assessment of health characteristics or risk factors and the study outcome (e.g., disease occurrence) as well as high rates of retention across all subjects are other key features of study quality. Differential assessment of risk factors or health characteristics and outcomes can lead to over- or underestimation of the true association between health characteristic and outcome (see the bibliography for references on features of study design that impact the interpretation of findings).

Because disease or health outcomes can occur in individuals without specific risk factors or health characteristics as well as individuals with the risk factor, use of a comparison group provides critical information about disease occurrence that is related to the specific risk factor under study. As a result, study designs that use control groups provide methodologically stronger estimates of the association between a risk factor and disease or intervention and outcomes. Finally, in observational studies where patients select treatment or health behaviors and the association with health outcome is measured, it is possible that unmeasured patient characteristics are associated with both behavior or treatment choice and outcome, thus clouding the interpretation of the observed association. Random assignment of treatment or prevention strategy to similar patients ensures that the health outcome is due to the treatment rather than underlying patient characteristics. Other techniques, such as use of propensity scores or the instrumental variable, can be used in observational studies to adjust for some of the bias associated with unmeasured patient characteristics.[35,36]

Features of study design (temporality of exposure and outcome, use of controls, and circumstance of exposure) are key components of the hierarchy of evidence for efficacy or effectiveness based on study design. The order of this hierarchy is RCTs, cohort studies, case–control studies, cross-sectional studies, and case series. This hierarchy is also used to assess the internal validity of the association between an intervention and outcome, with high internal validity in well-conducted RCTs and low internal validity in case series. The hierarchy is useful for choosing estimates of effectiveness for the model and is used more formally by the U.S. Preventive Services Task Force in developing recommendations for preventive services.[37]

This hierarchy is not absolute, however. Study quality plays a critical role in parameter estimation, and there may be situations where estimates of the association between an intervention and outcome from a well-conducted observational study are superior to those from a poorly conducted RCT. Similarly, an observational study may be more generalizable or provide information that is more directly applicable to a particular question.[37] Another related consideration is the external validity of a study. While usually considered to be synonymous with generalizability, in the context of a decision model, however, generalizability should be considered in relation to the target population. Thus, well-conducted, nationally representative cross-sectional surveys may have high external validity for estimating prevalence and for assessment of a strategy conducted in the general population, but estimates from this source may be less appropriate for a high-risk population.

In general, intervention efficacy parameters are best estimated with RCTs or, in the absence of data, from an RCT with data from cohort studies. Natural histories of disease parameters are best estimated with cohort studies and, in their absence, case-control studies; prevalence parameters are best estimated with data from cross-sectional studies. As discussed previously, because RCTs are conducted in highly select populations, baseline prerandomization information is usually not a good source of disease or risk factor prevalence data. Representative samples of well-conducted cross-sectional studies will provide better estimates of the prevalence of a risk factor or health characteristic. The specific study designs and their use in decision models are discussed in greater detail below.

Experimental Studies

The *RCT* is an experimental study in which subjects or communities are randomly assigned to groups where at least one group receives a therapeutic or other intervention and is compared to best usual care or placebo depending on the medical condition under investigation. Preferably, this assignment is unknown to the patients as well as the investigators (*masked* or *blinded assignment*), so that knowledge of assignment does not influence reporting of side effects or other symptoms, although there are some situations where status cannot be easily concealed.

However, as mentioned previously, despite strengths, subjects included in RCTs may be very different from typical subjects in the community (*limited generalizability*). Additionally, sample size and power are typically calculated for specific, primary outcomes that may result in insufficient power to assess secondary outcomes, limiting the use of these data for decision models. A decision analysis of a secondary outcome may be seriously limited by lack of power. Typically, RCTs take several years and are expensive to conduct, so data may not be available in a timely fashion for the model. Other interventions may not be assessed in a randomized trial setting because they are complex or the outcomes diffuse, requiring very long follow-up and extremely large samples. Further, some practices diffuse so rapidly into standard medical practice that assessing effectiveness can be very difficult. For example, the prostate-specific antigen (PSA) screening test for prostate cancer has become widely used despite the absence of definitive data for a reduction in prostate cancer mortality . However, in 1994, the multicenter Prostate Lung Colorectal and Ovarian Cancer screening trial was initiated to test, among other things, the effectiveness of prostate cancer screening.[38] Unfortunately, the usual-care control arm of the trial is likely to consist of men who use PSA screening as well, making the differences in screening practices and subsequent outcomes difficult to identify. Thus, absence of a strong impact of PSA screening on prostate cancer mortality may be a result of high utilization in the control group. The Multiple Risk Factor Intervention Trial examined the impact of intervention for multiple cardiovascular risk factors among men compared to a usual-care control group. The study was considered a failure because it could not distinguish between the outcomes of the intervention and the control groups. On closer examination, however, risk factors (and outcomes) were reduced in both the intervention and control groups.[39] Secular trends in cardiovascular risk factors were, in fact, a public health success. Finally, there are some conditions where subjects cannot ethically be randomized to a treatment or prevention strategy, such as the impact of cigarette smoking on lung cancer incidence. In these situations, observational studies are used to estimate effectiveness.

For some studies, in particular community-based intervention strategies, random assignment of communities or physician practice groups may not be feasible. *Concurrently controlled studies*, also called quasi-experimental studies, are a hybrid of RCTs and observational studies. This design introduces an intervention to one group and uses another, similar group as a control, but assignment to these groups is not randomized. Rates of study outcome are measured in both groups at baseline prior to the introduction of the prevention strategy and again following the intervention. Concurrently controlled studies offer some protection against bias due to secular trends.

Studies of the impact of gun control legislation on homicide and suicide have used time-series analyses to compare communities with and without changes in legislation.[40] These studies have been criticized, however, for appropriateness of the comparison areas and the period over which the intervention is evaluated.[41]

When historical controls are used for comparison to an intervention group, the design is also known as a *time series*. However, over time, even within the same system, data collection may differ in quality or usefulness for a research project. Results from these studies must be interpreted with caution when secular trends are known to affect the outcome. For example, several studies of interventions to increase mammography screening or clinical breast exams have used historical controls and reported increases in mammography use among eligible women following the intervention ranging from 10% to 25%.[42-44] However, in the past decade in the United States, mammography use in eligible women has risen from 54.3% in 1989 to 71.3% in 1997, an increase of 17% during the same periods the previous studies were conducted.[45] Thus, interpretation of intervention effectiveness within the context of increasing mammography use is limited.

When assignment of treatment or intervention is nonrandom, differences in characteristics between intervention and control groups may be responsible for any observed differences in outcome rather than the intervention itself. However, this design is useful for interventions that employ community outreach strategies, including the media and churches, where there is little control over the individuals reached within the community and, to minimize contamination, may be best compared to another similar community at baseline and during the post-study period.

Observational Studies

Observational studies are epidemiologic studies that do not involve any intervention to study participants but measure health characteristics or risk factors and health outcomes as they naturally occur in a defined population. Specific designs include cohort studies, case-control studies, cross-sectional studies, and case series, each of which will be described in further detail below. Within the category of observational studies, major distinctions between designs are related to the timing of risk factor or health characteristic measurement, outcome assessment and selection of control groups.

Cohort studies are longitudinal studies where data on risk factors or health characteristics are collected within a defined population before the occurrence of the health outcome of interest. Of the different observational studies, only cohort studies can generate incidence and relative risk estimates directly, although in studies where risk of disease is rare an odds ratio can approximate a relative risk. Examples of large cohort studies include the Framingham Study, the Nurses Health Study, and the Established Population for the Epidemiologic Study of the Elderly.[46]

A well-conducted cohort study is a good source of estimates of effectiveness in the absence of a well-conducted RCT. Cohort studies are also an excellent source of data for natural history of disease measures of association. For example, in a model of breast cancer screening in elderly women with and without comorbid conditions, estimates of excess mortality for women with high blood pressure or congestive heart failure were based on the Framingham Study.[47]

Like RCTs, cohort studies can be costly and estimates may not be available in a timely fashion since long-term follow-up of large numbers of subjects is usually required. Data on health characteristics can be collected prospectively or, if detailed records exist, retrospectively. However, retrospective cohort studies rely on the quality of previously collected data where forms may not have been developed for research purposes. Additionally, because a sample is selected from older records, tracking individuals for outcome assessment may be complicated.

The *case-control study* design identifies individuals with disease or the outcome of interest (cases) and individuals without disease or the outcome of interest (controls), as well as previous behaviors, risk factors, or characteristics. These data are collected retrospectively, typically by interview or medical record review, and the association between being a case and having a risk factor and being a control and having a risk factor is evaluated with an odds ratio. Case-control studies are especially good for rare diseases and are timelier than cohort or experimental studies.

However, this design has the potential for introducing bias in the process of choosing controls and measuring health behaviors or risk factors. Cases and controls are selected separately, following different procedures with different inclusion and exclusion criteria. Controls are typically selected from health-care settings, from communities by random-digit telephone dialing, or from historical records. Both approaches may have limitations since hospitalized controls may represent a select group with higher rates of comorbid disease and community controls may differ from cases in terms of socioeconomic status.

Retrospective assessment of risk factors or health behaviors may also introduce bias in measurement. Cases may have reflected more on their health behaviors or, as a result of a diagnosis, researched their family history of disease. Thus, disease-specific risk factors might be more frequently reported by cases than controls, potentially leading to differential assessment of risk (*recall bias*). Interviewers may also exert their opinions or beliefs during the interview process by questioning cases more rigorously than controls or differentially providing prompts (*observer or interviewer bias*). Risk factors might be more likely to be identified in cases because they are under surveillance as a result of having the disease. Finally, because outcome is measured after exposure, temporality cannot be established.

Cross-sectional studies collect data on health characteristics and health outcomes at the same time within the study population. These studies can be an important source of estimates of disease or health characteristic prevalence as well as generating hypotheses to identify associations between risk factors and health outcomes. The National Health Interview Survey (NHIS) and the National Health and Nutrition Examination Survey (NHANES) are examples of large, nationally representative, cross-sectional studies.[48] However, since temporality cannot be ascertained, cross-sectional studies reside at the other end of the spectrum from RCTs in terms of strength of evidence for causality. This design is, however, excellent for estimating risk factor, health behavior, or disease prevalence. Additionally, the NHIS and the NHANES are now linked with follow-up of subject mortality, creating cohorts for the assessment of risk factors and outcomes.

Case series are studies that focus exclusively on individuals with a disease or specific health event. Cases may be identified from medical records, disease registries, or administrative data. In the early phases of the identification of new forms of disease or disease in unexpected populations, findings from other study designs may be unavailable and case series may be the only source of data for modeling efforts. However, there are serious limitations in using estimates from case series to estimate the effectiveness of any intervention.

Synthesis Methods

Synthesis methods utilize a systematic review of the literature to identify studies that address a specific research question and, when appropriate, combine or integrate data from multiple studies for a summary effect estimate. Such methods may be particularly useful for increasing sample size and power when several similar but small studies have been conducted with consistent but statistically insignificant findings or in analyses of secondary outcomes where power to detect differences in the underlying study may be limited. Synthesis methods can be used to estimates most types of parameter in decision models.

Meta-analysis requires specification of a study question and systematic identification of relevant studies. Electronic databases are typically used; however, electronic indexing is imperfect, and searches may not identify all relevant studies. Review of multiple databases (e.g., MEDLINE, Psychlit) with multiple search engines (e.g., Ovid, PubMed) and reference lists as well as hand searches of journals can be used to supplement electronic indexing. Favorable studies are more likely to be published, so several investigators have suggested that identification of relevant unpublished studies and translation of non-English studies may reduce any bias associated with publication or language of publication.[49,50] Practically, however, identification of unpublished studies in a systematic manner is more complicated, although randomized trial databases (e.g., Cochrane Controlled Trials Register) and federal funding lists may provide some assistance.

Following identification of potential studies, well-defined criteria for selection and inclusion/exclusion criteria are necessary. Standardized methods for abstraction of data elements and use of multiple abstractors ensure consistent measurement of risk factors and health outcomes. Additionally, quality scoring, based on study characteristics such as design, description of blinding, loss to follow-up, outcome assessment in longitudinal assessment, or use of intention-to-treat analysis, can be performed as part of data abstraction.[51–54] A specific quality score can be developed or a more general ranking can then be used to exclude a study from analysis or for weighting studies by quality in sensitivity analysis.[55]

A key assumption for combining data from multiple studies is that the study effects are homogeneous. This is first assessed qualitatively through visual inspection and graphing and then quantitatively with formal tests of homogeneity, to ensure that data can be combined. These tests vary based, in part, on the method to be used for combining data from the separate studies. Data may be pooled directly from the primary studies[56] or abstracted and combined using specific meta-analytic statistical techniques.[57] When combining data from separate studies, assumptions about the different studies are made. Studies can be assumed to represent the same common effect (*fixed effects*) or to represent a random sample from an underlying group of studies where each study is different but shows a common effect (*random effects*). The assumption about underlying studies has an impact on the calculation of tests of homogeneity and variance for the summary estimate. Several references listed in the bibliography more thoroughly review the assumptions and statistical techniques underlying different meta-analytic techniques and models.

By combining studies conducted in different populations, meta-analysis may also increase the generalizability of results. However, any summary estimate will reflect the limits of the underlying studies as well as concerns about heterogeneity among studies. The limitations of meta-analysis are illustrated by a study comparing findings from large RCTs and meta-analyses that addressed the same clinical questions. Most findings were consistent, although in a portion of studies the results of meta-analyses and large randomized trials were divergent.[58] In situations where meta-analytic summary estimates reflected a positive association and RCTs did not, the authors were concerned about *publication bias*, that studies with positive findings are more likely to be published than studies with negative findings. In situations where RCTs reported a positive association but meta-analyses did not, authors were concerned about heterogeneity among studies, that variability among populations, age distribution, health status, differences in therapy, changes over time in medical practice, or underlying quality of studies overwhelmed any intervention effect. Thus, while meta-analysis is a useful tool for synthesizing data, its many potential limitations will influence the interpretation of findings, regardless of outcome.[58–61]

Bayesian methods are techniques of synthesizing data that employ empiric data and subjective probability.[62] One example is the confidence profile method, which can be used to estimate the probability distribution of a parameter.[63]

Expert Opinion or Consensus

In situations where there are few published data, expert opinion or consensus panel estimates may be an important source of data for decision models. Consensus panels have been used to develop clinical guidelines or to determine the appropriateness of specific procedures for clinical conditions.[64] Structured methods for eliciting opinions from experts include the Delphi method and the nominal group technique.[65] Briefly, the *Delphi method* solicits information from individuals anonymously, reports responses to the group, and then, based on summarized estimates, solicits information from the individuals again until a consensus is reached. This process can be time-consuming and does not allow for interaction among the panel. The validity of this process may vary based on the parameter being estimated. For example, clinicians may be able to accurately describe treatment patterns or standard practices in specific clinical settings, but they may be less accurate in their estimation of the effectiveness of specific prevention interventions.

Further limits of these methods include the selection of participants, which may be nonsystematic,[66] since results from expert consensus panels are often affected by the composition of the panel.[67–69] Additionally, as in all group settings, a single dominant member may disproportionately affect the outcome. Despite these limitations, recent studies have shown that the results of expert panels and surveys of practicing physicians generally agree on estimates of appropriateness of specific medical procedures in well-defined clinical situations.[70] They also show that expert panelists are internally consistent across methods of eliciting probabilities.[31] When estimates from consensus panels are included in decision analyses, sensitivity analysis can help the analyst understand the impact of opinions on overall model outcomes.

SPECIAL ISSUES AND CONSIDERATIONS IN ESTIMATING MODEL PARAMETERS

In the following section, additional considerations in the estimation of parameters for decision models of prevention strategies are reviewed.

Asymptomatic Screening

In models that assess the impact of asymptomatic screening of healthy populations for risk factors or early signs of disease, there are several specific issues to consider. First, screening tests are not perfect mechanisms for identifying individuals with and without risk factors or disease. In addition to correctly identifying individuals with and without disease, some individuals will test positive for the disease but upon further diagnostic testing will be found not to have the disease (*false-positive*), and some individuals will test negative for a disease that they actually have (*false-negative*). Screening test characteristics are referred to in the epidemiologic literature as *sensitivity*, the probability that a screening test will correctly identify an individual with disease or a risk factor, and *specificity*, the probability that a screening test will correctly identify an individual without disease. From the perspective of a screening model, it may not be possible to distinguish false-positives from true-positives; and as a result, all groups will undergo the cost of the screening test, and additional diagnostic testing or work-up. However, false-positives will also incur these costs and any psychological effects without any benefits of screening.[71,72]

Within a given population, the number of false-positive and false-negative results is based on the sensitivity and specificity of the screening test as well as the prevalence of disease in the underlying population. For a screening test with a given sensitivity and specificity, use in a population with high disease prevalence will yield higher *positive predictive value*, or the proportion of individuals with a positive test who have disease, and a lower *negative predictive value*, or the proportion of individuals with a negative test who do not have disease, compared to a population with lower disease prevalence. Because of the potential magnitude of the harms and costs associated with misclassifying individuals with screening tests, careful estimation of disease prevalence in the target population is essential. Additionally, the test sensitivity and specificity can vary across settings (particularly in situations where standards for test interpretation have not been implemented). For example, the sensitivity and specificity of lipid screening vary by type of test (high-density lipoprotein, low-density lipoprotein, and/or total cholesterol) as well as whether patients are tested at random or while fasting.[73] Evaluating the sensitivity and specificity of the screening test with sensitivity analysis will allow the analyst to understand the impact on variability in test characteristics on model findings (see Chapter 7).

A related consideration in the assessment of screening tests is that earlier diagnosis does not necessarily improve survival. Earlier diagnosis may only extend the length of time an individual has disease, with no disruption in the natural history of disease, particularly if treatment is not more effective earlier in the natural history of disease. Earlier detection without an improvement in mortality may also be associated with a decrement in well-being since patients may receive treatment for longer periods of time. This is referred to as a *lead time bias* and is an important reason for the assessment of mortality or survival based on stage of disease at diagnosis rather than survival from the point of diagnosis in studies of prevention strategies that assess screening.[74]

Surrogate Measures

The underlying goal of many prevention strategies is to disrupt the natural history of disease, to reduce the associated morbidity and mortality. However, prevention strategies that address safe sex practices or smoking cessation may not be able to assess the impact of these behavioral changes on the entire process of disease (sexually transmitted disease/HIV and lung cancer or cardiovascular disease, respectively) since development of disease may take many years and not all individuals with disease-specific risk factors will develop disease. As a result, short-term or surrogate measures of health behavior or factors within the disease pathway can also be used to measure the impact of health interventions or procedures. Surrogate measures include health-care process measures, intermediate end points, behavioral or environmental changes, and other health outcomes. Health-care processes reflect the experiences of patients in their interaction with providers (doctors, nurses, and other health professionals) within the health-care system.[75,76] Examples of process measures include documentation of a provider's discussion of treatment options, rehospitalizations, and rates of service use appropriate to patient age and health status. The value of surrogate markers is limited to situations where the presence of a particular marker is strongly associated with disease or outcome (sensitive) and the absence of a marker is strongly associated with the absence of disease or outcome (specific).

Intermediate end points are more typically variables that reflect events in the natural history of disease or injury. For example, patients with familial adenomatous polyposis have an extremely high risk of developing colon cancer, which may take many years.[77] These patients develop hundreds of colorectal polyps, which have a high probability of becoming cancerous, so randomized trials of chemopreventive agents have used the number and size of these polyps, as intermediate end points for assessing the effectiveness of therapeutic agents in preventing the development of colorectal cancer.[78] Other examples of intermediate end points used in assessing prevention of disease include cholesterol reduction for heart disease, lowered blood pressure for stroke, and earlier stage of disease at diagnosis for cancer. Other examples of intermediate end points used to assess the effectiveness of treatment in prolonging the development or recurrence of disease include viral load for HIV[79] as well as a variety of tumor markers,[80] such as PSA for prostate cancer.[81]

In the a decision model, surrogate outcomes can serve as a final outcome or the model can be used to estimate disease incidence or mortality. In the latter situation, sensitivity analysis should be used to assess the impact of assumptions about the relationship between the surrogate outcomes on model results.

Estimation of Prevention Strategy Impacts on Life Expectancy or Mortality

Models that assess the impact of a prevention strategy on the natural history of disease yield estimates of mortality or life expectancy. Because studies vary in the quality of disease-specific mortality assessment and it is useful to compare model findings across a common metric, most studies report all-cause mortality as an outcome. Race, gender, and age-specific life expectancy or mortality are routinely reported by the Centers for Disease Control and Prevention (CDC), National Center For Health Statistics (NCHS) for the general population.[13] However, if a prevention strategy has an impact on life expectancy or mortality, the analyst will need to estimate increased or decreased life expectancy or mortality associated with disease. This is also known as *excess mortality* and can be calculated with the declining exponential approximation to life expectancy (DEALE) model, where the decreased life expectancy for a population with disease is the reciprocal of all-cause mortality and cause-specific mortality.[82]

There are several limitations to this approach. Cause-specific mortality rates are estimated from death certificate data, where, for example, cardiovascular disease was reported as the underlying cause of death. Although cause of death on death certificates for some diseases is thought to be relatively accurate,[83] the sensitivity and specificity of death certificate data for stroke disease deaths is unknown (but thought to be poor).[84] Thus, estimates from death certificate data are of uncertain quality. The DEALE model has been reported to provide a good approximation for diseases where mortality is high and to be less useful when people may live with a disease for a long period, as in the case of most chronic diseases.[85]

Further, many chronic diseases occur together (e.g., diabetes, coronary heart disease),[86] and under the DEALE model, disease-specific mortality is considered to be additive. However, the majority of the underlying statistical models employed to report risk data in the medical literature use a multiplicative (e.g., logistic and Poisson regression, survival analysis), rather than an additive, approach. Multiplicative or additive models for estimating disease-specific life expectancy may overestimate or underestimate life expectancy;[87] sensitivity analysis of the method used to estimate life expectancy can explore the impact on model findings.

Another approach to estimating excess mortality is to calculate all-cause mortality rates directly using a large cohort with disease assessment and mortality follow-up. In practice, however, this approach is limited by the availability of a representative sample of sufficient size with chronic disease assessment and long-term mortality follow-up.

In the following section, sources of data for different study designs are reviewed.

DATA SOURCES

The data used to estimate parameters in decision models may be gathered from a variety of sources, including secondary data from the published literature or unpublished studies and primary data collected for the explicit purpose of the model. Additionally, specific analyses for parameters can be conducted using existing data. It is generally not feasible to conduct an RCT, cohort study, or case-control study within the time frame for the development of a decision model. More typically, estimates for these designs are collected from the published literature. Results from experimental studies can be identified using the search terms *clinical trial*, and *controlled clinical trials*, with the MEDLINE search engine. Similarly, the terms *cohort studies*, *case-control studies*, *cross-sectional studies*, and *meta-analyses* can be used to identify these study designs. Additionally, funding sources such as the National Institutes of Health, clinical trial registries, or networks (e.g., Cochrane Collaboration) can be used to identify ongoing studies that may not have been identified through a literature search or may have published preliminary findings in abstract form only. Organizations such as the National Health System Centre for Reviews and Dissemination in the United Kingdom compile a database of prior and ongoing meta-analyses (Database of Abstracts of Reviews of Effectiveness).

Published reports from the CDC, particularly the NCHS, are excellent sources of data for decision models. Mortality rates based on death certificates and estimates of the U.S. population for the underlying period are reported annually for all-cause and cause-specific mortality by the Vital Statistics branch of the NCHS.[13] Descriptive reports from nationally representative, cross-sectional surveys, such as the NHIS, and NHANES, are excellent sources of prevalence estimates.[48] Similarly, the state-based Behavioral Risk Factors Surveillance System conducted by the CDC provides nationwide and state data for prevention behaviors and risk factors.

There are also sources of public and other existing data that can be used specifically to estimate a parameter in a decision model. The NCHS makes available cross-sectional survey data in public formats, and the NCHS also makes longitudinal follow-up data available (e.g., the NHANES 1 Epidemiologic Follow-up Study). Other sources of existing data include administrative records from private insurers as well as Medicare and Medicaid, occupational records, hospital records, and tumor or other disease registries.

In some situations where studies cannot be identified from the published literature or existing data are insufficient, the analyst may consider primary data collection. Development of a case series, meta-analysis, or consensus panel specifically for a decision model is a feasible approach to estimating parameters, although, as described previously, there are limitations to these approaches.

Selection of the "best" data source will be based on the research question and target population, specific parameter to be estimated, availability and quality of existing studies, the strengths and limits associated with the study design for the available studies, and the availability of high-quality primary data. These aspects of data selection need to be considered simultaneously, and estimates where the data quality or underlying design is less than optimal should be assessed with sensitivity analyses.

Communication of Effectiveness Data for Policy or Program Planning

There is a significant body of literature that shows that patients do not fully understand concepts of risk and may react differently to identical information presented in different formats.[88–90] There is also evidence that researchers, analysts, and the scientific press may misinterpret or overstate risk estimates, particularly when dealing with relative and absolute estimates when underlying diseases or events are extremely common or very rare.[91,92] For example, if in an RCT rates of disease in the intervention group were 15 per 100 and rates of disease in the control group were 30 per 100, the absolute risk reduction would be 15% and the relative risk reduction would be 50%. If the rates of disease in the two groups changed to 15 per 1000 and 30 per 1000 or 15 per 10,000 and 30 per 10,000, the relative risk reduction would remain 50% in both scenarios, not reflecting the frequency of disease in the population; however, the absolute risk reduction would change to 1.5% and 0.15%, respectively. Thus, one advantage of presenting data as an absolute estimate is that the estimate reflects rates of disease in the underlying population.

Findings from decision models can also be presented in relative and absolute risk formats.[93] Denominator outputs are most commonly presented as life years saved and quality-adjusted life years; both are relative measures of population effects. Life years saved is an estimate of the average expected survival for a cohort receiving a prevention strategy compared to a baseline strategy, and quality-adjusted life years represent average expected survival combined with expected utility. Alternatively, the number needed to screen and the number needed to treat are absolute measures of intervention impact and represent the expected number of patients who must be treated or screened to identify a case or avoid or prevent adverse events compared to the group receiving the comparator or baseline strategy. These metrics may be particularly useful since policy analysts are often interested in information about the percentage incidence or mortality reductions that could be expected from the application of a specific intervention in a target population.

CONCLUSIONS

Decision models can be used to assess the impact of prevention strategies on the development of new disease, identify disease earlier in its natural history when treatment may be more effective, or reduce disease morbidity through improvements in medical care. This chapter highlights issues that need to be considered in constructing decision models, including estimating the values of model parameters and using measures of population effects and risk estimates, study design, and sources of primary and secondary data.

REFERENCES

1. Blondal T, Gudmundsson LJ, Olafsdoffir I, et al. Nicotine nasal spray with nicotine patch for smoking cessation: randomised trial with six year follow-up. *BMJ 1999;* 318:285–9.
2. Fiore MC, Smit SS, Jorenby DE, et al. The effectiveness of the nicotine patch for smoking cessation: a meta-analysis. *JAMA 1994;* 271:1940 7.
3. Jorenby DE, Leischow SJ, Nides MA, et al. A controlled trial of sustained-release buproprion, a nicotine patch, or both for smoking cessation. *N Engl J Med 1999;* 340:685–91.
4. Lancaster T, Stead L, Silagy C, Sowden A. Effectiveness of interventions to help peo ple stop smoking: findings from the Cochrane Library. *BMJ 2000;* 321:355–8.
5. Stapleton JA, Sutherland G, Gussell MAH. How much does relapse after one year erode effectiveness of smoking cessation treatments? Long term follow-up of randomized trial of nicotine nasal spray. *BMJ 1998;* 316:830–1.
6. Helzlsouer KJ. Early detection and prevention of breast cancer. In: Greenwald P, Kramer BS, Weed DL, eds. *Cancer Prevention and Control.* New York: Marcel Dekker, 1995: 509–35.
7. Mullooly JP, Bennett MD, Hornbrook MC, et al. Influenza vaccination programs for elderly persons: cost-effectiveness in a health maintenance organization. *Ann Intern Med 1994;* 121:947–52.
8. Weaver M, Krieger J, Castorina J, et al. Cost–effectiveness of combined outreach for pneumococcal and influenza vaccines. *Arch Intern Med 2001;* 161:111–20.
9. Lieu TA, Cochi SL, Black SB, et al. Cost–effectiveness of routine varicella vaccination program for US children. *JAMA 1994;* 271:375–81.
10. Chlebowski RT. Reducing the risk of breast cancer. *N Engl J Med 2000;* 343:191–8.
11. Ries LAG, Kosary CL, Hankey BF, et al. (eds). *SEER Cancer Statistics Review, 1973–1997.* Bethesda, MD: National Cancer Institute, 2000.

12. Cheng AK, Rubin HR, Powe NR, et al. Cost–utility analysis of the cochlear implant in children. *JAMA 2000;* 284:850–6.

13. Hoyert DL, Kochanek KD, Murphy SL. *Deaths: Final Data for 1997. Nat Vital Stat Rep 1999;* 47:1–104.

14. Karnofsky DA, Abelmann WH, et al. The use of nitrogen mustards in the palliative treatment of carcinoma. *Cancer 1948;* 1:634–56.

15. McGinnis JM, Foege WH. Actual causes of death in the United States. *JAMA 1993;* 270:2207–12.

16. US Department of Health and Human Services. *The Health Benefits of Smoking Cessation. A Report of the Surgeon General, 1990.* DHHS Publication (CDC) 90–8416. Rockville, MD: Public Health Service, Centers for Disease Control, Office on Smoking and Health, 1990.

17. Goldie SJ, Weinstein MC, Kuntz KM, Freedberg KA. The costs, clinical benefits and cost–effectiveness of screening for cervical cancer in HIV infected women. *Ann Inter Med 1999;* 130:97–107.

18. Col NF, Eckman MH, Karas RH, et al. Patient specific decisions about hormone replacement therapy in postmenopausal women. *JAMA 1997;* 277:1140–7.

19. Institute of Medicine. *Assessing Medical Technologies.* Washington DC: National Academy Press, 1985.

20. Chlebowshi RT, Bulter J, Nelson A, et al. Breast cancer chemoprevention. Tamoxifen: current issues and future perspective. *Cancer 1993;* 2 (suppl 3):1032–7.

21. Goodwin JS, Hunt WC, Humble CG, et al. Cancer treatment protocols: who gets chosen? *Arch Intern Med 1988;* 148:2258–60.

22. Thompson IM, Colman CA, Brawley OW, et al. Chemoprevention of prostate cancer. *Semin Urol 1995;* 13:122–9.

23. Cunningham WE, Bozzette SA, Hays RD, et al. Comparison of health-related quality of life in clinical trial and nonclinical trial human immunodeficiency virus–infected cohorts. *Med Care 1995;* 33(Suppl 4):AS15–25.

24. Walsh CR, Lloyd-Jones DM, Camargo CA Jr, et al. Clinical trials of unfractionated heparin and low-molecular weight heparin in addition to aspirin for the treatment of unstable angina pectoris: do the results apply to all patients? *Am J Cardiol 2000;* 86:908–12.

25. Horwitz RI, Viscoli CM, Berkman L, et al. Treatment adherence and risk of death after a myocardial infarction. *Lancet 1990;* 336:542–5.

26. Schwartz JS, Lewis CE, Clancy C, et al. Internists' practices in health promotion and disease prevention. *Ann Intern Med 1991;* 114:46–53.

27. McPhee SJ, Richard RJ, Solkowitz SN. Performance of cancer screening in a university general internal medicine practice: comparison with the 1980 American Cancer Society guidelines. *J Gen Intern Med 1986;* 5:275–81.

28. Burke LE, Dunbar-Jacob JM, Hill MN. Compliance with cardiovascular disease prevention strategies: a review of the research. *Ann Behav Med 1997;* 19:239–63.

29. Van Horn L, Kavey RE. Diet and cardiovascular disease prevention: what works? *Ann Behav Med 1997;* 19:197–212.

30. Lerman C, Hanjani P, Caputo C, et al. Telephone counseling improves adherence to colposcopy among lower-income minority women. *J Clin Oncol 1992;* 10:330–3.

31. Oddone EZ, Samsa G, Matchar DB. Global judgments versus decision-model-facilitated judgment: are experts internally consistent? *Med Decis Making 1994;* 14:19–26.

32. Young RC Jr. Rachal RE, Bailey SB, et al. Strategies for suppression, containment, and eradication of resurgent tuberculosis. *J Health Care Poor Underserved 1997;* 8:424–36.

33. Weis SE, Slocum PC, Blais FX, et al. The effect of directly observed therapy on the rates of drug resistance and relapse in tuberculosis. *N Engl J Med 1994;* 330:1179–84.

34. Dye C, Garnett GP, Sleeman K, Williams BG. Prospects for worldwide tuberculosis control under the WHO DOTS strategy. *Lancet 1998;* 352:1886–91.

35. D'Agostino RB. Propensity score methods for bias reduction in the comparison of a treament to a non-randomized group. *Stat Med 1998;* 17:2265–81.

36. McClellan M, McNeil B, Newhouse JP. Does more intensive treatment of acute myocardial infarction in the elderly reduce mortality? Analysis using instrumental variables. *JAMA 1994;* 272:859–66.

37. Harris RP, Helfand M, Woolf SH, et al. Current methods of the US Preventive Services Task Force: review of the process. *Am J Prev Med 2001;* 20(Suppl 3):21–35.

38. Prorok PC, Andriole GL, Bresalier RS, et al. Design of the Prostate, Lung, Colorectal, and Ovarian (PLCO) Cancer Screening Trial. *Control Clin Trials 2000,* 21:273S–309S.

39. Luepker RV, Grimm RH, Taylor HL. The effect of "usual care" on cardiovascular risk factors in a clinical trial. *Control Clin Trials 1984;* 5:47–53.

40. Loftin C, McDowall D, Wiersema B, Cottey J. Effects of restrictive licensing of handguns on homicide and suicide in the District of Columbia. *N Engl J Med 1991;* 325:1615–1621.

41. Britt CL, Kleck G, Bordua DJ. A reassessment of the DC gun law: some cautionary notes on the use of interrupted time series designs for policy impact assessment. *Law Soc Rev 1996;* 30:361–380.

42. Erwin DO, Spatz TS, Stotts RC, et al. Increasing mammography and breast self-examination in African American women using the Witness Project™. *J Cancer Educ 1996;* 11:210–5.

43. Kadison P, Pelletier EM, Mounib EL, et al. Improved screening for breast cancer associated with a telephone-based risk assessment. *Prev Med 1998;* 27:493–501.

44. Kohatsu ND, Cramer E, Bohnstedt M. Use of a clinician reminder system for screening mammography in a public health clinic. *Am J Prev Med 1994;* 10:348–52.

45. Blackman DK, Bennett EM, Miller DS. Trends in self-reported use of mammograms (1989–1997) and Papanicolaou tests (1991–1997)—Behavioral Risk Factor Surveillance System. *MMWR Morb Mortal Wkly Rep 1999;* 48:1–22.

46. Cornoni-Huntley J, Ostfeld AM, Taylor JO, et al. Established populations for epidemiologic studies of the elderly: study design and methodology. *Aging Clin Exp Res 1993;* 5:27–37.

47. Mandelblatt JS, Wheat ME, Monane M, et al. Breast cancer screening for elderly women with and without co-morbid conditions: a decision model. *Ann Intern Med 1992;* 116:722–30.

48. Massey JT, Moore TF, Parsons VL, Tadros W. Design and estimation for the National Health Interview Survey, 1985–94. National Center for Health Statistics. *Vital Health Stat 1989;* 2:110.

49. Dickersin K, Chan S, Chalmers TC, et al. Publication bias and clinical trials. *Control Clin Trials 1987;* 8:343–53.

50. Dickerson K, Min YI, Meinert CL. Factors influencing publication of research results: follow-up of applications submitted to two institutional review boards. *JAMA 1992;* 263:374–8.

51. Detsky AS, Naylor CD, O'Rourke K, et al. Incorporating variations in the quality of individual randomized trials into meta-analysis. *J Clin Epidemiol 1992;* 45:255–65.

52. Emerson JD, Burdick E, Hoaglin DC, et al. An empirical study of the possible relation of treatment differences to quality scores in controlled randomized clinical trials. *Control Clin Trials 1990;* 11:339–52.

53. Moher D, Jadad A, Nichol G, et al. Assessing the quality of randomized controlled trials: an annotated bibliography of scales and checklists. *Control Clin Trials 1995;* 16:62–73.

54. Schulz KF, Chalmers I, Hayes RJ, Altman DG. Empirical evidence of bias: dimensions of methodological quality associated with estimates of treatment effects in controlled trials. *JAMA 1995;* 273:408–12.

55. Moher D, Cook DJ, Jadad AR, et al. Assessing the quality of reports of randomized trials: implications for the conduct of meta-analyses. *Health Technol Assess 1999;* 3: i–iv, 1–98.

56. Lau J, Antman EM, Jimenez-Silva J, et al. Cumulative meta-analysis of therapeutic trials for myocardial infarction. *N Engl J Med 1992;* 327:248–54.

57. Laird NM, Mosteller F. Some statistical methods for combining experimental results. *Int J Technol Assess Health Care 1990;* 6:5–30.

58. LeLorier J, Gregoire G, Benhaddad A, et al. Discrepancies between meta-analyses and subsequent large randomized controlled trials. *N Engl J Med 1997;* 337:536–42.

59. Abramson JH. Meta-analysis: a review of pros and cons. *Public Health Rev 1990;* 18:1–47.

60. Antman EM, Lau J, Kupelnick B, et al. A comparison of results of meta-analyses of randomized control trials and recommendations of clinical experts. Treatment for myocardial infarction. *JAMA 1992;* 268:240–8.

61. Fleiss JL, Gross AJ. Meta-analysis in epidemiology, with special reference to studies of the association between exposure to environmental tobacco smoke and lung cancer: a critique. *J Clin Epidemiol 1991;* 44:127–35.

62. Brophy JM, Joseph L. Placing trials in context using Bayesian analysis. GUSTO revisited by Reverend Bayes. *JAMA 1995;* 273:871–5.

63. Eddy DM, Hasselblad V, Schachter R. A Bayesian method for synthesizing evidence: the confidence profile method. *Int J Technol Assess Health Care 1990;* 6:31–51.

64. Brook RH, Chassin MR, Fink A, et al. A method for detailed assessment of the appropriateness of medical technologies. *Int J Technol Assess Health Care 1986;* 2:53–63.

65. Fink A, Kosecoff J, Chassin M, Brook RH. Consensus methods: characteristics and guidelines for use. *Am J Public Health 1984;* 74:979–83.

66. Feinstein AR. Fraud, distortion, delusion, and consensus: the problems of human and natural deception in epidemiologic science. *Am J Med 1988;* 84:475–8.

67. Bickell NA, Earp J, Evans AT, Bernstein SJ. A matter of opinion about hysterectomies: experts' and practicing community gynecologists' ratings of appropriateness. *Am J Public Health 1995;* 85:1125–8.

68. Campbell SM, Hann M, Roland MO, et al. The effect of panel membership and feedback on ratings in a two-round Delphi survey: results of a randomized controlled trial. *Med Care 1999;* 37:964–8.

69. Murphy MK, Sanderson CF, Black NA, et al. Consensus development methods, and their use in clinical guideline development. *Health Technol Assess 1998;* 2:1–88.

70. Ayanian JZ, Landrum MB, Normand SL, et al. Rating the appropriateness of coronary angiography—do practicing physicians agree with an expert panel and with each other? *N Engl J Med 1998;* 338:1896–904.

71. Lerman C, Miller SM, Scarborough R, et al. Adverse psychological consequences of positive cytologic cervical screening. *Am J Obstet Gynecol 1991;* 165:658–62.

72. Lerman C, Trock B, Rimer BK, et al. Psychological and behavioral implications of abnormal mammograms. *Ann Intern Med 1991;* 114:657–61.

73. Pignone MP, Phillips CJ, Atkins D, et al. Screening and treating adults for lipid disorders. *Am J Prev Med 2001;* 20(Suppl 3):77–89.

74. Welch HG, Schwartz LM, Woloshin S. Are increasing 5-year survival rates evidence of success against cancer? *JAMA 2000;* 283:2975–8.

75. Brook RH, Cleary PD. Quality of health care: part 2. Measuring quality of care. *N Engl J Med 1996;* 335:966–70.

76. Starfield B. *Primary Care: Concept, Evaluation, and Policy.* New York: Oxford University Press, 1992.

77. Burn J, Chapman PD, Bishop DT, et al. *Susceptibility Markers in Colorectal Cancer. IARC Scientific Publication 154.* Lyon: International Agency For Research on Cancer, 2001, pp. 131–47.

78. Giardiello FM, Hamilton SR, Krush AJ, et al. Treatment of colonic and rectal adenomas with sulindac in familial adenomatous polyposis. *N Engl J Med 1993;* 328:1313–16.

79. Hughes MD. Analysis and design issues for studies using censored biomarker measurements with an example of viral load measurements in HIV clinical trials. *Stat Med 2000;* 19:3171–91.

80. Bast RC Jr. Ravdin P, Hayes DF, et al. 2000 Update of recommendations for the use of tumor markers in breast and colorectal cancer: clinical practice guidelines of the American Society of Clinical Oncology. *J Clin Oncol 2001;* 19:1865–78.

81. Kelly WK, Scher HI, Mazumdar M, et al. Prostate specific antigen as a measure of disease outcome in metastatic hormone-refractory prostate cancer. *J Clin Oncol 1993;* 11:607–15.

82. Beck JR, Kassirer JP, Pauker SG. A convenient approximation of life expectancy: validation of the method. *Am J Med 1982;* 73:883–8.

83. Percy C, Stanek E, Gloeckler L. Accuracy of cancer death certificates and its effect on cancer mortality statistics. *Am J Public Health 1981;* 71:242–50.

84. Corwin LE, Wolf PA, Kannel WB, McNamara PM. Accuracy of death certification of stroke: the Framingham Study. *Stroke 1982;* 13:818–21.

85. Holland RR, Ellis C, Geller BM, et al. Life expectancy estimation with breast cancer: bias of the declining exponential function and an alternative to its use. *Med Decis Making 1999;* 19:385–93.

86. Greenfield S, Aronow HU, Elashoff RM, Watanabe D. Flaws in mortality data: the hazards of ignoring co-morbid disease. *JAMA 1988,* 260:2253–5.

87. Kuntz KM, Weinstein MC. Life expectancy biases in clinical decision modeling. *Med Decis Making 1995;* 15:158–69.

88. Forrow L, Taylor WC, Arnold RM. Absolutely relative: how research results are summarized can affect treatment decisions. *Am J Med 1992;* 92:121–4.

89. Kahneman D, Tversky A. The framing of decisions and psychology of choice. *Science 1981;* 211:453–8.

90. Malenka DJ, Barron JA, Johansen S, et al. The framing effect of relative and absolute risk. *J Gen Intern Med 1993;* 8:543–8.

91. Kumana CR, Cheung BMY, Lauder IJ. Gauging the impact of statins using number needed to treat. *JAMA 1999;* 282:1899–901.

92. Schwartz LM, Woloshin S, Welch HG. Misunderstandings about the effects of race and sex on physician's referrals for cardiac catheterization. *N Engl J Med 1999;* 341:279–83.

93. Kerlikowske K. Efficacy of screening mammography among women aged 40 to 49 years and 50 to 69 years: comparison of relative and absolute benefit. *J Natl Cancer Inst Monogr 1997;* 22:79–86.

BIBLIOGRAPHY

Gold MR, Siegel JE, Russell LB, et al. *Cost–Effectiveness in Health and Medicine*. New York: Oxford University Press, 1996.

Gordis L. *Epidemiology*. Philadelphia: Saunders, 1996.

Kelsey JL, Whittemore AS, Evans AS, Thompson WD. *Methods in Observational Epidemiology*, 2d ed. New York: Oxford University Press, 1996.

Luce BR, Elixhauser A. *Standards for the Socioeconomic Evaluation of Health Care Services*. Berlin: Springer-Verlag, 1990.

Naglie G, Krahn MD, Naimark D, et al. Primer on medical decision analysis: part 3. Estimating probabilities and utilities. *Med Decis Making 1997;* 17:136–41.

Pettiti DB. *Meta-analysis, Decision-Analysis, and Cost–Effectiveness Analysis: Methods for Quantitative Synthesis in Medicine*, 2d ed. New York: Oxford University Press, 2000.

Sox H, Blatt MA, Higgins MC, Marton KI. *Medical Decision Making*. Boston: Butterworths, 1988.

4

Costs

ANNE C. HADDIX
PHAEDRA S. CORSO
ROBIN D. GORSKY

The costs of health care are essential components of economic evaluations of prevention-effectiveness programs. This chapter describes key concepts in cost analysis and discusses the collection and analysis of data needed to calculate the costs of interventions and health outcomes. The first section defines the types of costs typically included in a cost analysis. The second section presents methods for conducting a cost analysis of a health intervention. The third section describes the cost-of-illness approach to assessing the costs of health outcomes.

TYPES OF COST

In this section, we define some of the most common terms used to categorize costs. These definitions apply to both the costs associated with a health intervention and the costs of health outcomes.

Financial and Economic Costs

It is useful to distinguish between two concepts of cost: financial costs and economic costs. *Financial costs* are the real-money outlays for resources required to produce a program or intervention and to manage a patient's health outcome (e.g., salaries, rent, medical supplies). The *economic costs* of an intervention are the opportunity costs of the resources used to implement the intervention (i.e., the value of the resources if they had been used for another productive purpose). Economic costs include not only direct money outlays but also the value of resources for which no money was spent (e.g., volunteer time, space in the local public health department, donated brochures). Thus, economic costs provide a more complete estimate of intervention or health-outcome costs than financial costs because they include all of the resources used to implement a prevention strategy or manage a health outcome.

For many resources the economic cost is equivalent to the financial cost. The financial outlay (often the price) is sometimes assumed to be a measure of the opportunity cost of using a resource. In some circumstances, however, the economic cost of a resource may differ from the financial cost. A classic example is the distinction between costs and charges for medical services. The economic cost, measured as the opportunity cost of the resources used to deliver the medical service, is often substantially different from the reimbursement of the charge for the medical service, measured as the amount paid for the service. The distinction between costs and charges is explained in more detail later in the chapter. Because it is important to capture fully the value of the resources required for prevention–effectiveness studies, economic costs for an input should be used whenever possible.

Medical Costs, Nonmedical Costs, Productivity Losses, and Intangible Costs

Costs can also be classified as medical, nonmedical, productivity losses, and leisure losses resulting from morbidity and premature morality as well as intangible costs. *Medical costs* are the direct costs incurred to secure medical treatment or costs that accrue to the health system. Examples of medical costs include the costs of screening, counseling, hospitalization, diagnostic testing, prescription drugs, and visits to a clinician. *Nonmedical costs* are direct costs incurred in connection with the prevention activity or the health outcome of interest but for items and expenses not typically classified as medical or health expenditures. Examples of nonmedical costs include the cost of transportation for a patient or caregiver to visit a health-care provider, childcare expenses, and the cost of purchasing nonmedical equipment associated with an intervention (e.g., a bicycle helmet as a result of a bicycle safety education program) or outcome (e.g., a home air-filtration system to mitigate the effects of airborne particulates on a person with asthma). Caregiver time and patient time to participate in an intervention or to seek care are also considered nonmedical costs. These categories of cost are created, in part, to allow for disaggregation of costs by the study perspective. For example, only medical costs would be included in an analysis that incorporates the health-care system perspective, while a societal perspective would include all medical and nonmedical costs associated with an intervention.

Productivity losses are the measure of resources forgone to participate in an intervention, to seek care for a health condition, for caregiving, and as the result of morbidity or premature mortality. In cost–effectiveness analyses, productivity losses associated with participating in an intervention, seeking care, and caregiving are often categorized as nonmedical costs. Productivity losses resulting from morbidity and premature mortality are treated separately. These distinctions are explained below.

Productivity losses are often referred to as indirect costs in the literature. We use the term *productivity loss* because we are most interested in loss of work or leisure productivity, and we want to avoid confusion with the term *indirect costs*, which is used for accounting and contractual purposes. Productivity losses are typically defined as losses in earnings or wages or the imputed value of time spent to perform nonwage household activities and are frequently adjusted to account for lost leisure time as well.

Productivity losses can be incurred by a participant of a program or intervention (e.g., productivity losses associated with time spent away from work to seek medical care or clinical services), a caregiver (e.g., a parent's time missed from work to take a child to a pediatrician), or a person seeking care for a health condition. The Panel on Cost–Effectiveness in Health and Medicine recommends that these productivity losses be included as nonmedical costs in cost–effectiveness analyses that take the societal perspective.[1]

The inclusion of productivity losses that result from morbidity (e.g., work and leisure time lost due to a chronic illness that leaves one bedridden for a certain length of time) or premature mortality in a study depends on the perspective and the study design. For example, an economic evaluation conducted from a societal perspective may include productivity losses from morbidity, and premature mortality, although these costs would be omitted in a similar study taking the health-care system perspective. The inclusion of productivity losses also depends on what type of economic evaluation is being conducted. For example, if it is assumed that productivity losses associated with morbidity and premature mortality are imbedded in the utility weights in the denominator of a cost–utility analysis, then including them as part of overall costs in the numerator of the cost–utility analysis ratio would result in double counting (see Chapter 5 for more on this topic).

Other costs that one might consider in an economic evaluation are intangible costs. *Intangible costs* are the costs associated with a prevention activity or health condition for which it is extremely difficult to assign a monetary value. For example, intangible costs may include the costs of pain and suffering, emotional loss, and social stigmatization. Because they are difficult to measure directly, they are not typically included in cost–effectiveness studies. However, cost–benefit analyses should, at least theoretically, include all costs, even those that are intangible. This topic is addressed more comprehensively in Chapter 8.

Operating and Capital Costs

Costs for resources used to deliver health care can be categorized as operating and capital costs. *Operating costs* are the ongoing costs of a program required to deliver goods or services. They are generally considered to be the costs that accrue over the budget period, usually calculated on an annual basis. *Capital costs* are those costs used for the purchase of assets that have a useful life of longer than 1 year. Capital costs occur at a single point in time for an item that may be used throughout the life of a program. Examples of capital costs include vehicles, computers, and microscopes.

Fixed and Variable Costs

Costs can be further categorized by the relationship between their expenditure and the production of an output (e.g., a child vaccinated, an antismoking public service message delivered). In general, operating costs fall into two categories: *fixed* and *variable* costs. *Fixed costs* are those whose total remains constant (within a relevant range), even though the volume of the activity may vary. Examples include rent and the design and production of advertising media. In the short run, fixed costs do not change in response to the number of clients being served or the amount of product delivered. Capital costs are considered fixed costs. *Variable costs*, in contrast, are those that respond proportionately to change in the volume of activity. They vary with the number of clients served. Examples include test kits for human immunodeficiency virus (HIV), bicycle helmets, and condoms.

In some cost analyses, when the interventions being compared differ only in the type of output produced, it is possible to limit the collection of operating costs to variable costs. In such analyses, it is assumed that certain fixed costs remain constant, regardless of the type of output produced. In such cases, the analyst must be very careful to ascertain that there is, in reality, no change in the fixed costs needed for different outputs.

Total, Average, and Marginal Costs

Once costs are collected and categorized, one may want to analyze them in relationship to the outputs they are used to produce. In such cases, it is important to distinguish between the concepts of *total, average,* and *marginal* costs.

The *total cost* of an intervention or for treating a health condition is the sum of the accumulated costs of producing a given level of output. In prevention-effectiveness studies, *output* can be defined as either the result associated with the program or intervention under study or the health care and other resources provided to treat a health condition. For example, in a program designed to increase measles immunization rates in children, the intervention output may be a child successfully vaccinated. The output unit associated with treating the health condition would be the measles-related health-care services per patient. Total cost (TC) is expressed as follows:

$$(TC) = (Q_1 \times P_1) + (Q_2 \times P_2) + \dots + (Q_n + P_n) \qquad (1)$$

where:

Q_1 = quantity of resource 1
P_1 = value of resource 1

Estimates of total costs can be used for different purposes, such as ranking programs or health outcomes in terms of economic burden or measuring the true cost of a program relative to its budget. Because total cost is an aggregate measure, it can be difficult to interpret and use for comparison purposes when the level of output also needs to be considered. For example, comparing two programs based on their total costs can be informative only if it is known that both programs can achieve the same level of output. When units of output differ, the decision maker may feel more comfortable considering both costs and outcomes when making comparisons. In such cases, it is important to distinguish between average costs and marginal costs.

The *average cost* is the total cost divided by the total units of output:

$$average\ cost = TC/X \tag{2}$$

where

X = total outputs

Calculating the average cost to produce one unit of outcome is useful for comparison purposes across programs, population subgroups, etc. Such comparisons allow decision makers to differentiate between programs on the basis of technical efficiency, where a lower average cost reflects a more efficient use of resources. Average costs are also useful to compare various output levels within a program or intervention to determine economies of scale. Economies of scale occur when the average cost per unit produced decreases as the level of activity increases because in the short-term fixed costs can be spread over a larger number of units.

The *marginal cost* is the cost associated with producing one additional (or one less) unit of output. Marginal cost is calculated by subtracting the change in total costs that results from producing an additional unit of output from the original total cost:

$$marginal\ costs = (TC'' - TC') \tag{3}$$

where

TC' = original total cost of an intervention
TC'' = total cost of the intervention (TC') plus the cost of producing one additional unit of output

To determine the marginal costs for producing more than one additional unit of output, equation (3) can be modified as follows:

$$marginal\ costs = (TC'' - TC') / (X'' - X') \tag{4}$$

where

TC' = original total cost of an intervention
TC'' = total cost of an intervention after some marginal increase (or decrease)
X' = original output level of an intervention
X'' = new output level of the intervention after some marginal increase (or decrease)

Because marginal costs are a function of the level of output of a public health program, the marginal cost per unit of output can be greater than or less than the average cost per unit of output. When a marginal cost analysis of a program is conducted, it is important to consider whether the program is operating at its most efficient size. Because this is difficult to determine, prevention-effectiveness studies often implicitly assume that programs are operating at or close to optimal efficiency. The relationship between average and marginal costs at different levels of output is illustrated in Figure 4.1. In this example, the marginal cost is initially less than the average cost; however, as additional units are produced and additional fixed costs must be incurred to expand production, the marginal cost of an additional unit of output exceeds the average cost of that unit.

COST OF AN INTERVENTION OR PROGRAM

This section describes the process of estimating the costs of a prevention-effectiveness intervention. The methods described below can be used regardless of the type of intervention, including clinical and community-based health interventions and public policies designed to improve health. The steps are the same: (*1*) frame the cost analysis, (*2*) develop a cost inventory, (*3*) quantify costs, and (*4*) calculate summary measures.

Frame the Cost Analysis

As with any prevention-effectiveness study, the first step in conducting a cost analysis is to determine its scope and the key points that must be decided before the study begins. The 13 steps for framing a study presented in Chapter 2 should be followed for framing a cost analysis. This section presents material on framing studies specific to cost analyses.

Study Design
The strategy for estimating costs of an intervention depends on whether the cost study is designed as a retrospective study, a prospective study, or a component of a model of a prevention intervention. Prevention-effectiveness studies often rely on cost data generated as part of earlier and independent evaluations of interventions.

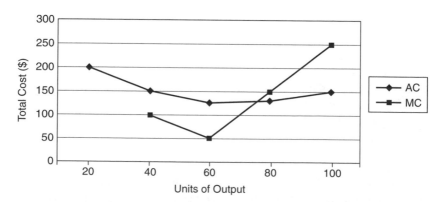

Figure 4.1   Average costs (AC) versus marginal costs (MC).

Thus, the choice of study design often depends on the information available and when in the planning and implementation of a prevention intervention the decision is made to conduct a cost or a prevention-effectiveness analysis.

In a *retrospective study*, the researcher attempts to identify costs after the program has begun or been completed. Often, no cost data have been collected for a program or the associated health outcomes, or they are imprecise and incomplete. Some costs, such as the costs to participants in the intervention (e.g., time and travel costs) and caregiver costs, may be impossible to estimate at this stage. In a *prospective study*, more consistent and reliable cost estimates may be obtained since actual cost data can be collected while the intervention program is in effect. The researcher decides in advance what cost information is needed for the study. Thus, complete and accurate cost data may be collected. Many prevention-effectiveness studies employ *models* designed to predict the most cost–effective strategy before a strategy is implemented. In the absence of detailed cost information, intervention costs in models are often the projected costs of an intervention. These costs may have been extrapolated from studies of similar programs or programs implemented on a smaller scale. Because specific cost data for the strategies under evaluation are not available, all assumptions regarding costs should be explicitly stated. Results of sensitivity analyses on estimates of intervention costs are generally presented with the study results as well as a discussion of the possible effects of using costs different from those of the model.

Study Perspective

Selection of the study perspective helps to determine which costs should be included. If the study takes a societal perspective, all cost categories will be relevant, including those of the health-care system, the participant, and other individuals affected by the intervention. However, if a health-care provider perspective is to be used, costs for participants or patients may be excluded. When conducting a study from multiple perspectives, it is helpful to construct a table of intervention costs with columns for each perspective.

Time Period

Costs are incurred at different points over the lifetime of the intervention. Three factors are important when selecting a time period over which to collect intervention costs: (*1*) the time period for the cost data collection must be contemporaneous with the time period for which clients are served, (*2*) the time period should be long enough to avoid any secular patterns (e.g., seasonal effects), and (*3*) the time period should be of sufficient length to capture program start-up and maintenance costs.

First, it is important that the cost data be collected for the same time period in which clients are served. In some facilities, cost data may be available for a fiscal year, whereas the number of tests or persons participating in programs may be available only by calendar year. The time period should allow matching of the cost data to client outcomes.

Second, selection of the time period depends on whether seasonality or other time patterns affect either costs or client participation. A time period of less than 1 year may have bias in the result due to seasonal effects on participation and behavior. A time period of at least 1 year is generally recommended.

Third, in addition to annual ongoing costs of the intervention, start-up costs should be collected since they must also be included when calculating the overall cost of an intervention. If the time period selected for study includes the start-up period for the intervention, an additional 1 year of cost data after the start-up period has ended should be included so that the cost data reflect ongoing costs. Often, for multiyear programs with significant start-up costs, an annual program cost is calculated to allow the use of a 1-year time frame in the prevention-effectiveness study. Construction of an annual cost requires annuitization of the program's capital resources that will not be exhausted during the lifetime of the program (see Chapter 6 for more details).

Often, there is an initial lag between when a program begins and the point at which it has reached full capacity. It may be necessary in such situations to plan a time period long enough to capture costs when the service delivery has reached a steady state. Consider, for example, a neighborhood outreach program designed to prevent sexually transmitted diseases (STDs) in adolescents. During the first year, the program may operate below capacity before community acceptance has been established. It is important to capture the costs of the program during the start-up year because it is likely that the costs would be replicated in new programs.

Costs also may change over the lifetime of an intervention. First-year costs associated with a smoke alarm giveaway program could include the costs for development of promotional materials and training of volunteers. Costs of the smoke alarms could be incurred during the second year. During the third and fourth years, in addition to smoke alarms, costs could include those for a battery replacement reminder program and for batteries.

Time periods greater than 1 year may require a decision about how to incorporate cost increases and changes in technology over time. Studies of interventions lasting longer than 1 year must also use discounting to account for the time value of resources expended in future years (see Chapter 6 for more details). A longer time period may also be appropriate because of the duration of the intervention or the time lag between the start-up of the intervention and the effect it creates.

Intervention Unit

Results of cost analyses must be summarized in a usable form for integration into prevention-effectiveness analyses. Generally, results of cost analyses are expressed as a function of output (i.e., cost per unit of production). This can also be referred to as the *unit cost*. One of the most common intervention units is the person receiving or beginning the intervention (e.g., cost per person exposed to the intervention).

Depending on the structure of the prevention-effectiveness study, more than one unit cost may need to be estimated from the intervention cost analysis. Most frequently, the need for multiple-unit costs occurs with programs that have varying degrees of participant completion. For example, consider a routine childhood vaccination program in which only 60% of participating children complete the three-dose series. Thirty percent receive only two doses, and 10% receive only one dose. The cost analysis for this study will be used to determine three unit costs: (*1*) the cost per child receiving three doses, (2) the cost per child receiving two doses, and (3) the cost per child receiving only one dose.

The unit costs are also useful in determining the net costs of the alternative strategies in prevention-effectiveness studies because most health-outcome rates are also expressed as some number per person exposed to or receiving the intervention. When prevention-effectiveness studies examine multiple interventions, comparability may depend on the use of a common intervention rate (e.g., cost per member of birth cohort, cost per clinic patient). Conversion of program costs to either a marginal or average rate allows comparison among several interventions of different sizes for the same health outcome.

Develop a Cost Inventory

Once the cost analysis has been appropriately framed, the next step is to develop an inventory of the resources required for an intervention or program. The cost inventory includes a comprehensive list of all of the resources required to carry out an intervention, the unit cost for each resource, and the total cost of the resource. Depending on the perspective of the analysis, this list will include (1) program costs, (2) costs to participants, and (3) costs to others affected by the intervention.

Program Costs
Types of program costs that may appear in the cost inventory include the following:

- Personnel costs, including salary or hourly wages and fringe benefits, categorized by the following:
  - Direct-provider time for each type of service or activity by provider type
  - Support staff
  - Administrative staff
  - Volunteers
- Supplies and materials associated with each type of service provided
- Laboratory costs for each service provided, including tests and controls
- Drug costs
- Facilities, including rent and utilities
- Maintenance for facilities and equipment
- Equipment
- Transportation costs and travel expenses
- Educational materials
- Media expenses, including production, air time, and space
- Training costs
- Outside consultant services
- Evaluation costs
- Other direct costs of providing services (e.g., courier services, uniforms or badges, additional insurance or permits, and construction and maintenance of a computer database)
- Participant time and expenses

Costs to Participants

The effectiveness of a prevention intervention may be influenced by out-of-pocket expenses incurred by a participant and a participant's time spent in receiving an intervention. Participant costs can be one of the largest costs associated with an intervention and should be included in intervention cost analyses conducted from the societal perspective. Costs incurred by participants fall into two categories: out-of-pocket expenses and productivity losses. *Out-of-pocket expenses* are costs that participants incur for items such as travel and childcare that are needed to allow participation in an intervention. Other out-of-pocket expenses include the purchase of items not accounted for in program costs, such as bicycle helmets, dietary supplements, or condoms. *Productivity losses* by participants measure the value of lost work that results when time is taken from work to participate in the intervention. Productivity losses include costs assigned to travel time, waiting time, and actual service time for the participant (e.g., the time costs associated with participating in a physical activity program).

Costs to Others

Depending on the perspective of the cost analysis, the cost inventory should include costs to others that may not be captured in program costs and costs to participants. For example, if an intervention causes an adverse event in those not directly participating, delineating these costs in the inventory is critical to assessing total program costs.

Quantify Costs

Once the inventory of all program resources has been completed, the next step is to measure the quantity of the resource utilized in the delivery of the program or health-care service and to assign a value or cost to the resource. In some circumstances, this is a straightforward exercise in which the amount of the resource utilized is multiplied by the price per unit of resource. In other circumstances, either measuring the amount of the resource utilized is a more complex undertaking (e.g., measuring the amount of provider time utilized per child vaccinated) or there is no apparent price for a resource (e.g., volunteer time). This section describes how to measure resource utilization and assign costs to inputs frequently found in prevention programs.

Fixed Program Costs

The fixed costs of a program or service are those that, in the short run, do not vary with the level of output. The most common fixed costs in the resource inventory for a program are those associated with the facility (e.g., rent and utilities) and personnel costs for support staff (e.g., receptionists and information services staff). One of the challenges in measuring fixed costs of health programs is identifying the portion of the resource that can be allocated to the program under assessment. For example, a peer counseling program designed to prevent adolescent drug abuse may be housed in a facility that also provides other community programs. The receptionist in a local public health clinic is responsible for registering clients for immunization programs as well as clients for other services. Methods for addressing some of the challenging issues associated with measuring fixed costs are discussed below.

Facilities, as a fixed cost, can be measured or quantified by including the cost of space, maintenance costs, and the cost of utilities. If a program is to be conducted in an existing facility, the cost of the additional space and time needed for the new intervention is based on the proportion of the total time the facility is in use. The proportion of time and space needed for the new intervention should be multiplied by the total cost of space (e.g., rent, ownership, taxes, insurance, maintenance) plus the cost of utilities. If neither additional facilities nor additional time is used (i.e., a marginal analysis is being conducted), then the facility cost can be ignored.

Costs for facilities are usually recorded as either the cost per unit (e.g., cost per square foot) or the total cost for the facility (e.g., monthly rent, utility costs, or insurance costs). When calculating costs within a portion of an existing facility, it is often useful to obtain the total square footage for the facility and to convert all facility costs to the cost per square foot. When the cost per square foot is not easily available (e.g., a clinic owned by the local health department), a proxy measure, such as the square foot rental rate for comparable commercial property, can be used.

The following equations can be used to determine the facility's costs for pro grams sharing space in an existing facility:

$$facilities\ costs = additional\ facility\ space\ used\ by\ the\ program \times cost\ per$$
$$square\ foot\ for\ space\ and\ utilities \tag{5}$$

or

$$facilities\ costs = (total\ facility\ cost\ for\ space\ and\ utilities \times total\ facility\ time$$
$$used,\ including\ program) \times facility\ time\ used\ by\ program \tag{6}$$

The costs of equipment and real estate as fixed capital can be measured in the following ways: computing the equivalent annual cost and the proportion of the equivalent annual cost that is assigned to the intervention. Two methods are recommended for computing the equivalent annual cost. The first and simplest is to determine whether market rates exist for renting comparable buildings or for leasing comparable equipment. These rates can be used to estimate the annual cost of capital equipment or real estate. The second and more accurate method is to annuitize the initial outlay over the useful life of the asset. The method for annuitizing capital costs is presented in Chapter 6.

Costs for administrative and staff support, as fixed costs, are calculated as a proportion of the staff time spent on this particular intervention. Salary and fringe benefits for each person who provides administrative and staff support are multiplied by the proportion of the person's time spent providing services for the intervention being studied.

The following equation is used to determine the cost of administrative and staff support associated with a program:

administration and support costs = [proportion of administrator's time spent
on intervention × (salary + benefits)] + [proportion of support staff time
spent on intervention × (salary + benefits)]   (7)

Variable Program Costs

The *variable costs* of a program are those that increase as the level of output in-creases. The measurement of certain variable costs is a straightforward process be-cause the quantity of the resources used is available in discreet units and the price per unit can be used as the cost. Other variable costs are not so disaggregated, and measurement of the quantity used to provide the service is required. Perhaps the most challenging is assessment of the amount of provider time utilized in a given service. Measurement of provider time and materials and of supply is addressed below.

Provider time, as a variable cost, can be measured by four methods: (*1*) direct observation of service duration, (*2*) random observations of provider activities (snapshots in time), (*3*) time diaries completed by providers, and (*4*) patient flow analysis using time forms that a client carries from provider to provider. The cor-rect sample sizes for estimating provider times can be derived from the statistical and epidemiologic references cited below.

While direct observation of services is considered the most accurate method, it requires that a trained observer who can differentiate among services follow each provider and correctly record the start time and stop time of each service. With di-rect observation, at least 25 and as many as 100 observations may be required to obtain a confident estimate of time durations.[2] To determine the number of obser-vations needed, a histogram may be constructed. If the histogram shows symme-try and small variation, 25 observations may be sufficient; however, a distribution with the mean equal to the standard deviation would suggest that 100 observations are needed to correctly estimate provider time.

Random observation uses the analogy that the proportion of observations on a particular service equals the actual proportion of time spent providing a particular service. In this method, providers are assigned a code number. The analyst chooses provider numbers from a random number table and prepares a list. This list is used to find, at fixed intervals, a specific provider and to note the service being provided at the exact moment of observation. At least five observations of each service type must be obtained for the proportionality assumption to hold, based on the multin-omial distribution.[3]

Time diaries allow self-observation by providers to record service to clients. Time diaries are generally kept on a sheet of paper carried by the provider for each day. The diary is divided into rows and columns. Rows represent new activities or services. Each row has a check list (columns) for the specific type of activity being performed, including personal time and a large final column for comments or ex-planations. To construct a check list that minimizes the provider time required to complete the diary, a pilot observation of a usual day must be made.

When using the time diary, the provider notes the start time of each activity (one activity = one row) in the first column. Since all activities are included in this continuous stream of activities, only the activity start time is needed. The start time of the next activity is the end time of the previous one. At least 25 self-observations or diary entries of each activity are required.[3]

Patient-flow analysis requires a time form that the client carries from provider to provider, beginning with the receptionist at the time the patient checks in for the program. Ideally, this form includes a space to note the times the client arrives at a program, is seen by the first service provider, leaves the provider, sees subsequent providers, and finally leaves the program. Again, data from at least 25 clients for each type of service are needed for an accurate analysis of provider time.

The cost of provider time is calculated by multiplying the time spent by the provider by the valuation of that provider's time. The hourly rate of compensation for the service provider, including fringe benefits, must be included. Employee fringe benefits are included as a cost of doing business and must be included in calculating the cost of an intervention. Information on salary and benefits can usually be obtained from the administrator or financial officer of the program.

Provider cost is determined for each provider type and service using the following equation:

$$provider\ cost = (provider\ salary + benefits) \times average\ duration\ of$$
$$service \times number\ of\ services\ provided\ in\ time\ period \qquad (8)$$

Other variable costs may best be measured by expert opinion or program personnel. For example, variable costs for materials and supplies can usually be obtained from the financial officer of the program. The cost of off-site laboratory tests can often be obtained from the state health department or the laboratory itself.

Material and supply costs, as variable costs per unit of service, are determined by the following equation:

$$material\ and\ supply\ costs = specific\ resource \times cost\ per\ unit \times number$$
$$of\ units\ used\ in\ time\ period \qquad (9)$$

In contrast to variable costs, fixed program costs are often paid in total and not per unit of service. For example, an X-ray machine may sit idle for some portion of every workday. If the X-ray machine was essential for screening, the same equipment cost would occur whether 10 or 20 participants were screened per day. (The cost of the film and supplies, of course, is a per-service variable expense.)

Valuing Resources not Traded in the Marketplace

Many population-based prevention programs rely on volunteers and donated goods, services, and facilities. Because these are considered inputs that are not traded in the marketplace, there is no price for them that can be used as the cost. Thus, a cost must be imputed based on values for other resources. Methods for valuing volunteer time and donated goods and services are presented below.

Volunteer time, as an economic cost can be measured using two approaches described in the health-care literature. The first approach assumes that a volunteer values his or her time spent in volunteer work as he or she would value leisure time. The most commonly used method for quantifying leisure time spent volunteering is to use the overtime equivalent of a volunteer's wage rate. However, this method can have distinct distributional biases. Programs that rely on volunteers who are middle- or upper-income earners may appear very expensive.

To cope with this problem and attempt to quantify volunteer time consistently, without regard to population characteristics, another method is recommended. With this method, the value of time spent in volunteer work is based on the equivalent wage rate of a person employed in a job that fits the description of the volunteer work.

In addition to volunteer time, programs frequently make use of other donated goods and services. These economic resources are also included in the cost inventory. The market value for these inputs is used as the cost of the resources. For example, resources for a bicycle helmet education program may include public service announcements for which both media production and airtime are donated. To estimate the cost of these resources, the actual price of purchased production services and the cost of airtime can be used.

When reporting the results of intervention cost analyses in which a portion of costs are allocated to volunteer time or other donated goods and services, these resources should be highlighted to indicate the extent to which a cost–effective intervention relies on nonfinancial inputs. Separate reporting of an intervention's financial and economic costs increases the generalizability of prevention-effectiveness studies by indicating the resources necessary to replicate an intervention.

Valuing Participant Costs

A cost analysis of a prevention program that takes the societal perspective will include the costs to the participants in the program. One method for quantifying participant costs is by a participant survey. Survey data can be obtained by interviewing participants when they arrive in a facility to participate in an intervention or with other survey techniques. Information can be collected about arrival time, service time, travel costs, and other out-of-pocket expenses. Questions asked of the participants can include the following:

- How far did you travel (miles)?
- Where did you begin your travel (home, work, school . . .)?
- What time did you leave that place?
- What time did you arrive at the intervention site?
- What time did you leave the intervention site?
- What expenses did you incur in order to come to the intervention site (e.g., bus fare, tolls, mileage, child care)?

To obtain total participant costs, participant productivity losses are added to out-of-pocket expenses (e.g., mileage or travel expenses, any child- or elder-care expenses, and any other cost paid by the participant). Depending on the study question, it may be desirable to present the out-of-pocket expenses and the participant productivity losses separately in the cost analysis.

Participant costs can be calculated using the following equation:

participation costs = (sum of time that participants spend traveling,
waiting, and participating in the service × median salary) + sum
of out-of-pocket expenses participants accrue for participation   (10)

Calculate Summary Measures

Once costs are identified and appropriately quantified, the final step in a cost analysis is to calculate summary measures. *Summary measures* can include total costs, annual costs, average costs, and marginal costs. The calculation of total, annual, average, and marginal program costs involves the following steps:

1. Multiply the cost per unit by the number of units used for each resource in the time period to obtain the sum of the variable costs.
2. Sum the fixed costs for the time period.
3. Annuitize and sum the capital costs for the time period (see Chapter 6 for more details).
4. Sum the subtotals from 1, 2, and 3; the participant costs for the time period; and any costs for side effects associated with the intervention. This sum is the total cost of the intervention.
5. To convert the total cost of an intervention with a multiyear time period to a shorter time frame, divide the total cost by the number of years to obtain the annual cost. [Note that annual intervention costs that occur in years following the base year of the analysis should be discounted. (see Chapter 6).]
6. Divide the total cost by the number of participants or other relevant intervention units to obtain the average cost of the intervention.
7. To calculate the marginal cost of the intervention, follow the steps above but exclude costs not relevant to the marginal analysis (i.e., fixed costs and capital costs).

Table 4.1 provides an example of how total annual costs and average costs were calculated for a hypothetical HIV counseling program.

MEASURING THE COSTS OF HEALTH OUTCOMES

The health outcomes in a prevention-effectiveness study include both the outcomes the prevention strategy is designed to prevent and any adverse health outcomes that may result from the intervention itself. This section describes the cost-of-illness (COI) method for estimating the costs of health outcomes. Other methods, such as those used in cost–benefit analysis, are described in Chapter 8.

The COI method is most often used to measure the cost of health outcomes in cost–effectiveness and cost–utility analyses. The COI method estimates the direct medical costs, the direct nonmedical costs, and the productivity losses associated with morbidity or premature mortality resulting from the health problem. Table 4.2 categorizes types of cost, which are discussed below.

Table 4.1 Total Annual and Average Annual Costs per
Client for a Hypothetical HIV Counseling Program

Resource	Quantity (A)	Cost/Unit (B)	Total Cost (A × B)
FIXED COST			
Personnel[a]			
Administrator	0.05 years	$64,421.00	$3221
Clerical worker	0.13 years	$14,375.00	$1869
Facilities			
Rent	12 months	$1485.00	$17,820
Maintenance	12 months	$240.00	$2880
Utilities	12 months	$150.00	$1880
Phone	12 months	$86.00	$1032
Supplies and equipment			
Office supplies	12 months	$450.00	$5400
Computer[b]	12 months	$1900.00	$1900
Subtotal			$35,922
VARIABLE COST			
Personnel[a]			
Counselor (4 hours/session)	980 hours	$22.44	$21,991
Supplies and miscellaneous			
Client education materials	4900 sets	$2.80	$13,720
Travel	11,000 miles	$0.28	$3080
Participant costs[c]			
Travel	58,800 miles	$0.28	$16,464
Subtotal			$55,255
TOTAL ANNUAL COST			$91,177
Participants per year (20 participants/session × 5 sessions/week × 49 weeks/year)			4900
Average annual cost per participant			18.61

[a] Includes benefits.
[b] Annuitized cost of capital equipment.
[c] Productivity losses not included.
Source: Gorsky.[4]

Prevalence- and Incidence-Based Costs

Prevalence-based costs are the total costs associated with the existing cases of a
health problem that accrue in a specific period divided by the total population.
Prevalence-based costs estimate the value of resources lost during a specific period
as the result of a health condition, regardless of when the condition became evident. Thus, in a prevalence-based prevention-effectiveness study with a time
frame of 1 year, all cases would be counted (including both new and existing cases);
however, only costs incurred during the 1-year period would be counted.

Prevalence-based costs are useful in prevention-effectiveness studies of health
problems of short duration. Generally, if the duration of the health problem does
not extend beyond 1 year, prevalence-based estimates can be used.

Prevalence-based costs are commonly found in the literature and frequently

Table 4.2   Examples of Costs Associated With Health Outcomes

DIRECT MEDICAL COSTS
Institutional inpatient care
  Terminal care
  Hospice
  Hospitalization
    specialized unit
    (e.g., ICU, CCU)
  Nursing home
Institutional outpatient
  services
  Clinic
  HMO
  Emergency room
Home health care
Physician services
  Primary care physicians
  Medical specialists
  Psychiatrists
Ancillary services
  Psychologists
  Social workers
  Nutritionist
  Physical and occupational
    therapy
  Ambulance
  Volunteer
Overhead allocated to
  technology
  Fixed costs of utilities
  Space
  Storage
  Support services:
    laundry, housekeeping,
    administration
  Capital costs (depreciated
    over life of equipment)
  Construction of facilities
  Relocation expenses
  Device or equipment
    cost
Variable costs of utilities
Medications (prescription
  and nonprescription)
  Drug costs
  Treating side effects or
    toxicity of medications,
    prophylaxis of side
    effects, ordering and
    inventorying
    preparation

Training in new
  procedures
Dispensing and
  administration
Monitoring
Devices and applications
  Prostheses, glasses
  Hearing aids
  Ostomy supplies
  Hypodermic needles,
    home urine and blood
    testing equipment
  Ordering and
    inventorying
Drugs, supplies, devices
  provided by household
Research and development
  Basic and applied research
Diagnostic test
  Community screening
    program
  Consumable supplies,
    personnel time,
    equipment
  Imaging
  Laboratory testing
  Costs of false-positive
    and false-negative
    cases
  Treating sequelae of
    undetected disease
Treatment services
  Surgery, initial and repeat
    Recovery room
    Anesthesia services
    Pathology services
    Acquisition costs for
      organ transplants
    Consumable supplies,
      personnel time,
      equipment
  Treatment of
    complications
  Blood products
  Oxygen
  Radiation therapy
  Special diets
Prevention services
  Screening space
  Vaccination, prophylaxis

Disease prevention in
  contacts of known cases
Rehabilitation
Training and education
  Health education
  Self-care training for
    patients
  Life-support skills for
    general population

**DIRECT NONMEDICAL
COSTS**
Public awareness programs
Social services
  Family counseling
  Retraining, re-education
  Sheltered workshops
  Employment services
Program evaluation
  Monitoring impact of
    program or technology
  Data analysis
Repair of property
  destruction
  (alcoholism, psychiatric
  illness, drug addiction)
Law-enforcement costs
Care provided by family and
  friends
Transportation to and from
  medical services
Time spent by patient seek
  ing medical services
Childcare
Housekeeping
Modification of home to
  accommodate patient

INDIRECT COSTS
Change in productivity
  resulting from change in
  health status
  Morbidity
  Mortality
Lost productivity while on
  the job
  Absenteeism
Foregone leisure time
Time spent by family and
  friends attending patient
  (e.g., hospital visitations)

Source: Adapted from Luce and Elixhauser.[3]

reported as annual costs of a health problem. If the problem does not extend beyond 1 year, the total cost of the health problem can be divided by the number of cases to obtain a cost per case of that health problem, which can be used in a cost–effectiveness analysis. However, care must be taken when converting prevalence-based costs of health problems with longer durations to incidence-based estimates.

Incidence-based costs are the total lifetime costs resulting from new cases of disease or illness that occur within a set time period. Prevention-effectiveness studies include incidence-based costs of new cases that occur within the time frame of the analysis or as the result of an exposure during the time frame of the analysis.

Incidence-based costs include those for medical care that is required for the duration of the illness, other costs associated with the illness, and lifetime productivity losses measured as lost earnings, resulting from morbidity or mortality related to the health condition. Because incidence-based costs often include costs that will occur in the future, discounting is performed to convert future costs to their present value in the base year of analysis.

Although incidence-based costs are more useful for the selection of cost–effective interventions, they are more difficult to obtain. Because lifetime costs are often necessary, incidence-based costs require knowledge of the course and duration of the health problem and its chronic sequelae on employment and earnings over the lifetime of an individual.

Recommendation 4.1: Incidence-based cost estimates of health outcomes should be used in cost–effectiveness analyses and cost–utility analyses unless the health problem being considered is of sufficiently short duration that prevalence-based estimates are equivalent to incidence-based estimates.

There are several means for obtaining incidence-based costs for prevention-effectiveness studies. A systematic review of the literature may provide reliable incidence-based estimates of the health outcomes. Sometimes it is possible to transform prevalence-based costs into incidence-based estimates. Several large public and private data sets are now available which report charges, reimbursements, or actual expenditures for medical services.

Sometimes it is possible to construct COI estimates by valuing the resource inputs. Although this method may produce the least reliable estimates, it can be used if no other estimates exist. To construct a COI estimate, develop an itemized list of all medical services (e.g., hospital days, number of visits to clinicians, pharmaceuticals) necessary to treat the person for the health problem. Average costs for medical services (e.g., cost per hospital day) can be obtained from the medical literature or from government or industry statistics. A list of costs found in COI analyses is shown in Table 4.2. Costs may also be obtained from reviews of medical records; however, it is important for the analyst to distinguish between costs and charges for medical services.

Costs versus Charges

When collecting medical costs, care should be taken to differentiate true economic costs from charges. *True economic costs* can be described as the value of forgone opportunities. If resources are used for one opportunity, such as a cholesterol-screening program, they are no longer available for another opportunity, such as a youth counseling program. The cost of the chosen option represents the opportunity cost of the option that was not chosen.

In a perfect marketplace, the charge or price for goods represents the true economic cost. In the health-care arena, the charge (or price) of a product or service does not generally represent the true economic cost of that product or service. The medical marketplace is not an efficient market for two reasons.[5] First, a "list price," or charge, for a medical good or service may not represent the true economic cost of that good or service. List prices are greatly influenced by the involvement of government (i.e., Medicare and Medicaid) and several large third-party payers (e.g., large insurers, managed-care organizations), which, because of their size and financial power base, may pay or negotiate discounted prices. Some suppliers of medical services may respond by instituting list prices that substantially inflate the true economic cost of goods or services in order to be compensated fully for the goods and services provided even when discounted payments are received. Self-payers and smaller insurance companies that are not able to negotiate discounts pay higher list prices for the goods or services. Thus, large discrepancies may exist among charges paid by large insurers, small insurers, and self-insurers.

The second reason for the discrepancy between costs and charges is that in the health-care setting some services and goods provided are profitable and some are not. Hence, providers often redistribute charges from less lucrative services to more lucrative services in order to make a profit. The result is that charges or financial (accounting) "costs" of a product or service may bear little resemblance to true economic costs. In addition, individual hospital bills may include charges for services outside the standard course of treatment. For example, a hospital bill for maternity services for a particular individual might include charges for a sterilization procedure. Inclusion of the unrelated sterilization procedure would distort the cost of service described as "maternity."

Health-care providers may shift costs from uninsured patients to insured patients to recover costs for unreimbursed medical services. All patients are charged for medical services at a rate above the actual cost to recover costs from that portion of the patient population that does not pay or fully pay for health care received. Thus, charges for medical goods and services frequently do not reflect the actual resource costs. With the distinction between costs and charges in mind, it is recommended that true economic costs be determined when possible.

Recommendation 4.2: Resource costs rather than charges should be obtained when possible.

Sources of Health Outcome Cost Data

In some circumstances, assessment of health outcome costs will be conducted as part of the study design. For example, it has become more common for cost data to be collected during a randomized controlled trial. However, estimates of the costs of health outcomes frequently are derived from secondary sources. Several of these sources are described below.

Medicare Reimbursement Data
Because the government is afforded a "discount" on health-care charges, its reimbursement data will more accurately reflect true economic costs than costs paid by small insurance companies or self-payers. However, Medicare reimbursement data are specific only to the elderly population and, therefore, may not represent societal costs in general. Medicare reimbursement data can be obtained from individual states or at the national level through such sources as *The DRG Handbook* or *The Federal Register*. Appendix F provides cost-to-charge ratios used by Medicare to reimburse hospitals and providers for delivery of health-care services.

Public and Private Data Sets
Several public and private data sets which are useful in constructing cost estimates for health outcomes are now available. These include public-use data sets available from the National Center for Health Statistics and the Agency for Healthcare Research and Quality and data sets available for purchase from private organizations. A list of data sets and information on where they may be obtained is given in Appendix E.

Charges Obtained from Hospital Records
Charges obtained from hospital records can be converted to cost data using Medicare conversion rates published in *The Federal Register*. *The Federal Register* publishes these conversion rates on a state-by-state basis each year, for both urban and rural populations (see Appendix F for current conversion rates by state). *The Federal Register* is available online from the Office of the Federal Register in the National Archives and Records Administration (www.gpo.gov/nara/index/html).

Physician Visits and Charges
Data on costs and the number of visits to physicians stratified by age group can be found in the most recent edition of the *Statistical Abstract of the U.S.* available either from the Government Printing Office or online (www.census.gov/statab/www). Costs can be updated, if necessary, using the medical component of the Consumer Price Index in Appendix G. These data reflect what is actually paid per visit to a physician and, therefore, will more closely represent true economic costs.

Panel of Experts
A panel of experts can be asked to estimate procedure costs. However, this method may yield an extremely broad range of results and is based on subjective judgment. Panel-of-experts estimates should be used only when no empirical data are available.

Outbreak Investigation Data
Data on illnesses from outbreaks of infectious diseases may be collected in conjunction with the investigation of the outbreak. Food- and waterborne disease out-

breaks are frequently investigated by state health departments, often with assistance from the Centers for Disease Control and Prevention. Because outbreak investigations generally are conducted by interviewing persons in communities or settings affected by the outbreak, questions may be added to the interview schedule to collect additional information on the duration and severity of the illness and the resource consumption associated with the illness.

Data on medical and nonmedical costs are available from several sources. Appendix E provides a list and description of several widely used sources that include literature indices, public-use tapes, annually published materials, and contractual services. If, however, cost information cannot be obtained from the literature or the other data sources specified in Appendix E, it may be possible to collect information directly from the source of the intervention. For example, if data are needed on medical costs of screening for gonorrhea, a clinic that does such screening might provide cost data related to cost of treatment, cost of tests, and cost of labor involved for the intervention.

Adjustments to Cost Data

When COI estimates are available for a year prior to the base year of the economic evaluation, cost estimates should be converted to base-year dollars, assuming, of course, that the services were similar in the two periods. The appropriate category of the Consumer Price Index can be used to make adjustments for inflation. The Consumer Price Index *all items* category and the major medical categories, including *medical care*, *medical-care services* (which includes professional services and hospital rooms), and *medical-care commodities*, for the period 1960–2000 are provided in Appendix H. Chapter 6 provides a more detailed explanation of accounting for the time differential of money, including how to use the Consumer Price Index to inflate dollars to the base year of the study.

Cost-of-illness estimates converted to base-year dollars enter the economic analysis in the year in which the health problem occurs. To determine the total lifetime COI, the COI that would occur in the future are discounted to the base year and summed. This sum is referred to as the *present value* of the illness. Discounting methods and values are discussed in Chapter 6.

Productivity Losses

The human-capital (HC) method, developed by Rice and others,[6-10] is used to assess the indirect costs or productivity losses from illness or injury, as measured by income forgone because of morbidity or mortality. Labor force participation rates and earnings of affected persons are used to calculate the value of productivity lost because of morbidity or premature mortality. Thus, the value of productivity losses from an individual's disability or death is the sum of the estimate of the present value of the individual's future income stream and the present value of future nonwage productive activity. Nonwage productive activity includes housekeeping activity, childcare activities, time caring for others, etc. Productivity losses associated with time to participate in an intervention program, caregiver time, or morbidity from side effects or adverse health outcomes associated with an intervention can also be calculated by the HC method.

The HC approach for assessing productivity losses associated with a health outcome is not all-inclusive.[7,9,10] The HC approach excludes the costs associated with pain and suffering, it values earnings and housekeeping services but not leisure time, and it may undervalue the productivity of groups whose productivity value is not reflected in earnings (e.g., volunteers). The category of earnings measures the value of employment but does not fully measure an individual's contribution to society.

Care should be taken in using productivity losses in cost–effectiveness analyses. Because of wage differentials and differences in the amount of time men and women spend performing nonwage activities, some age and gender may be valued more highly than others. For example, men may be valued more highly than women because men on average receive higher wages than women. Younger, working individuals would be valued more highly than older, retired persons. If productivity losses for specific gender and age groups are used in economic evaluations, it is possible that prevention programs targeted to men at the peak of their productive years will appear more cost–effective than similar interventions targeted to women and other age groups. To avoid this problem, productivity estimates, weighted by age and gender, are provided in Appendix I. Gender- and age-specific values can be used if appropriate for the study objectives and design.

Some questions have been raised about the appropriateness of attempts to assign a monetary value to human life.[8,11] This argument is used to oppose the inclusion of productivity losses in cost–effectiveness studies, regardless of whether the HC or other valuation approaches are used. However, taken in context, the HC approach calculates only the economic burden of illness and does not assign a value to a human life or to the pain and suffering associated with a health problem. Bearing this in mind, the HC estimation of mortality costs associated with a health problem should be considered the lower-bound estimate of the economic cost of mortality. Also, the willingness-to-pay approach does not place a value on a human life but on the value an individual or society places on reducing the risk of death.

Morbidity Costs
Productivity losses from morbidity are those that result from people being unable to work or perform normal housekeeping duties because of a health problem they have or one experienced by another individual for whom they must care (e.g., a child or elderly parent). The total cost of morbidity is determined by the number of days sick, hospitalized, or disabled multiplied by the daily wage rate associated with the value of lost wage-earning work and the imputed value of housekeeping and home-care activities. Daily wages can be used as an approximation for lost productivity. Unless data are available, assumptions can be made as to the number of recuperation days required per hospital day. For example, for every 1 day in the hospital, one might assume that 1 to 2 days of at-home recuperation are needed, depending on the severity of the illness. For instances in which there are insufficient data on the cost variables, a range of estimates should be used.

Appendix I gives the mean value of a lost work day in year 2000 dollars. This is calculated by dividing the average annual earning by 250 working days. If the days of morbidity reported do not distinguish between a work day and a non-work day, the mean value of an unspecified day should be used, calculated by dividing the same average annual earnings by 365 days. Morbidity costs can be updated to "years beyond 2000," using the increase in earnings reported annually in the *Employment and Earnings* March supplement, published by the U. S. Department of Commerce, Bureau of Labor Statistics. Chapter 6 explains this calculation. Appendix I also provides a complete description of the methods used for these calculations. These data assume that the entire population has productive potential, thus allowing adaptation to a base year without taking the 2000 unemployment rate into account.

Costs of Premature Mortality

The cost of mortality using the HC approach is the future productivity lost to society as the result of premature death. This value is derived by estimating the present value of future earnings lost by an individual who dies prematurely As in the calculation of morbidity costs, the HC approach applies labor force participation rates and earnings and the imputed value of housekeeping and caregiving time to persons who die prematurely as a result of an adverse health outcome.

The economic methods used to calculate morbidity costs are the same as those used to calculate mortality costs. Appendix I, Table 1.2 projects the present value of future lifetime earnings by age, using the recommended discount rate of 3% as well as the range in rates from 0% to 10%. It also presents the mean present value of lifetime earnings for the U.S. population, weighted by age or sex.

When assessing the costs of injury or disease averted, it is recommended that productivity losses be presented separately from other medical and nonmedical costs. Cost information may be interpreted in different ways depending on the decision maker's need. For example, a decision maker may be specifically interested in the impact of an intervention of the health-care system, in which case only direct medical and nonmedical costs (resources expended) should be included in the analysis. Therefore, it is recommended that two sets of results in a cost analysis be presented: (*1*) results that include direct medical and nonmedical costs only and (*2*) results that include both direct medical and nonmedical costs and productivity losses.

Recommendation 4.3: The human-capital approach should be used to estimate productivity losses for cost–effectiveness analyses.

CONCLUSION

This chapter has described the basic concepts, definitions, and techniques necessary to estimate costs in a prevention-effectiveness study as well as some of the issues associated with the design of prospective and retrospective studies and prevention-effectiveness models. The process of conducting a cost analysis of a prevention intervention has been described, including establishing criteria for a cost inventory, categorization and collection techniques for program and participant costs. The COI approach to assessing the costs of health outcomes was also explained.

Chapter 5 provides a detailed description of health-related quality of life measures designed to be used in prevention-effectiveness studies.

REFERENCES

1. Gold MR, Siegel JE, Russell LB, Weinstein MC. *Cost–effectiveness in Health and Medicine*. New York: Oxford University Press, 1996.
2. Drummond MF, O'Brien B, Stoddart GL, Torrance GW. *Methods for the Economic Evaluation of Health Care Programmes*, 2nd ed. Oxford: Oxford University Press, 1997.
3. Luce BR, Elixhauser A. *Standards for Socioeconomic Evaluation of Health Care Products and Services*. New York: Springer-Verlag, 1990.
4. Gorsky RD. A method to measure the costs of counseling for HIV prevention. *Public Health Rep 1996;* 111(Suppl 1);115–22.
5. Finkler SA. The distinction between cost and charges. *Ann Intern Med 1982;* 96:102–9.
6. Rice DP. *Estimating the Cost of Illness*. Health Economics Series 6. Publication 947–6. Washington DC: US Department of Health, Education, and Welfare, 1966.
7. Rice DP. Estimating the cost of illness. *Am J Public Health 1967;* 57:424–40.
8. Rice DP, Cooper BS. The economic value of human life. *Am J Public Health 1967;* 57:1954–66.
9. Rice DP, Hodgson TA, Kopstein AN. The economic costs of illness: replication and update. *Health Care Financ Rev 1985;* 7:61–80.
10. Hodgson TA. Cost of illness in cost–effectiveness analysis: a review of the methodology. *Pharmacoeconomics 1994;*6:536–52.
11. Landefield JS, Seskin EP. The economic value of life: linking theory and practice. *Am J Public Health 1982;* 72:555–66.

5

Quality of Life

ERIK J. DASBACH
STEVEN M. TEUTSCH

Improving health-related quality of life (QoL) is an important health-care goal. When evaluating health-care programs, accounting for QoL benefits is critical to demonstrating value. The literature on QoL measurement in health care is rich with instruments and applications. For the analyst faced with accounting for QoL benefits in a decision analysis, determining the best approach can be challenging. The purpose of this chapter is to provide guidance when incorporating QoL benefits into a decision analysis. Specifically, this chapter will focus on incorporating QoL benefits into economic evaluations. It will also discuss how QoL measures are used in other types of evaluation initiative such as clinical trials and population surveillance.

WHY MEASURE QUALITY OF LIFE?

One of the primary goals in health care is to improve QoL. Many definitions of QoL have been proposed over the years in the scientific literature. While there is no universally agreed-upon definition of health-related QoL, the Centers for Disease Control and Prevention (CDC) has defined it as "an individual's or group's perceived physical and mental health over time."[1] Key in this as well as other definitions is that QoL is a multidimensional construct incorporating the effects of both morbidity and mortality. For example, the dimensions might include physical, mental, and social functioning. Instruments that account for these broadly are typically referred to as *generic measures* of QoL. A well-known generic measure of QoL is the 36-item short form (SF–36) developed for the Medical Outcomes Study.[2] The SF–36 characterizes QoL using the following domains: physical function, role-physical, general health, vitality, social function, role-emotional, mental health, and reported health transition. Most of the dimensions consist of multiple items. For example, one of the items within the physical function domain asks the respondent "How does your health now limit you climbing several flights of stairs?" Sometimes the items comprising a generic measure are not sensitive to measuring the effect that specific forms of a disease have on a person's QoL. For example, a common condition experienced by persons with asthma is nighttime awakenings. How nighttime awakenings affect a person's QoL may not be adequately captured by the domains and items in a broad and general instrument such as the SF-36. As a result, *disease-specific measures* of QoL have been developed to address these disease-specific conditions. An example of a disease-specific instrument for measuring QoL in persons with asthma is the Asthma Quality of Life Questionnaire.[3] The domains comprising this questionnaire include activity limitation, asthma symptoms, emotional function, and environmental stimuli. Each of these domains contains items that are specific to asthma. An item represents a specific level or characteristic of the domain. For example, in the asthma symptoms domain, one of the items asks the respondent "How often during the past two weeks have you been awakened at night by your asthma symptoms?" A disease-specific item such as this would not be found in a generic measure of QoL.

In general, QoL measures can be classified in two ways: generic or disease-specific and preference-based or profile-based (Fig. 5.1).

Most instruments reported in the literature are the profile type. Both the SF-36 and the Asthma Quality of Life Questionnaire described above are profile-based measures. Later in the chapter, profile-based measures are differentiated from preference-based measures.

APPLICATIONS OF QUALITY OF LIFE MEASUREMENT

Both generic and disease-specific QoL instruments are used in a variety of applications in health care. These include clinical trials, population surveillance, and economic evaluations. Given the variety of QoL measures available, it is important to choose one that best matches the task because different instruments provide different levels of sensitivity to specific components of QoL and provide different absolute values of QoL. Different applications of QoL measurement and the types of instrument that are best suited for these applications are discussed.

	Generic	Disease-Specific
Profile Based	SF-36	Asthma Quality of Life Questionnaire
Preference Based	Quality of Well-Being Health Utilities index	Q-TWiST[4]

Figure 5.1   Classification of quality of life measures.

Clinical Trials

Measures of QoL are increasingly being included in clinical trials. A common objective in clinical trials is to measure the effect of an intervention on QoL. To maximize the likelihood that an effect can be detected, the right instrument needs to be matched to the task. As a result, it is not uncommon for disease-specific measures to be favored over generic measures in clinical trials. Moreover, it is often necessary that the disease-specific measure selected be responsive to changes in QoL over time. Many validated QoL instruments in the literature have been developed without determining whether the instrument is responsive to changes in QoL over time. As a result, such instruments may not be suitable for use in a clinical trial or may require further testing to determine responsiveness and a minimal clinically important QoL change. A more detailed account of QoL measurement in clinical trials can be found in Guyatt et al.[5]

Population Surveillance

Another application of QoL measurement is assessing the health of populations through QoL surveillance initiatives. The purposes of such initiatives include the following:

- Monitoring population health
- Planning programs and setting priorities
- Evaluating quality of care

An example of such an initiative is the CDC's survey-based population assessment of QoL using a generic measure, the Healthy Days measure.[1] The Healthy Days measure was developed specifically to monitor the health of populations and is based on four simple questions:

1. Would you say that in general your health is excellent, very good, good, fair, or poor?
2. Now thinking about your physical health, which includes physical illness and injury, for how many days during the past 30 days was your physical health not good?
3. Now thinking about your mental health, which includes stress, depression, and problems with emotions, for how many days during the past 30 days was your mental health not good?
4. During the past 30 days, for about how many days did poor physical or mental health keep you from doing your usual activities, such as self-care, work, or recreation?

The Healthy Days measure has been part of the Behavioral Risk Factor Surveillance System (BRFSS) since 1993 and the National Health and Nutrition Examination Survey (NHANES) since 2000. One of the primary uses of the Healthy Days measure is to support the two primary health objectives of the United States outlined in *Healthy People 2010:*[6] (*1*) to improve the quality and years of life and (*2*) to eliminate health disparities. In addition to conducting QoL surveillance at the national and state level, the BRFSS has been used for QoL surveillance at the community level.[7]

An alternative to the Healthy Days measure is the Years of Healthy Life (YHL) measure.[8] The YHL was developed in response to the need to monitor changes in the healthy life span as set forth in *Healthy People 2000*. The construct was developed using measures collected in the National Health Interview Survey (NHIS) and is based on two measures: perceived health status and activity limitation. Similar initiatives have also begun outside of the United States. For example, Statistics Canada uses the Health Utility Index (HUI) in population surveys to monitor population health trends in Canada.[9]

Another related and noteworthy initiative outside the United States is the Global Burden of Disease Study.[10] Initiated in 1992 at the request of the World Bank and in collaboration with the World Health Organization (WHO), this study is a comprehensive assessment of mortality and disability from diseases, injuries, and risk factors from 1990 and projected through 2020. A key measure is the disability-adjusted life year (DALY).[11] The DALY accounts for premature mortality, loss of QoL, and social values for allocating resources to health programs. Overall, the DALY is intended to serve as a measure of disease burden, which can be used both to assess the health of populations as well as to set priorities for allocating resources to health programs. Unlike the Healthy Days and YHL scores, DALY scores are not based on surveys of the general population but, rather, value judgments on disability and resource allocation made by regional representatives from around the world. The practicality of using the DALY to estimate disease burden has been questioned.[12] As a result, Hyder et al.[12] proposed a simpler alternative to the DALY, the Healthy Life-Year (HeaLY).

A similar use of QoL data as the Global Burden of Disease Study is the U.S. Preventive Services Task Force prioritization among recommended clinical preventive services.[13] This initiative prioritized 30 clinical preventive services recommended by the U.S. Preventive Services Task Force using quality-adjusted life years (QALYs).[14]

A final use of QoL in surveillance is for assessing quality of care. The Centers for Medicare and Medicaid Services (CMS) in conjunction with the National Committee for Quality Assurances (NCQA) uses the SF-36 to longitudinally evaluate the quality of care provided by Medicare managed-care plans.[15]

Economic Evaluations

The final application and focus of this chapter is the measurement of QoL for use in economic evaluations. One of the methodologic underpinnings of economic evaluation in health care is decision analysis. *Decision analysis* is a quantitative method from which to systematically analyze choices and the consequences of those choices under uncertainty. Fundamental to decision analysis is accounting for the preferences of the decision maker with respect to the consequences. Traditionally, this has been done using constructs that assign preference scores to the expected outcome(s), which are often referred to as *health states*. For example, two of the potential consequences of diabetes are blindness and end-stage renal disease

(ESRD). Choosing between two prevention programs, one of which is more likely to prevent blindness and the other of which is more likely to prevent ESRD, may depend on how an individual values these health states. For example, does the individual feel that being blind is less desirable than having ESRD or vice versa. A number of methods (e.g., standard gamble, time trade-off, and rating scale) are available to elicit such values from an individual.

With each of these methods, the details of which are discussed later in the chapter, the numerical score represents the relative preference of the individual for the given health state. Other profile (e.g., psychometric summated rating) non-preference-based instruments (e.g., SF-36) could be used to assign a numerical score to a health state. However, the resulting score would not be considered valid because it does not necessarily represent how an individual values the health state. For example, a non-preference-based instrument may assign the same health status rating to two individuals with ESRD; however, the way each individual values living with ESRD may differ considerably. A preference-based measure, however, would account for these differing values. A more detailed discussion of preference-based measures can be found in Neumann et al.[16]

Given that the other goal of health care is to improve survival, it is important that preferences for health states account for not only the desirability of the health state but also the length of time spent in the health state. For instance, to choose between the two prevention programs described earlier, an individual may want to know the duration of blindness and ESRD. One method for accounting for this is to weight the amount of time spent in the health state by the preference score assigned to the health state. The QALY is one such construct to account for both QoL and survival benefits in a single measure.[17]

The QALY construct is recognized as a universal metric given that it can be used to compare the benefits of different health programs aimed at preventing or treating different diseases. Despite the simplicity and intuitive appeal of the QALY construct, some of its simplifying assumptions have been criticized. This has led to the development and proposal of more complex elicitation methods and constructs: the Healthy Year Equivalent (HYE),[18] the Saved Young Life Equivalent (SAVE),[19] the DALY,[11] and Person Trade-Off (PTO).[20] Although these alternative preference measures and elicitation methods have theoretical merit, their adoption in economic evaluations by practitioners in the field has been minimal.

MEASURING PREFERENCES

The key to estimating QALYs in an economic evaluation is measuring preferences for the health states of interest. One well-established theory from the field of economics for guiding the measurement of preferences is the von Neumann-Morgenstern expected utility theory.[21] Utilities measured in accord with utility theory have interval scale properties, a necessary requirement for the calculation and use of QALYs in economic evaluations. Traditionally, when estimating a utility for a health state, the range of potential values for a given health state is bounded by 0 and 1, where 1 corresponds to the best imaginable health and 0 corresponds to death. A QALY is then calculated as the sum of the product of the expected number of years of life in the health state and the QoL experienced (i.e., preference score) in each of those years. For example, if an individual assigned a preference score of 0.5 to ESRD and the life expectancy with ESRD was 10 years, then the resulting number of QALYs would be 5 (0.5 × 10). A more detailed account of QALY measurement and utilities can be found in Torrance and Feeny.[22]

Given the influence of utility theory in decision analysis, *utility* has become the common term for these preference scores. However, a variant of this term is *value score*. Theoretically, the difference between utility and value preference scores is the method used to elicit the score. If the method involves uncertainty in the elicitation process, then the score is technically a utility measure; otherwise, the preference score is a value measure.

Preference Measurement Methods

The three traditional methods for measuring preferences are the standard gamble, time trade-off, and the rating-scale technique. The following describes in brief the mechanics of these methods. A more detailed description of the methods can be found in Froberg and Kane.[23]

Standard Gamble
The standard gamble descends directly from utility theory. Hence, the standard gamble is considered in theory to be the gold standard elicitation method because its theoretical foundations are rooted in the axioms of expected utility theory. If an individual's responses satisfy the axioms for calculating expected utility, the standard gamble elicitation method results in a measure with interval scale properties. Moreover, given that the score is elicited using uncertain outcomes, the measure represents a utility score.

Given that standard gamble accounts for uncertainty, the elicitation technique uses a lottery-based approach to measuring preferences. In this technique, an individual is asked to choose between a less desirable (but certain) chronic health state (e.g., blindness) and a gamble offering a certain probability of death or having an improved state of health (e.g., healthy with full vision). For example, a healthy patient with blindness might be given the following two options: (*1*) do nothing and remain blind and healthy for the remainder of life and (*2*) a new surgery that has a *p*% chance of surgical death and a (*1-p*%) chance of restoring vision for the remainder of life. To estimate the utility score for the state of being blind and healthy, the probability of death from surgery is varied until the patient is indifferent between the two options. Thus, if the patient felt that restoring vision was worth a 5% risk of surgical death, then the preference score for being blind and healthy would be 0.95.

Time Trade-Off
Because the standard gamble technique can be difficult to administer, the time trade-off technique, which many believe to be easier to administer, was developed.[24] The time trade-off technique is used to determine the maximum

number of years of life in excellent health an individual is willing to trade-off in order to avoid living the rest of his or her life in a less desirable health state. For example, the same patient with blindness would be asked to choose between the following two options. (*1*) remain blind for the remainder of life (*t* years) and (*2*) surgery that restores vision but with a life expectancy of *x* years (where $x \leq t$). Time *x* is varied until the individual is indifferent between the choice of surgery and no surgery. The preference score is calculated as the ratio x/t. Thus, if the patient felt that 10 years of being blind and healthy was equivalent to 8 years of having full vision and being healthy, then the preference score would be 0.8 (8/10). The time trade-off technique differs from the standard gamble in that the individual is presented with a choice that does not involve risk but certain outcomes. As a result, the preference score generated using the time trade-off technique is considered a value score.

Rating Scale
Another method to elicit health utilities is the rating-scale technique. In the rating-scale technique, an individual directly relates a health state to a linear scale, for example, from 0 to 1, where 0 corresponds to the least desirable health state (e.g., death), and 1 corresponds to the most desirable state of health (i.e., best imaginable health). This kind of scale is sometimes referred to as a "feeling thermometer." In addition to the feeling thermometer, a variety of cards are used to describe particular states of health (e.g., blindness and ESRD). The analyst instructs the individual to place the various cards on the scale such that each card's distance from the end points on the feeling thermometer corresponds to her or his feelings about the relative differences in desirability among the levels. If the individual places the card representing blindness at 0.8 and the card representing ESRD at 0.5, then the preference scores for these two health states would be 0.8 and 0.5, respectively. Like the time trade-off technique, the rating scale elicitation method does not involve uncertain outcomes. As a result, the preference score generated using the rating scale technique is considered a value score. A widely used rating scale technique that is available in a variety of languages is the EQ-5D visual analogue scale.[25]

The common theme in the measures described in this section is that they are intended to measure preferences that can then be used to construct a QALY. Moreover, the values elicited using these methods should preserve how individuals rank health states in terms of preference. They differ, however, in that the values elicited from an individual typically are not equivalent at an absolute level. Since each elicitation technique measures slightly different factors using strategies with different psychometric properties, it is not surprising that they may yield different QALY weights at an individual level as well as a population level. As a result, not all QALYs are measured equally if the values used to construct the QALY are based on sources that used different elicitation methods. Another criticism of these measures is that they measure only individual preferences, which when aggregated may not reflect how society would measure preferences. As a result, Nord[20] has recommended an alternative preference measurement method that measures social preferences, the person trade-off method. Despite the person trade-off method's theoretical merits, experience in the field with its application relative to the standard gamble, time trade-off, and rating scale has been limited. This primarily is attributable to the difficulty of administering the method. However, one example of where the person trade-off method has been used is in the construction of DALYs.

SOURCES OF PREFERENCE MEASURE SCORES FOR HEALTH STATES IN ECONOMIC EVALUATIONS

One of the primary challenges with estimating QALYs in an economic evaluation is estimating the preference scores for all of the health states in the decision analysis. Data for measuring preferences can be obtained through a variety of approaches: direct, indirect, surveys, and the literature.

Direct Approach

In the direct approach, one of the previously mentioned preference-measurement techniques (e.g., standard gamble) is applied in a sample of subjects that are representative of the economic perspective adopted in the analysis. For instance, if a societal perspective is adopted, then a sampling of the general population is required. Given that many of the subjects may not have experienced the health states of interest (e.g., blindness or ESRD), hypothetical health-state descriptions need to be developed to characterize the health states for the subjects. The disadvantage of this approach is that the process can be fairly resource-intensive, requiring trained interviewers, development of health-state scenarios, and recruitment of subjects.

Given the resource requirements associated with this approach, an alternative option has been commonly used to elicit preferences from a convenience sample of persons actually experiencing the health states (i.e., patients) or a surrogate familiar with the health states of interest (i.e., clinicians). The advantage of this technique is that it is less resource-intensive than measuring preferences in the general population. The disadvantage of the technique is that the representativeness of the scores with a societal perspective can be questioned.

Regardless of whether preferences are elicited from experienced or inexperienced subjects, many subjects have difficulty comprehending the tasks requested using a rating scale, the time trade-off, or the standard gamble. The task can be further complicated when the health states that are being rated are hypothetical. As a result, the analyst should critically assess the added value of directly assessing health-state utilities for the problem relative to other approaches to assigning utilities to health states (i.e., indirect approach, surveys, or the literature).

Indirect Approach

If societal preferences are necessary and a direct approach is not feasible or not warranted, then as an alternative the indirect approach can provide utility scores that are population-based and consistent with a societal perspective via an HUI. An HUI classifies a person's health state across a number of dimensions and then applies a mathematical model to assign a utility score to the health state.[26] This approach works by administering a questionnaire to a sample of persons experiencing the health states of interest. For example, the EQ-5D HUI questionnaire has five dimensions from which to classify a person's health: mobility, self-care, usual activities, pain/discomfort, and anxiety/depression. Each dimension has three levels of health. The mobility dimension, for instance, has the following three levels to categorize a person's ability to get around:

1. I have no problems in walking about.
2. I have some problems in walking about.
3. I am confined to a bed.

Collectively, the EQ-5D instrument has 243 different health states from which to classify a person's health state. Each of the 243 health states has a utility score associated with it ranging from 0 to 1. In addition to the EQ-5D, other HUIs are available in the literature: the Health Utility Index-Mark III [27] and the Quality of Well-Being (QWB).[28–29] While the advantage of the HUI approach is that it can provide population-based preference scores, the disadvantage is that it still requires primary data collection.

Data from Surveys

If primary data cannot feasibly be obtained, information from national surveys can be used.[30] The National Center for Health Statistics (NCHS) has developed a number of algorithms for mapping the National Health and Nutrition Examination Survey, the National Medical Expenditures Survey, and the National Health Interview Survey data into the QWB as well as into the HUI.[8,29,31]

Occasionally, an analyst may have access to QoL data collected using the SF-36 in the target population. A variant of this approach is to translate these SF-36 QoL scores into utility scores using translation functions reported in the literature. For example, Fryback et al.[32] reported a method for predicting QWB scores from the SF-36, and Nichol et al.[33] reported a method for predicting the HUI2 from the SF-36.

Data from the Literature

The final, and probably most common, approach to assigning preference scores to health states is to use data reported in the literature. Gold et al.[34] published catalogues of "off-the-shelf" preference scores for a variety of common health states. If these catalogues do not have the preference scores for the desired health states, then the final option is to search the literature. To assist with such a search, Tengs and Wallace[35] compiled a catalog of 1000 original preference scores reported in the literature, published databases, books, and government documents. A similar catalogue is available from Bell et al.[36]

In this section, we have outlined the different sources for preference-measure scores for health states in economic evaluations. Prior to investing considerable time into directly measuring preferences through primary data collection, it may be worthwhile for the analyst to determine how much the decision problem depends on the values assigned to the relevant health states. If the decision depends greatly on the preference scores, then it may be worthwhile to collect primary data if none are available for the health states of interest from the literature or surveys. Even when data are available for the health states of interest, the analyst should make certain that the methods used to elicit the preferences are consistent between the health states in the problem, to avoid constructing QALYs using different scales.

Recommendation 5.1: Utility assessment for use in QALYs should be preference-based and interval-scaled, on a scale where optimal health has a score of 1 and death has a score of 0. The health state classification system should be generic, that is, not disease-specific. Community preferences are desirable; however, when not available, patient preferences may be used.

EXAMPLE OF MEASURING QUALITY ADJUSTED LIFE YEARS FOR HEALTH PROGRAM EVALUATION

In this section, a simplified hypothetical example of a QALY analysis to evaluate a health program designed to prevent chronic disease at birth is presented. This example is intended to illustrate how QALYs may be incorporated into an economic evaluation of alternative health programs. The first step is to identify the options being evaluated. In this example, there are two options. Option A is a program that prevents chronic disease (X) at birth. Option B is a no-program option that would result in the natural progression of chronic disease (X) over an expected lifetime with the disease. The second step is to identify the health states that options A and B will follow. A minimum set of health states should include all those that result in a change in QoL. In this example, two health states are assumed: excellent health and chronic disease X.

Next, life expectancy should be estimated. In this example, two assumptions are made: (*1*) the life expectancy of an individual for whom chronic disease X has been prevented is 75 years (option A) and (*2*) the life expectancy of an individual with chronic disease X from birth is 30 years (option B). The utility of living in excellent health is assumed to be 1.0. In this example, it is assumed that the utility associated with living with chronic disease X (option B) is similar to living with type 2 diabetes. Thus, the corresponding utility found in Table 5.1 (i.e., 0.70) is used for the calculations.

Figure 5.2 depicts the results of the calculations used to determine the incremental gain in QALYs when option A is chosen instead of option B. Option A accrues 75 QALYs (75 years × 1.0). Option B, in contrast, accrues 21 QALYs (30 years × 0.70). Thus, option A gains 54 QALYs over option B.

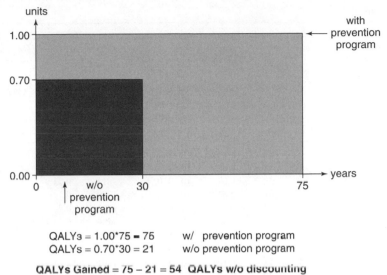

Figure 5.2   Measuring effectiveness with quality-adjusted life years (QALYs).

Table 5.1   Age-Adjusted Mean Scores on Quality of Well Being for Persons
Reporting Being Affected or Not by Various Health Conditions in the Past Year

Condition	Means for Person Affected by the Condition			Means for Persons Unaffected by the Condition		
	n	Mean Score[a]	95% Confidence Interval for the Mean	n	Mean Score[a]	95% Confidence Interval for the Mean
Arthritis	618	0.679	(0.68–0.70)	738	0.75	(0.75 0.76)
Gout	56	0.74	(0.72–0.77)	1300	0.72	(0.72–0.73)
Severe back pain	249	0.67	(0.66–0.68)	1107	0.74	(0.73–0.74)
Severe neck pain	103	0.68	(0.66–0.69)	1253	0.73	(0.72–0.73)
Migraine	73	0.70	(0.68–0.72)	1283	0.73	(0.72–0.73)
Angina	68	0.66	(0.64–0.69)	1283	0.73	(0.72–0.73)
Congestive heart failure	30	0.63	(0.59–0.67)	1326	0.73	(0.72–0.73)
Myocardial infarction	20	0.64	(0.60–0.68)	1336	0.73	(0.72–0.74)
Stroke	13	0.68	(0.62–0.73)	1343	0.73	(0.72–0.73)
Hypertension	495	0.72	(0.72–0.73)	861	0.72	(0.72–0.74)
Hyperlipidemia	110	0.74	(0.72–0.76)	1246	0.73	(0.72–0.73)
Cataract	327	0.71	(0.70–0.72)	1029	0.73	(0.73–0.74)
Glaucoma	68	0.70	(0.67–0.72)	1288	0.73	(0.72–0.73)
Macular degeneration	44	0.67	(0.64–0.70)	1312	0.73	(0.72–0.73)
Diabetes (insulin)	36	0.66	(0.63–0.69)	1320	0.73	(0.72–0.73)

(continued)

Table 5.1   Age-Adjusted Mean Scores on Quality of Well Being for Persons
Reporting Being Affected or Not by Various Health Conditions in the Past Year
(*continued*)

Condition	*n*	Means for Person Affected by the Condition		*n*	Means for Persons Unaffected by the Condition	
		Mean Score[a]	*95% Confidence Interval for the Mean*		*Mean Score*[a]	*95% Confidence Interval for the Mean*
Diabetes (noninsulin)	88	0.70	(0.68–0.72)	1268	0.73	(0.72–0.73)
Asthma	46	0.68	(0.65–0.71)	1310	0.73	(0.72–0.73)
Emphysema	40	0.67	(0.63–0.70)	1315	0.73	(0.73–0.74)
Chronic bronchitis	46	0.67	(0.65–0.70)	1309	0.73	(0.72–0.73)
Chronic sinusitis	95	0.72	(0.70–0.74)	1261	0.73	(0.72–0.73)
Depression	62	0.65	(0.63–0.68)	1294	0.73	(0.72–0.73)
Anxiety	54	0.68	(0.65–0.70)	1302	0.73	(0.72–0.73)
Ulcer	77	0.67	(0.65–0.69)	1279	0.73	(0.72–0.73)
Colitis	51	0.70	(0.67–0.73)	1305	0.73	(0.72–0.73)
Hiatal hernia	46	0.70	(0.67–0.72)	1310	0.73	(0.72–0.73)
Sleep disorder	136	0.68	(0.66–0.69)	1220	0.73	(0.73–0.74)
Thyroid disorder	88	0.70	(0.68–0.72)	1268	0.73	(0.72–0.73)
Miscellaneous allergies	280	0.72	(0.69–0.76)	1328	0.73	(0.72–0.73)

[a]All means adjusted to 64.0 years, the overall sample mean age; best = 1.0; worst = 0.0. Confidence intervals computed using Regress command in MINITAB Vax/VMS version 7.1, © 1989 Minitab, Inc.
Source: Fryback et al.[37]

An alternative to estimating a utility for a health state from the literature as described above would be to administer an HUI to a sample of patients experiencing the health state of interest. The following is an example from McDowell and Newell[38] of how this might be done using the EQ-5D instrument.

A 64–year-old diabetic woman has a small foot ulcer, early diabetic retinopathy, and hypertension but no other major health problems. She has difficulty in walking and experiences moderate pain. She is very concerned that her diabetes will progress and leave her with greater impairments. She completes the EQ-5D classifier as follows:

Mobility
I have no problems in walking about   ☐
I have some problems in walking about   ☒
I am confined to bed   ☐

Self-Care
I have no problems with self-care   ☒
I have some problems washing or dressing myself   ☐
I am unable to wash or dress myself   ☐

Usual Activities (e.g., work, study, housework, family or leisure activities)
I have no problems with performing my usual activities   ☒
I have some problems with performing my usual activities   ☐
I am unable to perform my usual activities   ☐

Pain/Discomfort
I have no pain or discomfort   ☐
I have moderate pain or discomfort   ☒
I have extreme pain or discomfort   ☐

Anxiety/Depression
I am not anxious or depressed   ☐
I am moderately anxious or depressed   ☒
I am extremely anxious or depressed   ☐

Each of the dimensions is scored as 1, 2, or 3 corresponding with the boxes checked. Her score is therefore 21122. The weight for each item can be determined from population-based preference weights which have been determined for specific populations. The "weight" is subtracted from 1 and an additional constant is subtracted if one or more scores are 2 and another if one or more are 3. One set of weights is shown in Table 5.2.

Her score would be $1.0 - 0.069 - 0.0 - 0.0 - 0.123 - 0.071 - 0.081 = 0.656$. If she were to live 5 years in this health state, she would lose $(1.0 - 0.656) \times 5$ years, or 1.72 QALYs. In other words, rather than 5 QALYs, she would have 3.28 QALYs for the 5-year period.

CONCLUSION

Incorporating QoL measures in economic evaluations can assist decision makers in two important ways. First, QoL measures can demonstrate whether or not the selection of a health program depends on preferences for the health states under consideration. Second, QoL measures can provide an assessment of whether or not the optimal health program is cost-effective relative to other health programs evaluated using QALYs as a common economic benchmark. The purpose of this chapter was to provide the analyst with guidance on how to incorporate QoL measurement into economic evaluations of health programs by identifying an assortment of tools that assign preference scores to health states. Ultimately, the selection of the best approach for assigning preference scores to health states depends on the research question of interest and the resources available to the analyst.

Table 5.2   Preference Weights for the EQ-5D

Dimensions	Item Weights		
	1	2	3
Mobility	−0.0	−0.069	−0.314
Self-care	−0.0	−0.104	−0.214
Usual activity	−0.0	−0.036	−0.094
Pain/discomfort	−0.0	−0.123	−0.386
Anxiety/depression	−0.0	−0.071	−0.236
Constants	−0.0	−0.081	−0.269

Source: McDowell and Newell.[38]

REFERENCES

1. Centers for Disease Control and Prevention. *Measuring Healthy Days*. Atlanta: CDC, 2000.
2. Ware JE, Sherbourne CD. The MOS 36-item short-form health survey (SF-36): conceptual framework and item selection. *Med Care 1992;* 30:473–83.
3. Juniper EF, Guyatt GH, Feerie PJ, Griffith LE. Measuring quality of life in asthma. *Am Rev Respir Dis 1993;* 147:832–8.
4. Rosendahl I, Kiebert G, Curran D, et al. Quality-adjusted survival (Q-TwiST) analysis of EORTC Trial 30853: comparing goserelin acetate and flutamide with bilateral orchiectomy in patients with metastatic prostate cancer. *Prostate 1999;* 38:100–9.
5. Guyatt GH, Jaeschke R, Feeny DH, Patrick DL. Measurements in clinical trials: choosing the right approach. In: Spilker B, ed. *Quality of Life and Pharmacoeconomics in Clinical Trials*, 2d ed. Philadelphia: Lippincott-Raven, 1996, 41–8.
6. Office of Disease Prevention and Health Promotion, Department of Health and Human Services *Healthy People 2010*. Available from www.health.gov/healthypeople.
7. Simon P, Lightstone A, Wold C, et al. Health-related quality of life—Los Angeles County, California, 1999. *MMWR Morb Mortal Wkly Rep 2001;* 50:556–9.
8. Erickson P, Wilson R, Shannon I. *Years of Healthy Life*. Statistical Note 7. Hyattsville, MD: National Center for Health Statistics, 1995.
9. Boyle MH, Furlong W, Feeny D, et al. Reliability of the Health Utilities Index-Mark III used in the 1991 cycle 6 Canadian General Social Survey Health Questionnaire. *Qual Life Res 1995;* 4:249–57.
10. Murray CJL, Lopez AD. Mortality by cause for eight regions of the world: global burden of disease study. *Lancet 1997;* 349:1269–76.
11. Murray CJL. Quantifying the burden of disease: the technical basis for disability-adjusted life years. *Bull WHO 1994;* 77:429–45.
12. Hyder AA, Rotllant G, Morrow R. Measuring the burden of disease: health life-years. *Am J Public Health 1998;* 88:196–202.
13. Coffield AB, Maciosek MV, McGinnis JM, et al. Priorities among recommended clinical preventive services. *Am J Prev Med 2001;* 21:1–9.
14. Maciosek MV, Coffield AB, McGinnis JM, et al. Methods for priority setting among clinical preventive services. *Am J Prev Med 2001;* 21:10–9.
15. Health Care Financing Administration. 2001. Available from www.hcfa.gov/quality.
16. Neumann PJ, Goldie SJ, Weinstein MC. Preference-based measures in economic evaluation in health care. *Annu Rev Public Health 2000;* 21:587–611.
17. Weinstein MC, Stason WB. Foundations of cost–effectiveness analysis for health and medical practice. *N Engl J Med 1977;* 296:716–21.
18. Mehrez A, Gafni A. Quality-adjusted life years, utility theory, and healthy-year equivalents. *Med Decis Making 1989;* 9:42–149.
19. Nord E. An alternative to the QALY: the saved young life equivalent (SAVE). *BMJ 1992;* 305:875–7.
20. Nord E. The person-trade-off approach to valuing health care programs. *Med Decis Making 1995;* 15:201–6.
21. von Neumann J, Morgenstern O. *Theory of Games and Economic Behavior*. New York: John Wiley and Sons, 1944.
22. Torrance GW, Feeny DH. Utilities and quality-adjusted life years. *Int J Technol Assess Health Care 1989;* 5:559–75.
23. Froberg DG, Kane RL. Methodology for measuring health-state preferences—II: scal-

ing methods. *J Clin Epidemiol 1989;* 42:459–71.

24. Torrance GW, Thomas WH, Sackett DL. A utility maximization model for evaluation of health care programs. *Health Serv Res 1972;* 7:118–33.

25. Kind P. The EuroQol instrument: an index of health-related quality of life. In: Spilker B, ed. *Quality of Life and Pharmacoeconomics in Clinical Trials*, 2d ed. Philadelphia: Lippincott-Raven, 1996: 191–201.

26. Torrance GW, Furlong W, Feeny D, Boyle M. Multi-attribute preference functions Health Utility Index. *Pharmacoeconomics 1995;* 7:503–20.

27. Feeny D, Furlong W, Boyle M, Torrance GW. Multi-attribute health status classification systems Health Utility Index. *Pharmacoeconomics 1995;* 7:490–502.

28. Kaplan RM, Anderson JP. A general health policy model: update and applications. *Health Serv Res 1988;* 23:203–35.

29. Andresen EM, Rothenberg BM, Kaplan RM. Performance of a self-administered mailed version of the Quality of Well-Being (QWB-SA) questionnaire among older adults. *Med Care 1998;* 36:1349–60.

30. Muennig PA, Gold MR. Using the Years-of-Healthy-Life measure to calculate QALYs. *Am J Prev Med 2001;* 20:35–9.

31. Erickson P, Kendall EA, Anderson JP, Kaplan RM. Using composite health status measures to assess the nation's health. *Med Care 1987;* 27:S66–77.

32. Fryback DG, Lawerence WF, Martin PA, et al. Predicting Quality of Well-Being scores from the SF-36, results from the Beaver Dam Health Outcomes Study. *Med Decis Making 1997;* 17:1–9.

33. Nichol MB, Sengupta N, Globe DR. Evaluating quality-adjusted life years: estimation of the Health Utility Index (HUI2) from the SF-36. *Med Decis Making 2001;* 21:105–12.

34. Gold M, Franks P, McCoy KI, Fryback DG. Toward consistency in cost–utility analyses: using national measures to create condition-specific values. *Med Care 1998;* 36:778–92.

35. Tengs TO, Wallace A. One thousand health-related quality of life estimates. *Med Care 2000;* 38:583–637.

36. Bell CH, Chapman RH, Stone PW, et al. An off-the-shelf help list: a comprehensive catalog of preference scores from published cost-utility analyses. *Med Decis Making 2001;* 21:288–94.

37. Fryback DG, Dasbach E, et al. The Beaver Dam Health Outcomes Study: initial catalog of health-state quality factors. *Med Decis Making 1993;* 13:89–102.

38. McDowell I, Newell C. *Measuring Health, A Guide to Rating Scales and Questionnaires*, 2d ed. New York: Oxford University Press, 1996.

BIBLIOGRAPHY

Torrance GW, Feene D, Furlong W. Visual analog scales: do they have a role in the measurement of preferences for health states? *Med Decis Making 2001;* 21:329–34.

O'Leary JF, Fairclough DL, Jankowski MK, Weeks JC. Comparison of time-tradeoff utilities and rating scale values of cancer patients and their relatives: evidence for a possible plateau relationship. Med Decis Making *1995;* 15:132–7.

6

Time Effects

PHAEDRA S. CORSO
ANNE C. HADDIX

Costs and benefits in prevention-effectiveness studies typically spread out over multiple years. Further, economic costs and benefits from published data are frequently available for years that are different from the study period under consideration. Because there are differences in the timing of costs and benefits or when information is available, they need to be converted to a common point in time to make them comparable. This chapter introduces the concept of differential timing of costs and benefits and the mechanics of discounting, inflation, and annuitization.

DEFINITION OF DISCOUNTING AND DISCOUNT RATE

In the delivery of health interventions, policies, and programs, the timing of costs incurred by the program or intervention may differ from the timing of benefits. In addition, individuals and society have preferences for when these costs and benefits occur. For example, program A has total costs of $100 in the first year but produces total benefits of $110 in the second year. Program B has total costs of $100 in the first year and yields total benefits of $105 in the same year. An initial comparison of these two programs might suggest that program A's net benefits (i.e., *total benefits – total costs*) outweigh program B's net benefits by $5. However, this initial comparison of net benefits ignores two main points: for program A, benefits and costs do not occur simultaneously; and benefits occur in the first year for program B, while benefits occur in the second year for program A. If society places a premium on when costs and benefits occur, then the initial comparison of net benefits for these two programs is incomplete.

Discounting is a technique to account for the differential timing of costs and benefits. The premium that society places on benefits received today versus the future is reflected in the rate at which an individual is willing to exchange present for future costs and benefits, typically in smaller versus larger quantities, respectively. This quantitative measure of time preference is known as the *discount rate*. Many different discount rates have been used. Conceptually, the appropriate discount rate depends on the perspective of the study and the question it poses. Rates may be based on such factors as the market interest rates, the marginal productivity of investment, the corporate discount rate, the government rate of borrowing, the individual personal discount rate, the shadow price of capital, or the social discount rate.

The discount rate for prevention-effectiveness studies that take the societal perspective is called *a social discount rate*. This is the rate at which society as a whole is willing to exchange present for future costs and benefits. The social discount rate has several determinants. First, individuals have different time preferences for benefits to society as a whole compared to benefits they pay to receive as individuals. Second, the social discount rate is based on the assumption that individuals in society get satisfaction from knowing that future society will "inherit" good health because of the current investment in prevention, even though spending money in the present requires consumption trade-offs. Because of individuals' attitudes toward society, consideration of children as part of future society, and feelings of altruism toward humanity, the social discount rate is sometimes lower than an individual's personal discount rate or a private sector discount rate. A low discount rate indicates that future benefits are also valued highly in the present. Because a social discount rate reflects the values of society as a whole, it is the most appropriate rate for public policy decisions. Others provide more thorough discussions on the types of discount rate and their application to economic evaluations of health-care programs.[1-3]

If a prevention-effectiveness study takes a perspective other than a societal one, however, a discount rate other than the social discount rate might be selected. For example, if a study of a prevention intervention is undertaken from the perspective of a purchaser of health care, such as a managed-care organization, a private-sector discount rate might be used. The selection of such a rate reflects the assumption that managed-care organizations may make investment decisions based in part on the opportunity cost of the intervention. For example, in a health plan where membership is fluid, a purchaser may have a higher discount rate, indicating that averting costs in the present is preferable to averting costs in the future.

Once the appropriate type of discount rate is selected, that is, the social, private, or individual discount rate, the value of the rate must be chosen. There has been wide variation in the choice of a discount rate for studies taking the societal or the federal government perspective. The Office of Management and Budget Circular A-94, *Guidelines and Discount Rates for Benefit-Cost Analysis of Federal Programs*, delineates the discount rates for use in economic evaluations that accompany proposed changes in federal regulations and programs.[4] These rates are based on the rate that the Treasury Department pays to borrow money for varying periods of time and are updated annually in conjunction with the president's budget submitted to Congress. While the Office of Management and Budget has suggested discount rates as high as 10% in the past, its suggested discount rates for 2000 ranged from 3.8% to 4.2% for cost–effectiveness analyses of 3-year and 30-year programs, respectively. These rates can be found on the Internet (http://www.whitehouse.

gov/omb/circulars/index.html). Other organizations that set discount rates for internal and external use include the International Monetary Fund and the World Bank.

Studies of health-care interventions, however, have consistently used a lower discount rate on the general premise that societal preferences for health improvements differ from consumer goods.[1,5] Following the lead of the U.S. Panel on Cost–Effectiveness in Health and Medicine,[3] most texts on the use of economic evaluation in health currently recommend 3% as the most appropriate discount rate and a 5% discount rate to allow for comparability between studies done in the past.[2,6,7] Smith and Gravelle[5] summarize recommended discount rates from primary international medical and public health sources.

This book recommends the use of a real discount rate for both costs and benefits. The term *real* indicates that the discount rate does not include the effects of inflation. When a real discount rate is used, all monetary costs and benefits are reported in real or constant dollars for a specific base year. Costs and benefits that will be incurred in the future are not adjusted for anticipated inflation (see Adjusting for Inflation, below). Because the selection of the discount rate can influence the decision result, wide sensitivity analysis on the discount rate should be conducted.[8]

Discounting Nonmonetary Benefits

Based on the economic principles stated above, it is reasonable to use the same discounting process for health gains as for costs. If health outcomes are not discounted but the costs are discounted in studies that report ratios as summary measures, the cost per health outcome prevented will decrease over time. This argument that inconsistencies arise when monetary costs are discounted and nonmonetary health outcomes are not discounted was first proposed by Weinstein and Stason[7] and formalized by Keeler and Cretin.[8] The following simple example summarizes the essence of the argument. Assume that an investment of $100 today would result in saving 10 lives (or one life per $10 of investment). If the $100 were invested at a 10% rate of return, then 1 year from now the $100 would be worth $110. With $110, it would be possible to save 11 lives. In 2 years, the $100 original investment would net $121, and it would be possible to save 12 lives. On the basis of these calculations and assuming that investments can be postponed indefinitely, the returns in the future look so appealing that one might never choose to save any lives in the present.

To attach greater value to the delayed benefits of prevention programs, some prevention-effectiveness practitioners argue that health outcomes should be discounted at a slightly lower rate than that used for costs.[10] When this is done, prevention programs can be made to appear more cost effective. However, there is no theoretical basis for this approach. The mechanism for discounting costs and benefits should be used to reflect society's time preference and opportunity costs, not to adjust the intrinsic value of health outcomes. Rather, if society values the benefits of prevention programs, values assigned to health outcomes that will occur in the future discounted at the same rate as costs should reflect this preference. Thus, discounting health outcomes at the same rate as monetary outcomes creates an "exchange rate" for dollars and health outcomes that is time-invariant.

In addition to issues of logical consistency, a growing body of literature captures the continuing debate on the treatment of future health outcomes; the appropriate discount rate for health outcomes; individual preferences for health improvements, environmental improvements, and improvements in education compared to consumption goods; societal versus individual preferences for health now versus later; and discounting intergenerational costs and benefits.[9,11-28] In this text, we present a discounting model that assumes a constant discount rate, whereby health in the long-term future is discounted at the same rate as health in the near-term future (i.e., the discount factor is not a function of how far in the future the benefits occur).

Recommendation 6.1: Future costs and health outcomes should be discounted to the present value.

Recommendation 6.2: Future costs and health outcomes should be discounted at the same rate.

Recommendation 6.3: A 3% real discount rate should be used. A 5% discount rate may also be used for purposes of comparability with older studies or studies from other settings. No adjustments for inflation in the future should be made because this is a real (not a nominal) discount rate. Perform sensitivity analysis on the discount rate over a reasonable range, for example, from 0% to 10%.

The Discounting Process

The concept of discounting is related to the concept of compounding interest. A compound interest rate is used to calculate the future value (FV) of money, that is, how much will a sum of money invested today be worth in the future. The discount rate is the reverse of this and is used to calculate the present value (PV) of a sum of money to be received (or paid) in the future. In addition to calculating the PV of money, the discounting process is used to calculate the PV of nonmonetary benefits received in the future.

The equation for discounting a stream of FV dollars (or future nonmonetary values) into PV dollars (or present nonmonetary values) is as follows:

$$PV = \sum_{t=0}^{T-1} FV_t (1 + r)^{-t} \tag{1}$$

or

$$PV = FV_0 + \frac{FV_1}{(1+r)^1} + \frac{FV_2}{(1+r)^2} + \dots + \frac{FV_{T-1}}{(1+r)^{T-1}} \tag{2}$$

where

PV = present value of investment
FV = future value of investment
r = discount rate
t = time period
T = time stream

The term $(1 + r)^{-t}$ represents the discount factor. For a given discount rate (r) and for a given year (t), the discount factor $(DF_{r,t})$ can be obtained from Appendix G, such that equations 1 and 2 can be modified as follows:

$$PV = \sum_{t=0}^{T-1} FV_t \times DF_{r,t} \qquad (1a)$$

$$PV = FV_0 + FV_1 \times DF_{r,1} + FV_2 \times DF_{r,2} + \ldots + FV_{T-1} \times DF_{r,T-1} \qquad (2a)$$

These formulas assume a constant discount rate over time and that monetary and nonmonetary outcomes occur at the beginning of each time period; that is, costs and benefits are not discounted in the first year of the time stream or analytic horizon. For example, suppose one wanted to calculate the PV of a program's costs that occur over a 3-year time stream or analytic horizon, such that costs initiated in the 3 years are $10,000, $15,000, and $5000. Using equation 2 above, where the discount rate (r) equals 3% and the time stream (T) equals 3, the PV of the future stream of program costs is calculated as follows:

$$PV = \$10,000 + \frac{\$15,000}{(1.03)^1} + \frac{\$5000}{(1.03)^2}$$

$$PV = \$29,276$$

It is also possible to have monetary and nonmonetary outcomes occur at the end of each time period, that is, costs and benefits are discounted in the first year of the time stream. In this case, equations 1 and 2 (and subsequently equations 1a and 2a) can be modified as follows:

$$PV = \sum_{t=1}^{T} FV_t (1 + r)^{-t} \qquad (3)$$

or

$$PV = \frac{FV_1}{(1 + r)^1} + \frac{FV_2}{(1 + r)^2} + \ldots + \frac{FV_T}{(1 + r)^T} \qquad (4)$$

Returning to the example above on calculating the PV of future program costs over a 3-year time stream, the following formula would be used if costs of the program occur at the end of each time period:

$$PV = \frac{\$10,000}{(1.03)^1} + \frac{\$15,000}{(1.03)^2} + \frac{\$5000}{(1.03)^3}$$

$$PV = \$28,424$$

If the stream of costs or benefits remains constant over time, that is, the annual cost or the annual benefit is unchanged for each time period within the analytic horizon and monetary and nonmonetary outcomes occur at the end of the year (as in equations 3 and 4), then equation 5 can be used to calculate the PV of that future stream.

$$PV = FV \left[\frac{1}{r} - \frac{1}{r(1 + r)^T} \right] \tag{5}$$

where

PV = present value of resource
FV = future annual value of resource
r = discount rate
T = time stream or analytic horizon

While assuming that outcomes occur at the beginning of the time period seems to be the most widely accepted approach,[3] it is also possible to discount outcomes midyear or use more sophisticated mathematical manipulations to discount outcomes continuously over the time stream. Regardless of the technique used, consistency in the discounting techniques used for monetary and nonmonetary outcomes is paramount.

ADJUSTING FOR INFLATION

When an economic analysis is done, cost data are often collected from years other than the base year of the evaluation. To ensure that all costs are comparable and that costs can be weighed against benefits that occur in the same time period, it is necessary to standardize costs to the same base year. Cost data reported for previous years can be adjusted for a specified base year using either the Consumer Price Index (CPI) or a relevant subindex, such as the medical care component of the CPI. The CPI is an explicit price index that directly measures movements in the weighted average of prices of goods and services in a fixed "market basket" of goods and services purchased by households over time. Appendix H presents the CPI for all items and for the medical-care component for the period 1960–2000. More information on how the CPI is calculated can be found on the CPI home-page (stats.bls.gov/cpihome.htm). Summary tables of the CPI are published annually in the *Statistical Abstract of the United States*[29] and can be found on the web (www.census.gov/statab/www/).

To adjust the cost of an item reported for a year before the base year, divide the index value for the base year by the index value for the year in which the cost was reported. Then, multiply the result by the unadjusted value of the item. The formula for this calculation is as follows:

$$Y_B = Y_P \left[\frac{D_B}{D_P} \right] \tag{6}$$

where

Y_B = base year value
Y_P = past year value
D_B = index value of base year
D_P = index value of past year

For example, if data are available for the 1990 cost of a visit to a clinician but are needed for a study using 1998 costs, the cost of the visit to the clinician can be inflated to 1998 dollars using the physician-services component of the CPI. The ratio of the 1998 to 1990 index values (229.5 and 160.8, respectively) is multiplied by the 1990 cost of a visit to a clinician ($45), and the result is the cost of a visit to a clinician in 1998 dollars ($64).

$$\$64 = \$45 \left[\frac{229.5}{160.8} \right]$$

Adjusting Earnings to Base-Year Monetary Units

Just as costs must be adjusted to base-year monetary units, earnings reported for past years must be adjusted to base-year monetary units. However, because earnings do not increase and decrease at the same rates as prices, the CPI should not be used. Instead, the adjustment of past years' earnings to base-year monetary units uses the estimated annual increase in average hourly earnings reported annually in the March issue of *Employment and Earnings* from the U.S. Department of Commerce, Bureau of Labor Statistics. These data can also be located in the most recent issue of the *Statistical Abstract of the United States*[28] or on the web.

The equation for adjusting earnings is as follows:

$$I_B = I_P \left[\frac{W_B}{W_P} \right] \tag{7}$$

where

I_B = income in base year
I_P = income in past year
W_B = average hourly wage in the base year
W_P = average hourly wage in the past year

For example, a cost–effectiveness analysis that includes productivity losses has a 1993 base year. The productivity losses data are based on 1990 income. The average hourly earnings for 1990 and 1993 were $10.01 and $10.83, respectively. Thus, income of $23,582 in 1990 would be adjusted to $25,514 for a 1993 base year by this calculation:

$$\$25,514 = \$23,582 \left[\frac{10.83}{10.01} \right]$$

ANNUITIZING CAPITAL EXPENDITURES

Several types of costs must be considered in evaluating prevention programs: direct program costs, direct medical costs, and indirect costs. Direct program costs can include the cost of personnel and materials categorized as ongoing costs or start-up costs. Ongoing costs, also referred to as maintenance, recurring, or operating costs, are the annual expenditures necessary to keep a program running (e.g., payroll costs). Start-up costs are the one-time capital expenditures necessary for the early implementation stage of a program. These costs may include capital equipment costs. Although the costs of capital expenditures occur at one time, the benefits accrue over their useful life. Because capital investments such as equipment are used over the duration of a project, the costs of capital expenditures may be spread out over that time period. This is done by annuitizing, that is, determining an annual value of the capital item for the life of the capital investment. The annual value can then be used with other annual costs to calculate costs for the duration of a project. This is especially useful for cost analyses for which it is desirable to show the annual value of resources in relation to the level of output produced.

Richardson and Gafni[30] use two criteria for calculating the equivalent annual cost of a one-time capital expenditure. Costs annuitization should be consistent with the PV method of calculation used in the analysis. First, if 3% is used in the calculation of the discount factor to estimate the PV of future costs, then 3% should be used in the calculation of the annuity factor to estimate the equivalent annual cost of a one-time capital expenditure. Second, when annuitizing costs, the equivalent annual cost should yield a constant cost value for each year of the useful life of the capital expenditure. The equivalent annual cost can then be used to calculate costs for the duration of the project.

The method described below meets both criteria. First, the present scrap value should be subtracted from the original purchase cost; the result should then be divided by the appropriate annuity factor. *Scrap value* refers to the resale value of the capital expenditure at the end of the project. Use of this method, which is simple and direct, avoids understatement or overstatement of annual costs, which could lead to incorrect decisions about the allocation of resources in health care. The equations for annuitizing a one-time capital expenditure are as follows:

$$C = \left[P - S\frac{1}{(1+r)^t}\right](AF_{r,t})^{-1} \qquad (8)$$

where

C = calculated equivalent annual cost of the unit
P = cost of purchasing the unit
S = the scrap value (after t years of service) of the unit
r = discount rate
$AF_{r,t}$ = annuity factor such that

$$AF_{r,t} = \left[1 - \frac{1}{(1+r)^t}\right]r^{-1} \qquad (9)$$

Notice that in calculating the annuity factor, $1/(1+r)^t$ represents the discount factor $(DF_{r,t})$ and can easily be determined from Appendix G. Once $DF_{r,t}$ is calculated, $AF_{r,t}$ can be calculated by subtracting $DF_{r,t}$ from 1 and dividing by the discount rate, as shown in equation 9. An annuity table, listing annuity factors for t years of service and for discount rates (r) from 1% to 10%, is also provided in Appendix G.

The following example demonstrates the use of these formulas. The purchase price (P) of a new six-test tube centrifuge is $950. Assume that the centrifuge will be used over 5 years and that its scrap value (S) after 5 years will be 20% of its original cost, or $190. The discount rate is 3%.

The first step is to calculate the PV of the scrap value. The PV of $190 in 5 years is $190/(1 + 0.03)^5$ or $164.

The next step is to calculate the appropriate annuity factor using equation 9:

$$A_{0.03,5} = \left(1 - \frac{1}{(1+0.03)^5}\right)0.03^{-1} = 4.57$$

Then, the annual cost is calculated using equation 8:

$$\frac{(\$950 - \$164)}{4.57} = \$172$$

When these methods are used to annuitize a one-time capital expenditure, a centrifuge purchased for $950 with a scrap value of $190 after 5 years has an equivalent annual cost of $172 over its 5-year life span. It is important to note that when capital expenditures have been annuitized, they should not be further discounted with other annual costs and benefits because this would result in double discounting.

CONCLUSION

This chapter has presented the three methods for adjusting costs and benefits, whether measured in monetary or nonmonetary terms, to the base year of the analysis. Discounting, adjusting for inflation, and annuitizing are methods used to adjust the costs of the intervention, the cost of the illness, and the costs of benefits for the effects of time.

REFERENCES

1. Krahn M, Gafni A. Discounting in the economic evaluation of health care interventions. *Med Care 1993;* 5:403–18.
2. Drummond MF, O'Brien B, Stoddart GL, Torrance GW. *Methods for the Economic Evaluation of Health Care Programmes*, 2d ed. Oxford: Oxford University Press, 1997.
3. Gold MR, Siegel JE, Russell LB, Weinstein MC. *Cost–Effectiveness in Health and Medicine*. New York: Oxford University Press, 1996.
4. Office of Management and Budget. Guidelines and Discount Rates for Benefit-Cost Analysis of Federal Programs. OMB, Circular No. A-94, 1992.
5. Smith DH, Gravelle H. The practice of discounting in economic evaluations of healthcare interventions. *Int J Technol Assess Health Care 2001;* 17:236–43.
6. Petitti D. *Meta-Analysis, Decision Analysis, and Cost–Effectiveness Analysis. Methods for Quantitative Synthesis in Medicine*, 2d ed. New York: Oxford University Press, 2000.
7. Russell LB. *Is Prevention Better than Cure?* Washington DC: Brookings Institution, 1986.
8. Weinstein MC, Stason WB. Foundations of cost–effectiveness analysis for health and medical practices. *N Engl J Med 1977;* 296:716–21.
9. Keeler EB, Cretin S. Discounting of life-saving and other non-monetary effects. *Manage Sci 1983;* 6:194–8.
10. Department of Health. *Policy Appraisal and Health*. London: Department of Health, 1995.
11. Gafni A, Torrance GW. Risk attitude and time preference in health. *Manage Sci 1984;* 30:440–51.
12. Lipscomb J. Time preferences for health in cost-effectiveness analysis. *Med Care 1989;* 27(Suppl):233–53.
13. MacKeigan LD, Larson LN, Draugalis JR, et al. Time preferences for health gains and health losses. *Pharmacoeconomics 1993;* 3:374–86.
14. Olsen JA. Time preferences for health gains: an empirical investigation. *Health Econ 1993;* 2:257–66.
15. Redelmeier D, Heller D. Time preference in medical decision making and cost–effectiveness analysis. *Med Decis Making 1993;* 13:212–7.
16. Weinstein M. Time-preference in the health care context. *Med Decis Making 1993;* 13:218–9.

17. Ganiats TG. Discounting in cost–effectivness research. *Med Decis Making 1994;* 14:298–300.
18. Redelmeier DA, Heller DN, Weinstein MC. Time preference in medical economics: science or religion? *Med Decis Making 1994;* 14:301–3.
19. Torgerson DJ, Donaldson C, Reid DM. Private versus social opportunity cost of time: valuing time in the demand for health care. *Health Econ 1994;* 3:149–56.
20. Chapman GB, Elstein AS. Valuing the future: temporal discounting of health and money. *Med Decis Making 1995;* 15:373–86.
21. Cairns JA, Van der Pol MM. Constant and decreasing timing aversion for saving lives. *Soc Sci Med 1997;* 45:1653–9.
22. Cairns JA, Van der Pol MM. Saving future lives. A comparison of three discounting models. *Health Econ 1997;* 6:341–50.
23. Meltzer M. Accounting for future costs in medical cost–effectiveness analysis. *J Health Econ 1997;* 16:33–64.
24. Van Hout BA. Discounting costs and effects: a reconsideration. *Health Econ 1998;* 7:581–94.
25. Torgerson DJ, Raftery J. Economics notes: discounting. *BMJ 1999;* 319:914–5.
26. Tasset A, Nguyen VH, Wood S, Amazian K. Discounting: technical issues in economic evaluations of vaccination. *Vaccine 1999;* 17:S75–80.
27. Harvey CM. The reasonableness of non-constant discounting. J Public Econ *1994;* 53:31–51.
28. Loewenstein GF, Prelec D. Anomalies in intertemporal choice: evidence and an interpretation. *Q J Econ 1992;* 107:573–97.
29. US Bureau of the Census. *Statistical Abstract of the United States: 2000,* 120th ed. Washington DC, US Bureau of the Census, 2000.
30. Richardson AW, Gafni A. Treatment of capital costs in evaluating health-care programs. *Cost Manage 1983;* 26–30.

7

Decision Analysis

SUE J. GOLDIE
PHAEDRA S. CORSO

This chapter provides an overview of decision analysis and its use as an analytic tool to inform difficult public health decisions. There are particular circumstances in which decision analysis is likely to be most useful, and such circumstances often characterize the decision making necessary in the field of public health. Decision-analytic methods may be applied to a wide range of problems from clinical decisions facing an individual to public health decisions that will affect a population. The aim of decision science is to develop and apply systematic and logical frameworks for decision making. Its defining characteristic is a focus on the outcomes of decisions, including characterization of the uncertainty about these outcomes that exists when decisions are made. In this discipline, consequences may be broadly defined, ranging from clinical and public health benefits (e.g., a clinical decision analysis or a prevention-effectiveness analysis) to both clinical benefits and economic consequences (e.g., cost–effectiveness, cost–utility, and cost–benefit analyses).[1,2]

DECISION ANALYSIS DEFINED

Decision analysis is an explicit, quantitative, and systematic approach to decision making under uncertainty. It encompasses a series of methods that have been developed to address the difficulties of identifying optimal solutions to problems with multiple alternatives; relevant to those in public health is the use of decision analysis to aid in decision making for the individual patient and for policy decisions affecting populations of patients.

MOTIVATION FOR DECISION ANALYSIS IN PUBLIC HEALTH

Consider the following simplified examples of four current public health concerns.

Example 1: 40-Year-Old Man with Hepatitis C

You are working in the state health clinic and a 40-year-old male recently diagnosed with chronic hepatitis C virus (HCV) requests information on treatment after reading an educational pamphlet on the potential long-term sequelae of this infection. The natural history of chronic HCV is uncertain, and there is conflicting information on the rate of progression to advanced liver disease. Although treatment is available, it is effective in fewer than 50% of patients and can be associated with moderate to severe side effects. What would you advise with respect to treatment alternatives? How would you explain the risks and benefits?

Example 2: Screening for Chlamydia in Adolescents

You are a state public health official responsible for the ultimate allocation of limited state funds for the control of sexually transmitted diseases. Additional unexpected federal funds have become available; however, they must be applied to the adolescent chlamydial control program. Currently, adolescent girls are screened annually in the state health clinic. These funds could be used to increase the frequency of screening to every 6 months, to improve partner notification efforts, or to develop improved methods to ensure prompt follow-up for girls with positive test results. If only one program can be implemented, which one would you choose?

Example 3: Allocating Resources to Control Human Immunodeficiency Virus in Sub-Saharan Africa

You have been appointed as the director of a 15-member international committee responsible for the allocation of a large donation by the Bill and Melinda Gates Foundation to "combat AIDS in Africa." One of the major responsibilities of the committee is to decide on the appropriate proportion of the fund that should be directed toward prevention efforts, treatment efforts, and human immunodeficiency virus (HIV) vaccine development. How will these different approaches be prioritized?

Example 4: Lead Removal in Subsidized Housing Complexes

You are the director of the public health department in Boston and unexpected state funds have become available to assist in the removal of lead from subsidized housing complexes. There are three strategies that may be used for lead removal. The method that is most effective is also the most expensive: given the available funds, only 80% of the houses could be treated. The method that is least costly is also the least effective; however, 100% of the houses could be treated. Which strategy would you choose?

Each of these decision problems is associated with important clinical, public health, and economic consequences; but what makes these decisions so difficult?

Complexity. Each presents a complex set of issues requiring consideration of all possible courses of action, multiple potential outcomes, and eventual consequences (costs and benefits) resulting from different outcomes. Decision analysis provides rigorous methods for organizing a complex problem into a structure that can be analyzed.

Uncertainty. A decision can be difficult because of the inherent uncertainty in the situation. For example, the decision whether to treat the 40-year-old man for HCV is complicated by the fact that the natural history of chronic HCV is uncertain. Despite the uncertainty, a decision will need to be made. A decision-analytic approach assists in identifying the most important sources of uncertainty, allowing them to be represented in a systematic manner.

Multiple Competing Objectives. A decision problem may have multiple competing objectives, making trade-offs inevitable. For example, important objectives in sub-Saharan Africa include preventing transmission of HIV between discordant partners, decreasing the rate of vertical transmission, and improving the quality of life of HIV-infected persons by providing treatment. A decision-analytic approach permits the potential gains from antiretroviral treatment to be quantitatively compared to the consequences of diverting funds now allocated to prevention activities.

Different Perspectives. Alternative perspectives may result in different conclusions. For example, public health officers and local government officials may have completely different viewpoints on the role of equity considerations with respect to different options for lead removal. By clarifying where the agreements and disagreements are, a decision-analytic framework allows for alternatives or choices to be reformulated and areas of conflict to be resolved.

In summary, these decisions have important consequences, are complex, and are characterized by uncertainty, inevitable trade-offs, risk, and the potential for multiple perspectives. Moreover, for a variety of reasons, it will not be feasible to conduct prospective randomized clinical trials to evaluate the different options within each situation.

DECISION ANALYSIS AS A DISCIPLINE

The risk and decision sciences, as subdisciplines of economics, have developed theories of how decisions "ought" to be made. Normative theories are distinguished from descriptive theories of how people and institutions actually behave. *Normative theories* explore how people ought to behave if they wish to be consistent with certain basic principles or axioms.[3–5]

The most widely accepted of the normative theories is expected utility theory.[6] Developed in the mid-twentieth century by von Neumann, Morgenstern, Savage, and others, the theory provides a method for making decisions that is consistent with the several basic axioms.[7] The axioms may be briefly stated as follows: (*1*) lottery A either is or is not preferred to lottery B, (*2*) preferences between two lotteries are not affected by any outcomes that have the same probability of occurring under both lotteries, and (*3*) no outcome is so good or bad that the possibility of getting it outweighs all other outcomes that may result from a lottery. Expected utility theory provides a method for evaluating decisions that can be established, through logical proof, to yield decisions that are consistent with these axioms. The method basically involves the following steps:

1. Assign a numerical value to each possible outcome that reflects the desirability of the outcome relative to other possible outcomes. This value is the *utility* of the outcome.

2. Assign a numerical probability that the outcome will occur, if the decision is taken, for each of the possible decisions.
3. Calculate the expected value of the utility (the *probability-weighted utility*) for each decision.
4. Choose the decision with the largest expected utility.

Decision analysis uses such mathematical tools to help decision makers choose the option that maximizes *expected value* or *utility*.[8] *Utility* is defined as the value of a preferred outcome when considered from a particular perspective. For example, many measures of health, such as quality-adjusted life years, and life expectancy, can be interpreted as utility functions. Decision analysis may be viewed as a technique for helping decision makers identify the option that has the greatest *expected utility* to an individual, society, or a particular community.

Most everyday decisions are not made using the particular logic and rationality of decision science. One reason for this is that some decisions are simple and straightforward. For decisions that are more complex, people may also rely on psychological shortcuts in thinking, or *heuristics*. Although heuristics can be useful, their use can also lead to suboptimal choices.[9] Decision analysis provides structure and guidance for systematic thinking in situations that are characterized as having uncertainty, multiple competing objectives, and several possible perspectives.[10] As opposed to a descriptive or normative approach, decision analysis generally adopts a "prescriptive approach"; application of tools from this discipline in such circumstances allows one to make effective decisions more consistently. Based on fundamental principles and informed by what we know about the limitations of human judgment and decision making in complex situations, decision analysis can offer guidance to public health providers working on hard decisions.

IS DECISION ANALYSIS APPROPRIATE?

Decision analysis is most useful in situations where multiple alternatives exist, information is incomplete, and it is uncertain what the most efficient choice would be. A fundamental question in designing a decision analysis is whether decision analysis is the best approach. If the answer to a question is straightforward, there is no reason for a decision analysis. If the consequences are trivial, the effort required to conduct the analysis may not be worthwhile. Decision analysis makes the most sense when the different alternatives, outcomes, and probabilities can be specified or at least estimated, and in the context of important consequences.

ELEMENTS OF A DECISION ANALYSIS

The core elements of a decision analysis can be classified into values and objectives, decisions, uncertain events, and consequences.[10] These elements are incorporated quantitatively into a *model* in order to structure a decision problem over time. Different types of model may be chosen to allow for a structure to suitably accommodate the complexity of the decision problem, and this chapter discusses three of them. Regardless of the type of model, however, the decision-analytic approach has six major components, which represent the building blocks of prevention-effectiveness analyses.

1. Specify the decision problem and objectives
2. Develop a model to structure the decision problem over time
3. Estimate probabilities
4. Value consequences
5. Analyze the base case
6. Evaluate uncertainty

Specify the Decision Problem and Its Components

The starting point in a decision analysis is a decision that must be made on behalf of an individual, group of persons, or population. The first step is to therefore explicitly state the question that the decision analysis is being constructed to evaluate. The problem should then be broken down into its component parts: objectives, alternatives, and outcomes. Understanding one's objectives is a prerequisite to defining the alternatives, choosing the relative outcomes, and deciding on the kinds of uncertainty that need to be considered in the analysis.[11,12] Chapter 2 provides a complete discussion of framing a study question. The component parts particularly applicable to decision analysis are described briefly below.

Perspective
Depending on the perspective adopted by the analyst, the objectives, alternatives, and valued outcomes will likely differ. Public health decisions may involve the viewpoints of communities, nations, individuals, interest or advocacy groups, public health agencies, or society at large. A decision analysis of a public health problem will almost always include population measures of health as relevant outcomes. In such analyses, the broadest perspective is the societal perspective, which incorporates all health outcomes and all economic outcomes regardless of who obtains the effects and who pays the costs.[1] In some cases, where the decision is being made on behalf of a specific group or entity, a more limited perspective may be appropriate.

Target Population
The *target population* is the population for whom the program being evaluated is intended. If the focus of the analysis is decision making for an individual, such as in our first example of HCV, the target population might be described as a hypothetical cohort of identical 40-year-old men or women infected with HCV. In other analyses, the relevant target population may be a population subgroup, for example, adolescents seeking health care from a state health clinic. Depending on the nature of the analysis, important subgroups to consider might include individuals of a given age or sex, those living in a specific geographic region, or those with certain risk factors.

In many analyses, the target population will be heterogeneous. Consider the example of allocating funds for the control of HIV in Africa. The target population includes groups of people in different countries, each with a distinct infection prevalence and incidence pattern, level of health infrastructure, language, culture, and level of education. It is important in framing a decision analysis to identify relevant subgroups and to determine the extent to which subgroup analyses should be undertaken. Alternative interventions may affect different population subgroups differently. For example, treatment for chronic HCV may be less effective in HIV-infected patients compared with HIV-uninfected patients. Chapter 3 discusses the specification of the target population in decision modeling and measures of population effects, including incidence, prevalence, and characteristics of morbidity and mortality.

Finally, a target population may not always involve human beings. For example, in the program designed to remove lead from subsidized housing complexes, the target population consists of the houses themselves, even though it is the health of the individuals inhabiting the houses that has motivated the program.

Alternatives

The range and number of alternatives will differ depending on the nature of a study, but all relevant options must be identified. In our first example, there are at least two main options facing our 40-year-old patient: treatment for HCV and no treatment for HCV. Realistically, there may be other options as well. For example, a third option might be to defer the treatment decision and obtain more information (e.g., a liver biopsy), or wait for the development or discovery of more effective therapies.

Time Frame and Analytic Horizon

The *time frame* of an analysis is the specified period in which the intervention strategies are actually applied. The *analytic horizon* is the period over which the health and economic consequences of the intervention are considered. Often in public health decision modeling the analytic horizon will be longer than the time frame. For example, an aggressive behavioral intervention and educational program to reduce risky sexual behaviors associated with HIV transmission might be implemented in a middle school system in Zimbabwe (i.e., the time frame), while the benefits of that program would include the averted future cases of HIV that would have occurred in the absence of the program over the ensuing years of sexually-active adulthood (i.e., analytic horizon).

Develop a Model to Structure the Problem over Time

Models are the fundamental analytic tools used in decision analysis to display the temporal and logical sequence of a decision problem.[10] Influence diagrams, decision trees, and state-transition Markov models are three examples of models that may be used to perform decision analyses.[13–16] Models are increasingly being used to address clinical issues in national and international health policy planning, to develop computer algorithms for clinical information and decision support systems, to evaluate clinical pathways, to establish practice guidelines, and to conduct epidemiological research.[17]

Classification of Models

Models may be classified several ways; this may cause confusion since these classifications are not mutually exclusive.[1] First, models can be classified according to the structure they employ to account for events that occur over time (e.g., decision trees, state-transition models). Second, models can be classified according to the nature of the target population (e.g., longitudinal cohort models, cross-sectional population models). Third, models may be classified by the method of calculation (e.g., deterministic, probabilistic). This chapter is organized by the first classification system, with separate sections on decision trees and state transition models.

Regardless of the choice of model, decision analysis is characterized by a set of core elements. We will introduce these core elements within the context of a decision tree, one of the simplest and most transparent of these tools.

Developing a Simple Decision Tree

A *decision tree* is a simple visual tool to represent how all of the possible choices relate to the possible outcomes.[10,18] The decision tree depicts graphically all of the components of the decision problem and relates actions to consequences. It consists of nodes, branches, and outcomes. There are three kinds of nodes: decision nodes, chance nodes and terminal nodes.

Decision Node. The first point of choice in the decision tree, and often the focus of the analysis, is represented as a decision node. It is represented in the decision tree as a small square (Fig. 7.1). This node represents the two alternatives that may be chosen by the patient with chronic HCV in our first example, although any number of options could be specified. At this decision node, the only alternatives are to treat or not to treat chronic HCV.

Regardless of the decision that is ultimately chosen, the patient's final outcome is determined by a series of chance events. Even if the patient is treated for HCV, there is a chance he may suffer progressive liver disease. Likewise, if the patient is not treated, there is a chance he will not experience progressive liver disease.

Chance Node. A chance node represents a point in time at which chance determines which of several possible events that are beyond the control of the decision maker may occur. A line attached to the circle denotes each outcome of a chance event, and each line is labeled with the event. There is no limit to the branches allowed on a

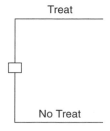

Figure 7.1 Decision node in a decision tree.

chance node, but the events at a chance node must be mutually exclusive and collectively exhaustive. Therefore, at the chance node in this simplified example, the branch "moderate hepatitis" represents the hypothetical patient(s) who will never develop cirrhosis. Similarly, the branch "cirrhosis" represents those patients who ultimately do develop end-stage liver disease regardless of any past history of moderate hepatitis. Both patients with cirrhosis and, to a lesser degree, patients with moderate hepatitis have a chance of developing liver cancer (i.e., hepatocellular carcinoma). For each possible event, a numerical probability must be assigned that represents the chance that an individual will experience the event. At any given chance node, the sum of the probabilities of the events must be equal to 1. The assignment of probabilities is discussed below (see Estimate Probabilities).

Terminal Node. By convention, a decision tree is developed from left to right, starting with the initial decision node on the extreme left and moving to the final outcomes on the extreme right. The sequence of chance nodes from left to right usually follows the temporal sequence of events. A terminal node indicates the end point of each sequence of events and represents the outcome (e.g., life expectancy or quality-adjusted life expectancy) resulting from that particular pathway. In this example, we focus on a decision facing an individual patient. A decision tree, however, may be used to calculate the expected outcomes of alternative prevention strategies for a single person or for a cohort of individuals (Fig. 7.2).

Estimate Probabilities

There are several justifiable approaches to the baseline set of parameters for the model. At a minimum, the selection of probabilities should include a systematic

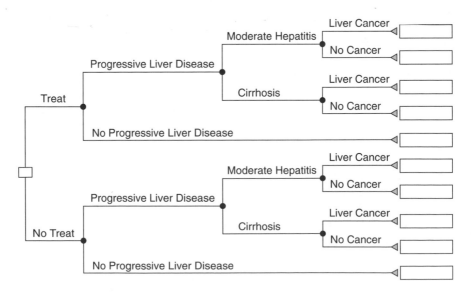

Figure 7.2   Terminal nodes in a decision tree.

process for the identification of information, the documentation of sources of information excluded, and an explanation of how the point estimate or probability distribution (see Monte Carlo Analysis, below) for each parameter was chosen. When decision analyses target populations as opposed to individuals, it is important to specify how the members of the cohort differ from one another. The more precisely demographic and socioeconomic characteristics can be specified, the more precisely the data requirements for the model can be selected. Chapter 3 provides a more complete discussion on specifying population parameters for use in decision modeling and a description of the types of study (e.g., randomized controlled trials, cohort studies) that can provide the necessary data.

In our first example, a decision analysis would require data on the risk of progression to advanced liver disease. The uncertainty with respect to the natural history of HCV is a good example of how the use of only certain types of studies would lead to biased results.[19] Several studies have considered patients with chronic HIV and established liver disease and either followed them prospectively or evaluated them retrospectively to estimate the time of infection. Data from such studies reveal a relatively high rate of progression to cirrhosis and hepatocellular carcinoma but are subject to *referral bias* since they were generally performed at tertiary referral centers, which attract persons with existing chronic liver disease. Data from prospective cohort studies starting with disease onset describe a slower and more heterogeneous rate of progression, with a much lower probability of severe liver disease.

Value Consequences

Outcomes are the consequences of the events represented in the decision tree. A value must be assigned to each outcome on the decision tree. The most straightforward outcomes to value are those that occur naturally in appropriate units of measure (e.g., costs or life expectancy), and these may be inserted directly into the model. When quantitative outcomes are used (e.g., the cost of a medical outcome or the life expectancy associated with liver cancer), the expected values of the decision alternatives are calculated. It is possible to consider more than one quantitative outcome at the terminal node in a decision-tree model. For example, if one is interested in costs and life expectancy, one can first include costs at the terminal nodes and calculate the expected value and then include life expectancy at the terminal nodes and calculate the expected value. Comparison of these two expected-value calculations is the basis for cost–effectiveness analysis discussed in the subsequent chapters.

Valuing health outcomes is more complicated when no natural units are available and when more than two final health outcomes are possible. In this case, we need to consider the strength of preferences among possible health outcomes and express this preference quantitatively.[12] A decision analysis that incorporates measures of the preferences of individuals or society for different health states is referred to as *utility analysis*. When the health outcomes are expressed as utilities, the *expected utility* for the decision alternatives is calculated by multiplying the health outcomes expressed as utilities by their probabilities of occurrence. The process of calculating expected value and expected utility is identical.

Utility Assessment for Health Outcomes

Several methods can be used to express preferences for different health outcomes quantitatively, but only utility assessment yields a numerical scale (called a "utility scale") that is theoretically appropriate for the calculations required in a decision model.[20,21] Chapter 5 provides a thorough examination of three methods to ascertain utilities, including the standard gamble technique, the time trade-off method, and a rating scale.

A discussion of combining preferences for quality of life (i.e., using utilities) with preferences for longevity, using the quality-adjusted life year (QALY), is also provided in Chapter 5. The QALY is a measure of health outcome that assigns to each period of time a weight, ranging from 0 to 1, corresponding to the quality of life during that period, where a weight of 1 corresponds to perfect health and a weight of 0 corresponds to death. The number of QALYs, then, represents the number of healthy years of life that are valued equivalently to the actual health outcome.

For the decision-tree example (Fig. 7.3), 15 QALYs were used for a health outcome of moderate hepatitis (i.e., the average quality-adjusted life expectancy for a 40-year-old male with moderate hepatitis is 15 QALYs), 5 QALYs were used for cirrhosis, and 0.8 QALYs were used for liver cancer. Twenty-five QALYs were used for a patient with chronic HCV who does not develop liver disease. Because a person with mild chronic hepatitis who is treated but not destined to develop progressive liver disease experiences the side effects and toxicity of treatment, the expected QALYs are 24.6. These values may be substituted into the decision tree for the outcomes.

Analyze the Base Case

Expected utility, or *expected value,* is a way of expressing in numbers which decision option would provide the highest value, cost, or other unit of measurement. When

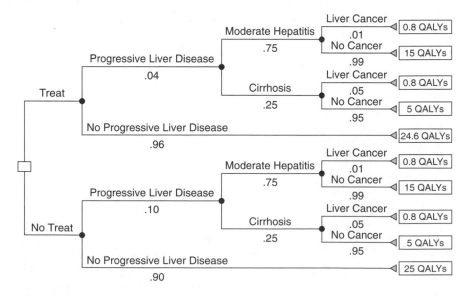

Figure 7.3   A decision tree.

outcomes are expressed as utilities, by definition, the decision option with the highest expected utility should be preferred. Other decision rules may apply in different circumstances. After all possible outcomes are quantified, the expected utilities or expected values for each strategy can be calculated. This calculation process is the subject of this section.

The process of calculating the expected value or utility of a decision-tree model is referred to as *averaging out and folding back*. The expected value or utility is the sum of the products of the estimates of the probability of events and their outcomes.

Averaging Out and Folding Back

Averaging out and folding back starts at the tip (right) of the tree and works back to the root (left) of the tree. Beginning with the outcomes on the right, the value of the outcome at each terminal node is multiplied by the probability of that event occurring. On branches of a chance node, products for each terminal node are summed. This is the expected value of the chance node. For example, calculate the expected value of the chance node at the top far right branch of the "Treat" option in the tree in Figure 7.4. In step 1, (Fig. 7.5) each of the two outcomes is multiplied by its respective probability of occurring; the products are then summed to obtain the expected value of the chance node (14.86). The averaging-out-and-folding-back process continues to work toward the left side of the tree until the main decision node (the *root node*) is reached. In complex decision trees, this process may be completed quickly using computerized decision-making software. This decision tree has been presented very simply, to illustrate the calculation process. In many

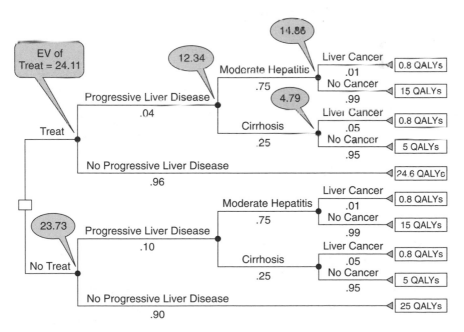

Figure 7.4 Averaging out and folding back to obtain expected values in a decision tree.

Expected Value of Treat
Step 1: [(0.8* .01) + (15*0.99)] = 14.86
Step 2: [((0.8*0.01) + (15*0.99))*0.75] + [((0.8*0.05) +
(5.0*0.95))*0.25] = 12.34
Step 3: [(12.34*0.04 + (24.6*0.96)] = 24.11

Expected Value of No Treat
Step 1: [(0.8* .01) + (15*0.99)] = 14.86
Step 2: [((0.8*0.01) + (15*0.99))*0.75] + [((0.8*0.05) +
(5.0*0.95))*0.25] = 12.34
Step 3: [(12.34*0.10) + (25*0.90)] = 23.73

Figure 7.5   Calculating the expected values of outcomes using the process of averaging out and folding back.

decision problems, there will be more than one decision. When a decision tree contains additional decision nodes in addition to a root node, only the branch with the product of the highest numerical value is folded back. Branches with products of lower numerical values are "pruned" (i.e., temporarily removed or ignored) from the tree.

For decision analyses with multiple outcomes (e.g., costs and QALYs), averaging out and folding back is done twice: the expected value in costs and the expected value in terms of clinical benefits are calculated separately. These two outcomes are expressed as a cost–effectiveness ratio, which is described in detail in Chapter 9.

Evaluate Uncertainty

A critical part of any decision analysis is to evaluate the uncertainty in the model structure, parameter estimates, and assumptions. In general, sensitivity analysis involves varying key model parameter values to evaluate their impact on model outcomes. For example, in the chronic hepatitis example, there is a great deal of uncertainty as to the probability of progression to advanced liver disease and one could easily find evidence of both lower and higher estimates.[19] A sensitivity analysis is a test of the stability of the conclusions of an analysis over a range of parameter estimates and structural assumptions.

Sensitivity analyses address the following types of question:

- If the numerical estimate of a probability or an outcome is changed, how does expected utility or expected value change? (e.g., If the risk of liver disease progression is much lower than estimated, how does the expected value, as measured in QALYs change?)
- Do the conclusions change when the probability and outcome estimates are assigned values that lie within a reasonable range? (e.g., Is treatment for HCV still the most attractive strategy when the range of treatment effectiveness is varied between 30% and 60%?)

- How much would an estimate have to change to produce a different result? (e.g., How low would the risk of progressive liver disease have to be for the expected value of no treatment to be higher than the expected value of treatment?)
- What value would a variable have to have for two strategies to be of equal expected value (i.e., threshold analysis)?
- What happens to the results of the model if the "best-case-scenario" or "worst-case-scenario" estimates are used?

Parameters with the greatest level of uncertainty, the greatest degree of variation, or the greatest influence on outcomes must be included in sensitivity analyses. The range of values used for a sensitivity analysis can be based on statistical variation for point estimates or on probability distributions. Alternatively, expert opinion can be used to evaluate the range of values. To maintain the model's transparency, an analyst should disclose the rationale for the choice of values.

One-Way versus Multi-Way Sensitivity Analysis

A sensitivity analysis can be done by varying one parameter in a decision tree or by simultaneously varying two or more probability or outcome estimates. When one value is changed (a one-way or univariate sensitivity analysis), the decision maker can see the effect of one variable on the results of the decision model. When several values are changed simultaneously (a multi-way or multivariate sensitivity analysis), the decision maker can examine the relationships among the various estimates used in the decision-modeling calculations. An example of a one-way sensitivity analysis is described below.

Assume that in the decision analysis for HCV treatment the plausible range for the probability of liver disease progression over a 10-year period ranges from 1% to 25%. A one-way sensitivity analysis can be conducted by recalculating the expected value of the treat and no treat strategies, first using a 1% progression risk and then using a 25% progression risk. If the treat option continues to be preferable (i.e., has a higher expected value), the analyst and target audience can have confidence that the results are stable despite the uncertainty in this parameter. Figure 7.6 illustrates the results of this sensitivity analysis. The probability of progression to advanced liver disease needs to be at least 5% (over the 10-year time horizon) for the treat strategy to remain the preferred option when maximizing health regardless of costs.

Threshold Analysis

Threshold analysis is a type of one-way sensitivity analysis that is also useful to determine and describe the conditions under which alternative decisions have equivalent consequences. Using a threshold analysis, one can determine how much a probability or outcome value would have to change for the decision tree to yield a sufficiently different value so that a different decision alternative should be chosen. Threshold analyses are also useful to determine the plausibility of a decision being altered; i.e., a parameter would have to be at least greater (or less) than $X\%$, which is (or is not) a plausible scenario. Consider the uncertainty about the effec-

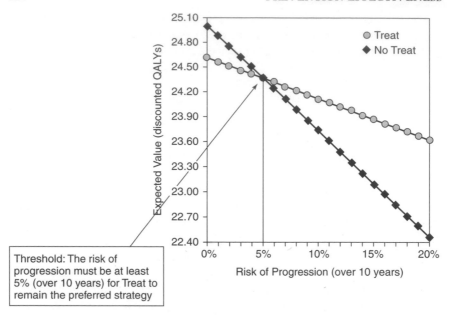

Figure 7.6   One-way sensitivity analysis varying the risk of progression to advanced liver disease (over 10 years) in patients with chronic HCV infection.

tiveness of treatment for HCV. A reasonable question to pose is "How effective must treatment be in order to remain the preferred strategy?" In a threshold analysis, the first step is to identify the best and next-best strategies (since there are only two strategies in this simplified example, these are *treat* and *no treat*); the second step is to identify the uncertain parameter of interest, e.g., effectiveness of treatment for HCV (defined as the reduction in the probability of progressive liver disease); and the third step is to determine the value of the parameter such that the expected values of the two strategies are equal.

A threshold analysis is shown in Figure 7.7. Treatment needs to reduce the probability of progression to advanced liver disease by at least 30% over the 10-year time horizon before the *treat* strategy would no longer be the preferred option.

Threshold analyses can also be used to plan strategies for public health intervention programs. For example, in the chlamydial screening example presented earlier, an initial strategy of screening every 6 months might be preferred in a high-risk adolescent population. Over time, however, as the prevalence of chlamydia decreases in response to screening and treatment, a less frequent or a more selective screening strategy may be more effective. Threshold analyses in this situation could help to identify the prevalence at which one screening strategy is preferred over another. While two–way and multivariable sensitivity analyses (varying multiple parameters simultaneously) permit greater exploration of variability, the results can be more difficult to interpret. Other approaches to evaluating parameter uncertainty, such as probabilistic approaches, are discussed in the next section.

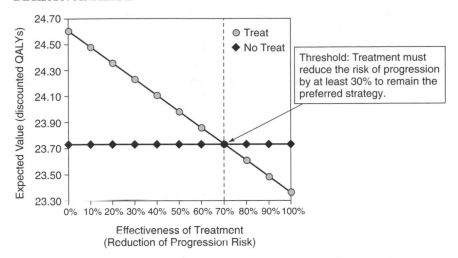

Figure 7.7   One-way sensitivity analysis varying the effectiveness of treatment for hepatitis C virus at reducing the probability of liver disease progression.

Best- and Worst-Case Scenarios

In best- and worst-case-scenario sensitivity analyses, the decision-tree model can be analyzed using low- or high-range estimates of variables that favor one option and can be reanalyzed using estimates that favor another option. If a decision is unchanged at extreme levels, the decision maker may gain confidence in the results of the decision analysis.

Second-Order Monte Carlo Simulation

A *second-order Monte Carlo analysis* is when a hypothetical cohort of people is run through a decision model, allowing the computer program to randomly select from a probability distribution specified at each chance node. Statistical results of the accumulated computer runs provide information for further interpretation and analysis. For a given structure and set of parameter values, the distribution of results gives a measure of central tendency and variance of results which could be expected across members of a cohort. The information about the distribution of results obtained from either type of Monte Carlo analysis is very useful for understanding the robustness of the results to changes in parameter values and for estimating the range of results that cohort members might experience. Several software programs described in Appendix C have Monte Carlo analysis capabilities.

LIMITATIONS OF DECISION-TREE MODELS

Decision trees work well for relatively straightforward clinical problems with short-term outcomes. A decision-tree framework becomes less useful for diseases

in which ideal events occur repeatedly (e.g., multiple episodes of pelvic inflammatory disease resulting from chlamydial infection and reinfection) or over a long
time period (e.g., risk of chlamydial infection from the start of sexual activity
through the fourth decade). In addition, a decision tree mandates a fixed time horizon (e.g., the HCV decision-tree model was specified to have a 10-year time horizon). In reality, when evaluating populations, one would accommodate multiple
time horizons. Complex public health problems that involve preventive strategies
require both a more complex model and a long time horizon. One such model is
generically referred to as a "state-transition" model. State-transition models have
been used to represent the natural history of many chronic diseases such as coronary heart disease, HIV, and colorectal, breast and cervical cancers. [22–25] These
natural history models have been used to evaluate both primary and secondary
preventive health interventions.

STATE-TRANSITION MODELS

State-transition models allocate and subsequently reallocate members of the
population into one of several categories, or "health states." [15,26] Health states are
defined according to factors such as disease stage and treatment status. Transitions
occur from one state to another at defined recurring intervals of equal length according to transition probabilities. Transition probabilities can be made dependent
on population characteristics such as age, gender, and chronic disease by specifying the probabilities as functions of these characteristics. Through simulation, the
number of members of the population in each health state at each point in time
can be estimated. Model outcomes can include life expectancy and quality-
adjusted life expectancy, as well as other intermediate outcomes. A special type of
state-transition model in which the transition probabilities depend only on the
current state and not on the previous states or the pathway by which the state was
entered is a Markov model. [27]

The general decision-analytic approach and key elements described for a
decision-tree model apply to the development of a Markov model as well. In this
section, we will briefly review the development steps of a Markov model and highlight its unique attributes and limitations.

Specify the Decision Problem and Its Components

Similar to the development of a decision tree, our first step is to define the decision
problem and identify the major issues; objectives need to be defined clearly, alternatives identified, and outcomes specified. In addition, the perspective, target
population, target audience, analytic horizon and time horizon, need to be explicitly defined.

Develop a Model to Structure the Problem over Time

A very simple Markov model is developed below to illustrate its components.

Step 1: Delineate a Set of Mutually Exclusive Health States
A Markov model is made up of a set of mutually exclusive and collectively exhaustive health states, or Markov states, that persons might reasonably experience within the context of the clinical problem. Each person in the model resides in one and only one health state at any point in time. Consider a simple example in which only three health states are possible: well, disease, and dead.

Step 2: Specify Transitions
The next step is to specify the ways in which persons in those health states might behave during some brief time interval. For example, persons in the well state may stay well, may acquire disease, or may die during any given time interval. Each of these "movements" is referred to as a *state transition*. Figure 7.8 is an example of a state-transition diagram. Arrows connecting two different states indicate allowed transitions. Arrows leading from a state to itself indicate that the patient may remain in that state in consecutive cycles. Only certain transitions are allowed. Health states can be transient (persons can revisit the state at any time), temporary (persons can stay in the state for only one cycle), or absorbing (once persons enter the state, they can never exit).

Step 3: Specify the Cycle Length
The analytic horizon of an analysis is divided into equal increments of time, referred to as *Markov cycles*. During each cycle, a person can make a single transition from one state to another. The length of a cycle is chosen to represent a clinically meaningful time interval. For example, a cycle length of 1 year might be required for a model that spans the patient's entire life. However, the cycle time might be shorter, for example, monthly or even weekly, if the model needs to represent very frequent events or events that occur at a rate which changes over time. Often, the cycle time will be determined by the available data.

Identify Probabilities

In a Markov model, each of the transitions between health states is governed by an associated transition probability (Fig. 7.9). Transition probabilities can be either constant over time or time-dependent. An important limitation of Markov models is the *Markovian assumption*, which states that knowing only the present state of

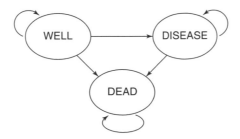

Figure 7.8   State-transition diagram of a simple Markov model in which only three health states are possible.

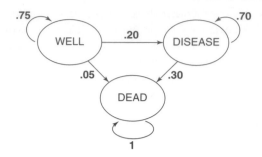

Figure 7.9   State-transition diagram of a Markov model with the associated transition probabilities.

health of a patient is sufficient to project the entire trajectory of future states. In other words, the transition probabilities depend only on current health state residence and not on prior health states. It is possible to get around this assumption by expanding the number of health states so that each represents persons with a unique history. Creating these separate health states allows one to model the event rates dependent on clinical history. As a result, however, the probabilities required for the model also increase. If the public health problem being modeled is so complex, it may be preferable to consider running a Monte Carlo analysis as described below.

Value Consequence

To incorporate quality and length of life in a single measure, each health state is assigned a quality weight or quality factor, which represents the quality of life in that health state relative to perfect health. For example, quality weights or utility weights of 1.0, 0.5, and 0.0 could be assigned to the well, disease, and dead states (i.e., a year spent in the disease state is equivalent to 0.5 years in the well state). If a quality weight of 1.0 is assigned to all states except dead (which is assigned a value of 0.0), then the model will calculate life expectancy (Fig. 7.10, top equation). If the utility or quality weights

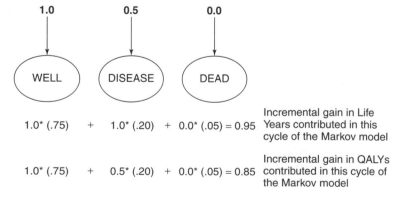

Figure 7.10   Each health state is associated with a quality factor representing the quality of life in that state relative to perfect health.

represent a health-related quality adjustment for each health state, then the model will calculate quality-adjusted life expectancy (Fig. 7.10, bottom equation.).

Analyze the Base Case

The two most commonly used methods of evaluating a Markov model are a cohort simulation and a first-order Monte Carlo simulation.[16]

Cohort Simulation

In a cohort simulation, a hypothetical cohort of people enter the model according to a prevalence distribution specified by the analyst. This distribution will vary depending on the objective of the analysis. For example, in a Markov model developed to simulate chlamydial screening in adolescents, one might start an analysis with an entire cohort of uninfected 10-year-olds (i.e., everyone in the cohort starts in the well state). However, one might want to distribute the cohort upon entry into the model into different health states according to age-specific prevalence of disease. After specifying where people start, a hypothetical cohort of patients transition through the model simultaneously. For each cycle, the fraction of the cohort initially in each health state is divided among all health states according to a set of defined transition probabilities (Fig. 7.11). For example, assume that 100% of the cohort starts in the well state (i.e., 1000 patients). Cohort members face an annual probability of acquiring disease of 0.20 and an annual probability of dying of 0.05. In the second cycle of this analysis, 75% would be in the well state (750), 20%

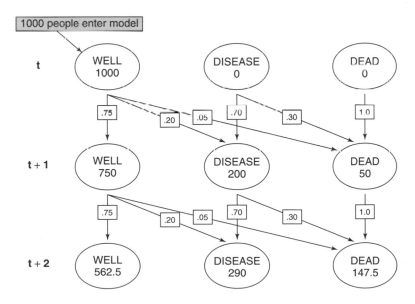

Figure 7.11   Distribution of a cohort of 1000 people in three cycles of a simple Markov model.

would be in the disease state (200), and 5% would be in the dead state (50). In each subsequent cycle, there will be a new distribution of the cohort among the various health states.

Figure 7.12 shows the distribution of the cohort after four cycles. The simulation is terminated when the entire cohort is in the dead health state (also called an *absorbing state*).

Calculation of a Markov process yields the average amount of time spent in each health state. If the only attribute of interest is duration of survival, then average amounts of time spent in individual states are added together to set the expected survival. If both attributes of quality of life and length of life are used, then the quality-adjusted time spent in each health state is added up to arrive at an expected quality-adjusted survival time. The units in Figure 7.12 would therefore be 4.33 QALYs. The advantages of a cohort simulation are that it is a relatively fast method of evaluation and relatively transparent.[15–17] For example, one could simulate a cohort of sexually active U.S. adolescents and run the model until everyone in the cohort is dead. It would be relatively simple to look at the 5-year, 10-year, and 15-year cumulative incidence rates of chlamydial infection in a model like this. The main disadvantage of a cohort simulation is that it requires each health state definition to describe all relevant current and past clinical information.

Monte Carlo Simulation
In a first-order Monte Carlo simulation randomly selects a patient from the hypothetical cohort and each person transitions through the model one at a time.[15–18] The characteristics (age, sex, risk factors) of each person are randomly drawn from distributions derived from the data. Using simulation, the model tracks patients individually, one after the other, from entry into the model until death. By examin-

Cycle	Well	Disease	Dead	Cycle Utility	Cumulative Utility
0	1 0	0		0	0
1	0.75	0.2	0.05	0.85	0.85
2	0.5625	0.29	0.1475	0.7075	1.5575
3	0.4219	0.3155	0.2626	0.5796	2.1371
4	0.3164	0.3052	0.3784	0.4690	2.6061
N	0	0	1	0	4.3333

A cohort simulation produces a Markov trace which shows the movement of a cohort through the health states and the cumulative utilities and costs assigned. This table illustrates the Markov trace for the first 4 cycles.

Figure 7.12   Cohort simulation using a Markov model.

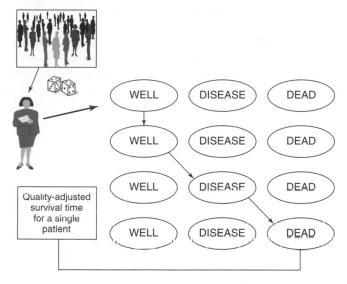

Figure 7.13   Generation of quality-adjusted survival using Monte Carlo simulation.

ing the clinical course of a disease, one person at a time, the model can generate a quality-adjusted survival time for that individual (Fig. 7.13). By running large numbers of simulated cases (e.g., 1,000,000), a distribution of survival values is obtained. The mean value of this distribution will approximate the expected utility (quality-adjusted life expectancy) or expected value (life expectancy) of a cohort simulation. The advantage of a Monte Carlo simulation is that since each individual's prior history is traced specifically for that individual as he or she transitions through a model, it requires only that health states describe the current clinical situation. The disadvantages of this type of simulation are that it takes much longer to run the model and examining the cohort at certain intervals over time is not as transparent as in a cohort simulation.[16]

Evaluate Uncertainty

Parameter uncertainty and sensitivity analyses were addressed earlier in the chapter. Probabilistic sensitivity analysis can be performed for a state-transition model using a decision tree or a Markov model using a second-order Monte Carlo simulation.[16, 28]

ADVANTAGES OF STATE-TRANSITION MODELS

Evaluating prevention effectiveness for many interventions is difficult. Consider cervical cancer screening. The optimal cervical cancer screening policy for a particular target population mandates consideration of different screening tests, alternative reactions to abnormal results, and alternative treatment options for precancerous lesions. In addition, evaluating program effectiveness requires specification of the underlying natural history of disease, an understanding of the heterogeneity of risk in the target population, information on the performance and effectiveness of screening and treatment, and accessibility, compliance, and feasibility in the target population of interest. No clinical trial or single longitudinal cohort study will be able to consider all of these components and assess all possible strategies for all possible populations. Mathematical models can be a useful way to evaluate alternative strategies by extending the knowledge from empirical studies to other screening situations. They can also extrapolate costs and health effects beyond the time horizon of a single clinical study. These models can also provide quantitative insight into the relative importance of different components of the screening process and investigate how cost–effectiveness ratios will change if values of key parameters are changed. Accordingly, they can also be used to help prioritize and guide data collection.

OTHER MODELS

It is beyond the scope of this chapter to comprehensively review all types of models, but there are other models that may be used to structure a decision problem over time. For example, Markov models analyzed as a cohort simulation cannot incorporate infectious disease transmission dynamics. Therefore, one could not use such a model to assess the impact of HIV antiretroviral treatment in Africa on the transmission of disease. To capture this potential benefit, one might use an epidemic model. In an epidemic model, difference equations are used, in which the numbers of susceptible, immune, and infected persons in a population are modified in each time period according to an equation that relates the change in the number of persons in each category to the number of persons in each category in the preceding time period as well as to variables that may be modified by intervention, such as contact rates and infectivity rates.[29-31]

SUMMARY

Decision analysis can be used in public health to help decide what should be done in a particular set of circumstances so that our decisions will be consistent with our understanding of the decision problem, our assessment of the uncertainties, and our estimates of the valued outcomes. Decision analysis is used in public health to assist policy makers in thinking systematically about complex problems and to improve the economic efficiency in the allocation of scarce resources.

REFERENCES

1. Gold MR, Siegel JE, Russell LB, Weinstein MC, eds. *Cost–Effectiveness in Health and Medicine.* New York: Oxford University Press, 1996.
2. Drummond MF, O'Brien B, Stoddart GL, Torrance GW, eds. *Methods for the Economic Evaluation of Health Care Programs.* New York: Oxford University Press, 1997.
3. Bell DE, Raiffa H, Tversky A. *Decision Making: Descriptive, Normative, and Prescriptive Interactions.* New York: Cambridge University Press, 1988.
4. Raiffa H. *Decision Analysis.* Reading, MA: Addison-Wesley, 1968.
5. Raiffa H. *The Art and Science of Negotiation.* Cambridge, MA: Belknap, 1982.
6. French S. *Decision Theory: An Introduction to the Mathematics of Rationality.* London: John Wiley and Sons, 1986.
7. von Neumann J, Morgenstern O. *Theory of Games and Economic Behavior.* Princeton: Princeton University Press, 1947.
8. Howard RA, Matheson J, eds. *The Principles and Applications of Decision Analysis.* Palo Alto, CA: Strategic Decisions Group, 1983.
9. Kahneman D, Slovic P, Tversky A. *Judgment Under Uncertainty: Heuristics and Biases.* New York: Cambridge University Press, 1982.
10. Weinstein MC, Fineberg HV, eds. *Clinical Decision Analysis.* Philadelphia: Saunders, 1982.
11. Keeney RL. *Decisions with Multiple Objectives: Preferences and Value Trade-Offs.* New York: John Wiley and Sons, 1976.
12. Keeney RL. *Value-Focused Thinking.* Cambridge, MA: Harvard University Press, 1992.
13. Clemen RT, Reilly T. Making Hard Decisions. Pacific Grove, CA: Duxbury, 2001.
14. Halpern MT, Luce BR, Brown RE, Geneste B. Health and economic outcomes modeling practices: a suggested framework. *Value Health 1998,* 1.131 47.
15. Sonnenberg FA, Beck JR. Markov models in medical decision making: a practical guide. *Med Decis Making 1993;* 13:322–38.
16. Kuntz KM, Weinstein MC. Modelling in Economic Evaluation In: Drummond M. McGuire A, ed. *Economic Evaluation and Health Care Merging Theory and Practice.* New York: Oxford University Press, 2002: 141–171.
17. Tom E, Schulman KA. Mathematical models in decision analysis. *Infect Control Hosp Epidemiol 1997;* 18:65–73.
18. Sox HC, Blatt MA, Higgins MC, Marton KI. *Medical Decision Making.* Stoneham, MA: Butterworth-Heinemann, 1988.
19. Seeff LB. Natural history of hepatitis C. *Hepatology 1997;* 26:21S–8S.
20. Torrance GW. Measurement of health state utilities for economic appraisal: a review. *J Health Econ 1986;* 5:1–30.
21. Torrance GW, Feeny D. Utilities and quality-adjusted life years. *Int J Technol Assess Health Care 1989;* 5:559–75.
22. Goldie SJ, Kuhn LK, Denny L, et al. Cost–effectiveness of alternative screening strategies to decrease cervical cancer mortality in low resource settings. *JAMA 2001;* 285:3107–15.
23. Weinstein MC. Methodologic issues in policy modeling for cardiovascular disease. *J Am Coll Cardiol 1989;* 14:38A–43A.
24. Freedberg KF, Losina E, Weinstein MC, et al. The cost–effectiveness of combination antiretroviral therapy for HIV disease. *N Engl J Med 2001;* 344:824–31.
25. Frazier AL, Colditz GA, Fuchs CS, Kuntz KM. Cost–effectiveness of screening for colorectal cancer in the general population. *JAMA 2000;* 284:1954–61.

26. Weinstein M, Stason W. Foundations of cost–effectiveness analysis for health and medical practices. *N Engl J Med 1977;* 296:716–21.
27. Beck JR, Pauker SG. The Markov process in medical prognosis. *Med Decis Making 1983;* 3:419–58.
28. Doubilet P, Begg BC, Weinstein MC, et al. Probabilistic sensitivity analysis using Monte Carlo simulation: a practical approach. *Med Decis Making 1985;* 5:157–77.
29. Anderson RM, Garnett GP. Mathematical models of the transmission and control of sexually transmitted diseases. *Sex Trans Dis 2000;* 27:636–43.
30. Stover J. Influence of mathematical modeling of HIV and AIDS on policies and programs in the developing world. *Dex Transm Dis 2000;* 27:572–77.
31. Kaplan EH, Brandeau ML, eds. *Modelling the AIDS Epidemic: Planning, Policy and Prediction.* New York: Raven, 1994.

8

Cost–Benefit Analysis

MARK MESSONNIER
MARTIN MELTZER

Cost–benefit analysis (CBA) is considered the preeminent method of economic evaluation because it allows for the direct comparison of different types of outcomes resulting from a variety of actions. If done correctly, it provides the most comprehensive monetary measures of the positive (beneficial) and negative (costly) consequences of a possible course of action, such as recommending the routine vaccination of restaurant employees against hepatitis A.[1] With CBA, one can compare two or more different public health strategies, such as using whole- cell pertussis vaccine versus acellular vaccine for routine childhood immunizations.[2] It can also be used to compare health-related interventions to those in the nonhealth sector. For example, assume that policy makers have to choose between funding a vaccination program for the elderly or a preschool enrichment program. A CBA would provide the policy makers with an understanding of the economic consequences of enacting each program (i.e., the returns on investing societal resources). The program with the best economic return would be the logical option to receive funding. The CBA is widely used to answer questions of this type in public and private decision-making settings and has a long history in the study of environmental effects and natural resource use in the United States.

COST–BENEFIT ANALYSIS DEFINED

Cost–benefit analysis has its theoretical roots in the subdiscipline of economics called welfare economics. *Welfare economics* is the study of the changes in the well-being, or welfare, of both individuals and society. Changes in welfare occur when decisions are made regarding the allocation of resources to produce, distribute, and consume goods and services of all kinds. As this subdiscipline has evolved, theories have been developed to address more than just the arithmetic calculation of the monetary value of costs and benefits. Issues of equity and justice can be addressed as well. That is, a CBA has the potential of identifying who gains and who pays as well as the amount of gain or loss.

In a CBA, all costs and benefits associated with a program are measured in monetary terms and then combined into a summary measure. Examples of such measures are the net present value (NPV) and the benefit–cost ratio (BCR). The NPV is calculated by adding all of the dollar-valued benefits and then subtracting all of the dollar-valued costs, with discounting applied to both costs and benefits as appropriate (see Chapter 6).

The formula for calculating NPV is as follows:

$$NPV = \sum_{t=0}^{N} \frac{(benefits - costs)_t}{(1 + r)^t}$$

where

t = year (from 0 . . . N)
N = number of years being evaluated
r = discount rate

Whenever the benefits are greater than the total costs, a CBA will yield an NPV that is greater than \$0. This means that if the project being analyzed was to be initiated, there would be a net benefit to society.

For a BCR, the total benefits are divided by the total costs to provide a ratio.

The formula for calculating BCR is as follows:

$$\frac{PV_{benefits}}{PV_{costs}}$$

where

$PV_{benefits}$ = present value of benefits
PV_{costs} = present value of costs

For example, a CBA may produce a BCR of 1.10:1, which would commonly be interpreted by stating that for every \$1 invested (costs), society would gain (benefits) \$1.10. Again, when using BCR, both costs and benefits are discounted as appropriate. There are other summary measures, and some experts have argued that these alternatives are superior to others under certain decision-making contexts. Therefore, we will discuss these alternative measures in more detail later in the chapter. Calculation of PV is discussed in Chapter 6.

As a final note on the formal definition of CBA, when a CBA produces a positive NPV, or a BCR greater than 1, decision makers may consider it desirable to initiate the proposed intervention. That is, a positive NPV, or BCR greater than 1, is not an automatic or absolute mandate to invest resources. No matter how comprehensively done, a CBA can only produce data. Regardless of the result from a CBA, society and public health decision makers are never absolved from carefully considering all aspects related to a new project or the alteration of an existing program.

HISTORY OF COST–BENEFIT ANALYSIS IN HEALTH

The CBA was first proposed as a technique to assist public policy decision making in 1844 in the essay "On the Measurement of the Utility of Public Works," by Jules Dupuit.[3] In the United States, the use of CBA as a tool for decision making began when Congress passed the United States Flood Control Act of 1936. The act stated that benefits, "to whomsoever they may accrue," generated by federally funded projects must exceed the costs. The first guidelines for conducting CBAs were issued in 1950 by the Subcommittee on Benefits and Costs of the Federal Inter-Agency River Basin Committee in *Proposed Practices for Economic Analysis of River Basin Projects*, the so-called Green Book.[4] Ever since, CBA has been widely used as a policy tool by the federal government, particularly in the funding of public works projects and environmental regulations.

Early efforts to quantify health benefits and the value of life in monetary terms date from the seventeenth century.[5] The application of CBA in the health arena began in earnest in 1966, when Dorothy Rice published her work on methods to estimate the cost of illness.[6] During the 1970s and early 1980s, applications of CBA for medical decision making appeared frequently in the literature.[7–11] Controversy over the valuation of health benefits, particularly the value of life, resulted in cost–effectiveness analysis (CEA) becoming the dominant analytic method for evaluating health care projects and health technologies. However, due to the inability of CEA to fully capture all of the benefits associated with improving health, interest in CBA has been renewed. Since the early 1990s, many researchers in the area of health-care economics have concentrated on refining CBA methodologies and providing worked examples.[12–15]

WHEN TO USE COST–BENEFIT ANALYSIS

Recall that a CBA measures changes in societal and individual welfare due to changes in the allocation of resources used to produce, distribute, and consume goods and services. Thus, CBA is the most appropriate form of analysis to use whenever a policy maker has a broad perspective and is concerned about the potential changes in welfare associated with a health-related project (i.e., who will pay, who will benefit and by how much). It is also an appropriate methodology when there is concern about economic efficiency. Assume, for example, that there is a defined health-related objective, such as eradicating an infectious disease. It would be logical for a policy maker to choose a program that uses the least resources to achieve the stated goal. Often, a CBA is done before a public health program is implemented, but the method can also be used to evaluate what existing programs have accomplished. Further, because CBA converts all costs and benefits into a common monetary metric, it is the best method to use when an intervention produces several very different outcomes. For example, a community-based lead-abatement program to reduce blood-lead levels in children may also increase local property values. The increased property values can readily be included in a CBA. It is not difficult to imagine situations where nonhealth benefits, such as increased property values, may be an important factor when policy makers and communities decide whether or not to implement a public health intervention.

In summary, it is best to use CBA when a policy maker has a broad perspective and is faced with one or more of the following situations: (*1*) must decide whether to implement a specific program, (*2*) required to choose among competing options, (*3*) has a set budget and must choose and set priorities from a group of potential projects, or (*4*) the interventions under consideration could produce a number of widely differing outcomes. For the first situation, if a CBA could be used to show that implementing a single program would result in a net gain in social welfare, then it may be judged acceptable to start the program (but, as discussed earlier, this is not an absolute mandate). If, as in the second situation, there are multiple options for achieving a desired outcome, then the project with the largest NPV (gain in welfare) is preferred. When allocating a fixed budget among a group of projects, a policy maker should choose the combination of projects that would result in the largest NPV.

COMPARING COST–BENEFIT ANALYSIS TO OTHER FORMS OF ECONOMIC ANALYSIS

In contrast to CBA, CEA and cost–utility analysis (CUA) produce summary measures in terms of cost per unit of health outcome, such as dollars per life saved or dollars per quality adjusted life year (QALY) saved (see Chapters 5 and 9 for further details). While such outcome measures may intuitively seem appropriate to a public health practitioner, policy makers must still decide if the cost per unit outcome is worthwhile. For example, how would a policy maker choose between an infant vaccination program that costs $2000 per life saved and an influenza vaccination program for middle-aged persons that costs $1500 per life saved? If the summary measure used were dollars per QALY saved, the policy maker would still face the decision of whether a QALY saved among 50-year-olds is equal to a QALY saved among 5-year-olds (i.e., are all QALYs saved equal?). Even if the policy maker is not comparing potential programs, there is the issue of deciding what are "acceptable costs" per unit outcome and what is too expensive. That is, what is the maximum, or threshold, cost per life or cost per QALY saved that society should accept? A summary measure, such as NPV or BCR, avoids such questions because a CBA includes all costs and benefits (within practical limitations) of an intervention program in monetary terms. That is, the value of a life saved, or quality adjustment to a life, is included in a CBA. Consequently, CBA answers one question that CEA and CUA cannot: "Will this program generate net savings?"

Another important difference between CBA, CEA, and CUA is that, although all three methods allow comparison among various health-program options, CBA is the only method that allows comparison of a health program with a nonhealth program (recall the hypothetical example of a vaccination program versus pre-school enrichment classes). Further, unlike CEA and CUA, CBA can readily combine both health and nonhealth outcomes that may be associated with a single program. The need to value a wide variety of outcomes was illustrated in the lead-abatement program example, which produced both health benefits and increased property values.

WHAT ARE COSTS AND BENEFITS?

When we measure costs and benefits, we are actually measuring economic concepts that aid us in understanding the consequences of decisions made regarding the use of limited resources (and there is some limit on every resource). What, for example, are the consequences of a policy maker deciding to fund a children's vaccination program instead of one targeting middle-aged adults? Various methods of classifying and measuring costs were presented in Chapter 4. Now, we will consider the economic principles and methods needed to measure and classify benefits.

Classifying an item as either a cost or a benefit may seem like a simple task, but it can depend on a number of factors. The case of lead-paint pollution presents an example of how classification of inputs and outcomes can impact the final result of a CBA. Assume that a proposed program to eliminate lead based paint in a public housing project is to be analyzed using a CBA. Some of the inputs, outcomes, and their assigned values are listed below (Table 8.1). The values represent an evaluation of the program relative to a "no program" alternative and were determined after appropriate discounting (discussed in Chapter 6).

From the above data, we can calculate the following total benefits and costs:

Total Benefits = $9,000,000 + $13,000,000 = $22,000,000
Total Costs = $11,000,000 + $4,000,000 + $6,000,000 = $21,000,000

We see that benefits are greater than total costs by $1,000,000. This suggests that a policy maker, taking the societal perspective, would consider the project acceptable and may recommend its implementation. That is, the policy maker may recom-

Table 8.1 Classification of Costs and Benefits Associated with a Lead-Removal Program in Rental Housing

Item	Dollar Value	Cost	Benefit
Removal of old paint	$11,000,000	Yes	
Temporary housing for residents	$4,000,000	Yes	
New paint (materials and labor)	$6,000,000	Yes	
Property value increase	$9,000,000		Yes
Learning disabilities averted	$13,000,000		Yes

mend that public funds (i.e., tax revenues) be used to pay for the rehabilitation of the houses.

Direct, Indirect and Intangible Benefits

Just as there are direct and indirect costs (discussed in Chapter 4), there are also direct and indirect benefits. In the lead-paint removal example, the increase in housing values would be considered a direct, tangible benefit of the paint-removal program. A dollar value of this benefit can be easily obtained by examining sales of similar property. That is, the benefit can be valued using market-based data. The learning disabilities that can be averted by the program represent indirect benefits.

In addition to the direct and indirect benefits, there may be other benefits. Have you ever said, on a hot summer afternoon, "I'd pay 10 dollars for a cold glass of water?" If so, then you have voiced an example of an important economic concept, *consumer surplus*. The difference between the value placed on a good or service (the price the person is willing to pay) and the price that must actually be paid (say $1 for a bottle of water) represents the consumer surplus for the water. When conducting a CBA, economists are interested in determining both the financial value (the $1 per bottle) and the consumer surplus associated with an output. Sometimes the consumer surplus can be notably larger than the face value, or financial cost, of producing an output; and it is also easy to imagine situations where *intangible benefits* (consumer surplus) could be the most important outcome from implementing a public health program. We did not discuss intangible benefits in the lead-paint example, but parents may value peace of mind knowing that the program would reduce health-related risks faced by their children. This reduction in anxiety is an example of an intangible benefit that could have been estimated and included in the CBA of the program.

STEPS IN CONDUCTING A COST–BENEFIT ANALYSIS

We have now discussed the following important concepts related to CBA: when to use CBA, NPV, and BCR; perspective; classification of costs and benefits; and three types of cost and benefit (direct, indirect, and intangible). We will now discuss how to apply these concepts when conducting a CBA, using the following basic steps:

1. Define the problem in terms of question, audience, perspective, time frame, analytic horizon, and discount rate.
2. Identify the prevention interventions to be evaluated.
3. Identify the effects of the interventions for all health and nonhealth outcomes and classify them as either benefits or costs.
4. Assign values (usually dollars) to the prevention interventions and their outcomes.
5. Determine and calculate the summary measure to be used.
6. Evaluate the results with sensitivity analysis.
7. Prepare the results for presentation.

Define *the Problem*

Chapter 2 discussed the importance of defining the problem. Several items in the list of key points presented there are decided at this step. The study question must be clearly stated. The audience, perspective, time frame, analytic horizon, and even the discount rate should be specified at this step. The identity of the primary audience can dictate the answers to some of these questions.

Consider the simple example of the lead-paint removal program (Table 8.1). From the perspective of society, benefits were evaluated to be greater than costs. A different audience or perspective, however, can cause an analyst to reclassify some of the items. Suppose that the public health officer in charge of environmental health proposes that, to reduce public expenditures, a private property developer should be encouraged to purchase the property and (as a condition of the sale) take on the task of removing the lead-paint. Thus, the purchase of the property and potential increase in property value would be part of the incentive for the developer to invest in the lead-paint removal. The question then becomes: "What are the costs and benefits from the perspective of the developer?" From the developer's perspective, it is easy to classify the removal of old paint, temporary housing of existing residents, and new paint as costs associated with the project (i.e., the classification of these items remains the same as for the societal perspective). However, consider that, while an increase in property value would be an obvious benefit, it could also result in a potential cost due to higher property taxes. Much would depend on whether or not the developer could pass on the increased property taxes to the tenants. Further, note that the developer will not gain from the benefits labeled "learning disabilities averted" and, thus, would value such benefits as $0. Therefore, from the developer's perspective the costs and benefits from the project would be as follows:

Total Benefits = $9,000,000 + rents
Total Costs = $11,000,000 + $4,000,000 + $6,000,000 = $21,000,000 + *cost*
of purchase + potential costs associated with increased
property taxes

Thus, costs exceed benefits by at least $11,000,000. The developer, to recoup the investment in purchasing and rehabilitating the property, must obtain at least $11,000,000 from rents. Rents may have to be raised to cover the costs associated with the rehabilitation. Increased rents would, of course, make the rehabilitated housing that much less affordable to people with low or fixed incomes. This potential net impact may be the exact opposite of what policy makers want to see as an outcome of the project, i.e., safe, affordable housing for the existing tenants.

The time frame, analytic horizon, and discount rate are not just abstract choices dictated by mathematics. The values chosen for these variables are often dictated by practical, political, and regulatory considerations. A study conducted from a private business perspective, for example, will probably use a higher discount rate than a study conducted from a societal perspective. For example, when evaluating vaccinating restaurant workers against hepatitis A, a CBA conducted from a restaurant owner's perspective may use an annual discount rate of 7%–10%.[1] This is notably higher than the rate of 3%–5% typically used when a societal perspective is taken. The higher rate reflects factors facing the restaurant owner such as the cost of commercial financing and rates of return available from other market-based investment options. Even when comparing studies that consider only a societal perspective, readers may find a difference in the values used for the discount rate. This is because some federal agencies are required by law to use a higher discount rate than recommended in this book, even when human health issues are at stake.

Identify the Interventions to be Evaluated

The choice of intervention(s) to be analyzed is often specified by someone other than the analyst performing the CBA. The analyst's first step, therefore, is to determine the scope of the analysis, which can be done by answering the following questions:

1. What is the general problem?
2. What specific questions need to be answered by the CBA?
3. What are the intervention options? Even if there is no stated alternative to the intervention being considered, a CBA should compare the proposed project with the *status quo*.
4. What differences among the options may affect comparability?
5. Is CBA the appropriate technique to answer the specific questions?

The last question is not always answered or even asked. In addition to the answers provided earlier in the chapter (see When to Use Cost–Benefit Analysis), the following points may help an analyst decide if CBA is the appropriate technique. The size of the project can determine the need for a CBA. Some government agencies, for example, are mandated to conduct a CBA if the project is expected to have an economic impact exceeding a legally set threshold value. The number and degree of uncertainties in terms of outcomes may prevent an analyst from conducting a rigorous CBA. The analyst must also consider the reaction of an audience to the monetary valuations of the inputs and outcomes.

Identify the Outcomes of the Interventions

When taking a societal perspective in a CBA, it is important to identify all potential outcomes. This includes all types of cost and benefit: direct, indirect, and intangible. However, is it realistic or even desirable to include all possible outcomes? If not, how inclusive should the analyst be in the effort? Any prevention activity can have far-reaching, multiple impacts and the analyst will have to decide at what point to "draw the line" in trying to capture the full range of health and nonhealth outcomes. Accounting for all of the ripple effects caused by an intervention can be both extremely difficult and costly to measure. Further, many of the potential impacts not directly associated with the program may in fact be rather small, and their existence may not really be an important factor in the decision-making process.

It is also true that some proponents or opponents of an intervention may place particular emphasis on an outcome that others may consider residual or "minor." In such a situation, an analyst may wish to include a minor outcome specifically to demonstrate its relative importance. For example, the authors of a CBA examining interventions to combat the next influenza pandemic specifically included the cost of treating the vaccine-related side effect Guillain-Barré syndrome, which is very rare. The resultant net increase in vaccination costs due to the syndrome was less than $0.20 per person vaccinated.[16] The syndrome, however, has been negatively associated in the past with influenza pandemic vaccination and prevention programs. Therefore, failure to specifically include the syndrome as a cost associated with vaccination may cause some to think that public health officials are deliberately undervaluing the true costs of the proposed interventions.

In summary, unless there is some compelling reason to do otherwise, it is generally advisable to include only those outcomes that can readily be associated with the program. [17, 18]

Outcomes versus Direct, Indirect, and Intangible Costs and Benefits

Although we have already classified costs and benefits in terms of being direct, indirect, or intangible, many public health analysts and audiences readily classify the impact of an intervention in terms of health, nonhealth, and intangible outcomes. This reclassification does not impose any real problems to an analyst, and using terms such as *health outcome* may make it easier for the intended audience to understand the results of a CBA. The analyst must remember, however, that terms such as *health outcome* can include direct and indirect costs and benefits. An example of a direct cost that may be classified as a health outcome would be that of treating clinical side effects such as the headaches and sore arms following vaccination. Vaccination campaigns, of course, have a number of health-related benefits, including the potential generation of "herd immunity" or an "umbrella" effect. The savings associated with having to treat fewer unvaccinated persons due to this herd immunity is an example of a health outcome that could be considered an indirect benefit, while the savings associated with not having to treat those actually vaccinated would be classified as a direct benefit. Both benefits are positive health outcomes.

Health Outcomes

Even when a decision has been made to restrict a CBA only to those inputs and outcomes directly associated with an intervention, identification of the "correct" outcome may not be straightforward. For example, when considering the benefits of a program to alleviate the impact of arthritis, rather than attempting to value additional life years saved, it would probably be more appropriate to place a monetary value on the reduced pain and suffering. Conducting CBAs on diagnostic technologies is another example of the challenge of identifying the appropriate outcome to use in a CBA. For diagnostic tests, the available epidemiological and clinical data describing the effectiveness of the test often report an intermediate outcome, such as the number of cases correctly identified (and sometimes the number misdiagnosed). Factors such as a long time lag between identification and improved health outcomes make it very difficult to value the impact of a diagnostic test on the incidence, prevalence, and pattern of disease. The analyst would have to work very closely with clinicians and epidemiologists to choose the most appropriate outcome and may choose more than one. The health-related outcomes that may be appropriate in a CBA include the following:

1. Increased life expectancy
2. Decreased morbidity
3. Reduced disability
4. Improved quality of life
5. Averted medical costs
6. Increased worker productivity

Nonhealth Outcomes

Often, public health programs produce benefits other than improved health. Such nonhealth outcomes might include increases in property values, as in the lead-paint example, or reductions in time lost from work or community activities. The value of these outcomes should also be included in a CBA. When nonhealth outcomes are not fully captured in the analysis, a CBA will not accurately reflect the total economic value of the proposed public health intervention. If problems of valuation prevent important nonhealth outcomes (both costs and benefits) from being included in the monetary calculations, they should be highlighted in the presentation and discussion of the results. As discussed earlier, different audiences may have different definitions of the term *important nonhealth outcomes*.

Intangible Outcomes

Recall the earlier statement that intangible outcomes, such as a reduction in pain and suffering, may be seen as an important reason to start an intervention. Thus, it is logical to include the value of such intangible outcomes in a CBA. Analysts, however, face the practical problem that some intangible outcomes cannot be valued easily. Economists have devised and tried several different methods of valuing intangibles, and some of these methods are discussed below. Again, as in the case of indirect outcomes, if a value cannot be placed on some intangible outcomes, they should at least be listed and included in the discussion of the results.

Assign Values to Interventions and Outcomes

Valuation of Intervention Costs and Benefits
After the outcomes of the program are identified and quantified in their natural units (e.g., clinical cases averted), dollar amounts must be assigned to each outcome and input. Comprehensive CBAs include values for: (*1*) the cost of conducting the intervention program, (*2*) any side effects associated with the intervention,

(3) the illness or injury prevented, (4) nonhealth outcomes, and (5) intangible outcomes. For a complete discussion of determining the costs of the intervention, see Chapter 4. Further, any benefits or costs that occur after the first year of a program must be adjusted by discounting (see Chapter 6).

A common pitfall encountered when listing different costs and benefits is double counting. Much of the criticism of early CBAs was that some analysts counted benefits more than once, usually in an effort to account for all possible outcomes of a project.[17] Benefits and costs should be counted only once. For example, to calculate the cost of a participant's time in a clinical drug trial, it is tempting to include both the participant's lost wages and the participation fee paid to the volunteer. Using both measures would be considered double counting, and only one of the two measures should be used. Since the volunteer is willing to participate for the participation fee, this might be considered one estimate of the value of volunteer time (the fee may also include an inducement to overcome the discomfort of undergoing a procedure or the risk associated with participation in the study). If lost wages were selected as the means for valuing the participant's time, an analyst may decide not to use the total wages lost. This is because most people do not expect to receive their full wages while engaged in volunteer activities.

Valuation of Health Outcomes

Many health outcomes of a clinical nature, such as the medical care costs avoided due to the use of bicycle helmets, can often be valued using much the same techniques described in the chapter on cost analysis (Chapter 4). Problems arise when there are direct and indirect health outcomes for which there are no readily available methods for obtaining a value. For example, what is the value of the reduction in swelling and sore joints associated with an arthritis treatment program (an example of a direct health benefit)? The program might reduce the number of doctor visits, which could be valued using existing standard costing techniques; but how do we value the reduced pain, which surely some would regard as a direct health outcome? Suppose that an influenza-vaccination program among retirees notably reduces the number of sick days in bed. How would we value the extra time that vaccinated retirees will have available to volunteer for community based projects (an example of a nonhealth outcome)?

Some of the methods available to value nonmarketed outcomes include the following:

1. Expert opinion: a consensus of experts can be used to obtain the best estimate of value.
2. Past policy decisions: estimates from previous legislative or regulatory decisions may imply a certain baseline value.
3. Court awards and regulatory fines: these may seem a logical source of data for valuing some outcomes, particularly intangibles such as pain and suffering.
4. Cost-of-illness (COI) approach: a method for determining the economic cost of disease by summing the direct and indirect costs of the disease-related morbidity or premature mortality (see Chapter 4 for more details).
5. Contingent valuation method (CVM): a method for determining how much

people are willing to pay to obtain an intervention or avoid contracting a disease; it can also be used to obtain a value of what people would have to be paid in order to give up an existing intervention or the promise of such an intervention.

A disadvantage of the first three approaches is that it is difficult to validate the estimates. Two other problems with using regulatory fines and court awards to value nonmarketed outcomes is that such data are often not readily available and when they are available, they may not be representative. For example, many law-suits are settled out of court, and the terms of settlement may prohibit either party from publicly disclosing the amount. Perhaps the most serious problem with the first three methods is that all are indirect methods of valuation and, thus, violate the economic tenet that consumers are the best judges of the value of outcomes. Although the COI approach can be validated, it usually limits the value of life to an individual's potential to produce and earn a wage. As can be readily appreci-ated, this may notably underestimate the total value of the nonhealth outcomes as-sociated with an intervention (see Chapter 4).

Contingent Valuation Method

The CVM was developed by economists in direct response to the problems of ob-taining reliable estimates of the value of outcomes that are not routinely traded in any easily observed market place. Much of the initial development of CVM was done by natural resource economists, who needed to value outcomes such as clear, nonsmoggy skies above the Grand Canyon or keeping a remote lake free from pol-lution by acid rain. Analysts have reasoned that, in concept, there is a great deal of similarity between the type of natural resource outcome valued by resource econo-mists and the intangible health outcomes that must be evaluated in a health-intervention CBA. There is a growing body of literature that uses CVM to value intangible and other nonmarketed health outcomes associated with medical inter-ventions (both clinical medicine and prevention).

The CVM estimates the value individuals place on intangible health outcomes by directly asking them to value a hypothetical, or a contingent, change in the risk of death, injury, or illness due to disease or accident. For example, suppose a per-son living in a New England state faces an average annual risk of 1 in 200 of con-tracting Lyme disease. Further, suppose there is a vaccine being developed that will reduce the risk of contracting Lyme disease to 1 in 1000. A researcher con-ducting a CBA on the vaccine could use the COI approach to valuing that reduc-tion in risk. The COI approach (as discussed above and in Chapter 4) can be used to estimate the medical costs associated with treating a case of Lyme disease as well as the time lost from work due to illness. However, the COI approach would en-tirely omit intangible outcomes associated with reducing the risk of Lyme disease, such as reducing the anxiety associated with going for a walk in a heavily wooded area or even working in a garden adjacent to a wooded area. (In areas where Lyme disease is prevalent, both activities represent some risk of contracting it).

To value this potentially important intangible outcome (reduced fear of con-tracting a disease), a researcher may use the CVM to conduct a survey, during which individuals would be asked if they were willing to pay, for example, $100 per year to reduce the risk of contracting Lyme disease from 1 in 200 to 1 in 1000. The hypothetical scenario described for the respondents should explain clearly that they would have to completely pay for the medical care and time lost from work (i.e., assume that there is no insurance or other party paying for the direct or indirect costs), either to obtain the vaccine or if they were to contract the disease. Also, the bid amount presented should be considered in excess of all other expenditures related to Lyme disease, including any risk-reduction activities they are already taking. These restrictions are put into place so that, to the extent possible, the consumer surplus associated with the vaccine is the only thing being measured.

It is most important to realize that some people may not place a positive value on the intervention. Someone placing a value exactly equal to zero may be indifferent to receiving the vaccine. Analysis of the supplemental questions answered in the survey (see Conducting a Contingent Valuation Survey, below) can shed light on whether a zero value reflects indifference. Other respondents may place a negative value on the intervention. This would imply that such persons answering the survey would essentially have to be paid to be vaccinated. There could be many reasons why a person would have a net negative valuation of using an intervention. In the case of a vaccine, the person answering the survey could have a fear of needles that is far greater than the fear of Lyme disease. Including negative values in the analysis can depend on the nature of the responses from the intervention. Receiving a vaccination for Lyme disease is voluntary, so the analyst may want to consider omitting those with such a fear of needles when calculating the mean willingness to pay. However, if vaccination were mandatory, as is the case for many other vaccines, the negative values should be included.

The CVM can also be used to value a quantity change in a health outcome. For example, an analyst could conduct a CVM survey to obtain valuations of an intervention that would reduce the discomfort associated with arthritis by 50%. The problem, however, is that each individual will have a different perception of the level of discomfort associated with arthritis before and after the intervention. The 50% reduction in discomfort will not really be a consistent measure of health outcome (i.e., 50% of what?). As a practical matter, it is far easier to conduct a CVM survey in which the risk of a health outcome is altered due to an intervention, such as in the Lyme disease vaccine example.

Studies that use the CVM to estimate the value of a change in risk are commonly called *willingness to pay* (WTP) studies, which is probably the reason the CVM is called the WTP method in much of the health economics literature. However, the term *willingness-to-pay* is not a technically correct description of the CVM; it is just one way of estimating the economic concept of consumer surplus and should never be confused with a marketing survey, such as asking people if they would pay $5 for a bottle of aspirin or shampoo. In that type of survey, the researcher is not seeking an estimate of the intangible value of the product but typically attempts to determine the price that would maximize gross sales (price × volume). In a CVM WTP survey, a researcher is not interested in maximizing gross sales but in determining consumer surplus and total valuation of all benefits (direct, indirect, and intangible). Unfortunately, perhaps because CVM is still relatively new to health and public health economics, it is not uncommon to find published WTP surveys that really are marketing surveys.

In fact, WTP is not always the appropriate concept to be valued. Sometimes, willingness to accept (WTA) is the theoretically and ethically appropriate welfare measure. For example, an analyst might conduct a WTA survey to determine the value of placing a nuclear waste storage site in a community. The community typically will not pay to have the facility sited near them but may accept it if the residents receive some form of compensation (e.g., for improved recreational facilities or school buildings). However, economists have identified conceptual problems with implementing WTA studies, and they are consequently seldom used.[19]

The CVM can also be used to assess the value of a statistical health outcome, such as a statistical life, by determining what society as a whole is willing to pay to reduce the risk of the adverse outcome an individual faces (e.g., death). The following example is taken from Fisher and colleagues:[15] "If each of 100,000 persons is willing to pay $20 for a reduction in risk from 3 deaths per 100,000 people to 1 death per 100,000 people, the total WTP is $2 million and the value per statistical life is $1 million (with 2 lives saved)." Here, we see that the individual valuations are aggregated to find a society-level value.

Conducting a Contigent Valuation Survey

A thorough description of all of the possible methods of conducting a WTP (or WTA) survey is beyond the scope of this book. Readers interested in learning more of the technical and theoretical aspects of CVM are recommended to read Mitchell and Carson.[19] Most economists would consider a CVM survey "well done" if it contained most or all of the following elements: (*1*) a brief, introductory set of questions designed to obtain an understanding of the knowledge, attitudes, and beliefs of survey respondents regarding both the health outcome and the intervention. If a survey respondent either has had the outcome in question (e.g., Lyme disease) or knows of somebody who has had the outcome or condition, he or she may value an intervention differently from persons who have never experienced or seen first hand the effects of the disease. (*2*) a short scenario describing the risk of contracting the disease or condition (e.g., 1 in 200 risk of contracting Lyme disease), the impact of the disease (e.g., mentions Lyme disease–related arthritis), and the possibility that an intervention would reduce the risk of disease (e.g., Lyme disease vaccine). It would also be appropriate to briefly mention any notable side effects associated with the intervention. (*3*) a set of questions asking respondents whether they would pay a specified amount for a specified reduction in risk for a specified time period. For example, a survey respondent may be asked "Would you pay $100 per year for a vaccine which reduces your annual risk of contracting Lyme disease from 1 in 200 to 1 in 400?" (*4*) random variation in both the amount offered and the potential reduction in risk. In the Lyme disease vaccine example, some respondents may be asked if they would pay $150 for the same reduction in risk, while others may be asked if they would pay $75 for a reduction in risk from 1 in 200 to 1 in 600. (*5*) a set of questions determining the socioeconomic status of the respondent, typically including questions concerning age, gender, marital status, occupation, type of health insurance (including copayments and deductibles for medical care), level of education, and household or personal annual income. Any one of these variables could markedly impact a respondent's stated willingness to pay. Compared to a respondent with a low income, a respondent with a high income may be more ready to state that "Yes, I would be willing to pay $100 per year for a stated reduction in risk of a health outcome."

In item (3) in the list above, the respondent was offered a preset amount, or bid, for a preset reduction in risk ($100 for an annual reduction in risk from 1 in 200 to 1 in 400). Other surveys have used an "open bid" type of question, such as "How much would you pay for a reduction in risk from 1 in 200 to 1 in 400?" The debate to determine which method is best continues. Other economists have focused efforts on determining if the answers obtained during a CVM survey are genuine (i.e., some form of validation). One of the methods used is to ask a set of double-bounded questions. If respondents say "yes" to the first bid, they are then asked if they would pay a higher amount (e.g., if "yes" to $100, would they pay $125?). If they say "no" to the first bid offered, they are asked if they would pay a lower amount (e.g., if "no" to $100, would they pay $75?). Obviously, the amount of increase/decrease is an important factor, and it is common when the double-bounded method is used to adjust all initial bids by a set percentage, such as ± 25%.

The number of persons interviewed and the type of person interviewed are also vital elements in a well-done CVM survey. To ensure that the results of the survey are representative of a larger population, the researcher should employ standard statistical survey-design techniques. Standard texts on the statistical elements of survey design will provide the reader greater detail. In principle, the survey should be designed so that all potentially important subgroups, such as different levels and combinations of levels of education and income, are adequately sampled. Given the need to randomly ask, within each subgroup, a different combination of price and reduction-in-risk questions, an adequate sample size can be quite large. The question of sample size also relates to the question of how many combinations of reductions in risk and initial bid prices are needed (e.g., $50, $100, $150 for reductions from 1 in 200 to 1 in 400, 1 in 600, and 1 in 800 creates nine possible combinations that must be included in the survey). Unless the researcher accepts a marked reduction in the statistical power and accuracy of the survey, the more combinations of prices and risks, the larger the required sample size. Sample size considerations can make a properly conducted CVM survey comparatively costly.

Some Problems with the Contingent Valuation Method
The primary disadvantage of CVM is that estimates are derived on the basis of what people say rather than what they may actually do. Just because people state that they are willing to pay $100 per year for a vaccine to notably reduce the risk of contracting Lyme disease does not mean that, if presented with the opportunity, they will actually pay. That is, how reliable are the results? This potential problem is obvious to most who read the results of such surveys, including those who may consider using the results as part of a policy-making process. Part of this problem stems from the fact that many individuals have health insurance and, thus, do not pay the full direct and indirect medical costs of their illnesses. Individuals with health insurance may also overuse (a form of undervaluation) medical services because they pay only a fraction of the actual costs (economists call this problem

"moral hazard"). Further, individuals who have fully paid sick days as part of their work-related benefits package do not pay all of the indirect costs associated with an illness. The net result is that individuals with health insurance and paid sick days may overemphasize the value of the intangible outcomes associated with a disease.

The fact that a well-done CVM survey often requires a complex questionnaire and a complex survey design means that analyses of the data are often not simple or direct. Simple mean values of the stated WTP would not account for the influence of factors such as age, income, and education. Data collected in a CVM survey often have to be analyzed using rather sophisticated statistical techniques, such as multivariable regression techniques. These complexities mean that CVM surveys often cannot be planned, executed, and analyzed quickly. Furthermore, the degree of complexity requires that the research team conducting the survey be specialists trained in this area. The potential complexity of CVM surveys is one possible reason that some published studies do not adequately measure consumer surplus.

Once regression techniques have been used to estimate a weighted mean or median WTP (weighted by influence factors such as age and income) for individuals, that mean or median value can be multiplied by the population to obtain a societal-estimate of the WTP for the intervention. Some economists, however, have pointed out that the "well-being of society is not necessarily an aggregation of individual well-being."[20] Often, it is the distribution of the estimated individual values, rather than a single or even an aggregated value, that provides the most important information for policy makers.

Another problem that impacts the reliability of the results of a CVM survey is that many individuals have a hard time readily understanding probabilities. While most can easily understand the difference between a 1-in-2 chance and a 1-in-10 chance, how many really understand the difference between a 1-in-100,000 and a 1-in-1 million chance? Probabilities of rare events, however, may be crucial in evaluating both the health outcome and the intervention. Recent research has shown that problems in understanding probabilities can be overcome, to a large extent, if respondents are given some examples of the relative rarity of various outcomes.[21] However, it takes time and additional resources to prepare and present such material, adding to the cost of correctly doing a CVM study. Yet another problem in determining the reliability of the results of a WTP study is that different individuals with different backgrounds and resources may value outcomes quite differently. Wealthy individuals, for example, may be willing to pay more than economically disadvantaged individuals, simply because they both are able to pay more and value money differently. As mentioned earlier, the impact of differences in income on average WTP can be controlled by including it as a factor in the regression analysis, but the analyst will still implicitly assume that money has the same value for everybody, though this may not be the case.

There is also the possibility of a price indifference/threshold effect. That is, as long as a respondent believes that the risk of disease exists and the intervention can work and that the offered bid (e.g., $50 annually for a vaccine against Lyme disease) is below some threshold, he or she will tend to say "yes" without really evaluating the reasons. There are many potential reasons for the existence of such a threshold: health insurance (which tends to mask the true costs of medical care and prevention to an individual), the misunderstanding of the probabilities involved (perhaps undervaluing the cost of the intervention and overvaluing the cost of treatment), and the fact that a CVM survey addressing the concept of health addresses a potentially very emotional subject. Thus, it is difficult to value objectively when the bid amount seems small. The potential existence of a threshold can be empirically shown when the data for a WTP survey show almost no decline in the percentage of persons saying "yes" as the bid increases. Being insensitive to changes in price can readily be explained by the classic economic demand and supply theory. However, recall that a CVM study is not meant to measure price-related demand; it is meant to measure consumer surplus. If respondents are insensitive to a relatively large increase in the bid (say $10–$30) in a WTP survey, can analysts really feel confident that they have accurately measured the value of consumer surplus and intangible outcomes?

In general, for CBA, it is suggested that the CVM should be used only when adequate survey instruments can be developed, reliable and comparable estimates are not available in the literature, and the method is judged to be the best for capturing important nonmarket outcomes. An example of the latter is when a regulatory program to reduce food borne illnesses (e.g., improved compulsory meat inspection programs) could produce nonmarketed outcomes (e.g., consumer confidence in the food supply), which may be the main reason for implementing such a program.

Other Techniques for Valuing Nonmarketed Outcomes

Required Compensation. The required-compensation approach attempts to obtain value for interventions that reduce risk by measuring the difference in wages for persons in occupations associated with higher health risks than other occupations. For example, again from Fisher and colleagues:[15]

> Suppose jobs A and B are identical except that workers in job A have higher annual fatal injury risks such that, on average, there is one more job-related death per year for every 10,000 workers in job A than in job B, and workers in job A earn $500 more per year than those in job B. The implied value of a statistical life is then $5 million for workers in job B who are each willing to forgo $500 per year for a 1-in-10,000 lower annual risk.

Viscusi has published some well-known work using such methods.[22,23]

This approach, like every other, has drawbacks. Workers may not be aware of the actual risk associated with their jobs and, thus, may not be able to evaluate risk-based differences in wages. Further, if alternatives to a worker's current job do not exist, his or her wage may not reflect the true value of the risk associated with the job. Some workers may not be able, due to lack of training, or willing to switch jobs because of risk. This lack of mobility reduces employers' need to pay higher wages even if the occupation in question is relatively risky. Some would argue that most wage differences exist because of reasons other than risk. Consider how wages for computer programmers rose rapidly in the United States in the late 1990s because demand for their skills exceeded the supply of programmers. The increase in average wage had nothing to do with increased job-related health risks. Allowing for such nonhealth risk factors in an analysis of "pay for risk" can be very difficult. Finally, a person's wage is never the sum valuation of that person to either society or that person's family and friends. When was the last time you heard somebody admit that they were paid the full measure of what they were worth? Thus, while required compensation may be a good "first guess" of the value of a life, it may not be that accurate.

Consumer-Market Studies. The value of nonmarket inputs or outcomes can be calculated by studying the market for similar inputs or outcomes. This method is similar to required compensation and suffers from the same limitations.

Common Mistakes in Assessing and Valuing Benefits

Although there are limitations associated with all of the techniques presented above, the unsatisfactory alternative to using them is to not value outcomes (direct, indirect, and intangible) for which market-based prices are not readily available. Therefore, it is always a good idea when conducting a CBA to explicitly identify problems associated with valuation and how such problems may have impacted the calculated results.

In addition to excluding outcomes whose value cannot easily be determined, other common mistakes in valuing outcomes include the following:

1. Using dollar valuations of costs or benefits blindly without asking if the valuations are relevant or correct (e.g., using hospital charges to represent medical costs (see Chapter 4)
2. Failing to account for all costs and benefits relevant to the study
3. Making assumptions about the effectiveness of the intervention that are not supported by available data; when there is uncertainty regarding effectiveness, sensitivity analyses must be conducted
4. Including benefits or costs that are not linked to the intervention (i.e., costs and benefits that occur whether or not the intervention is implemented)
5. Double counting of costs and benefits
6. Extrapolating from a small, potentially biased sample to the whole population or from a nonrepresentative sample (similar to making unsupported assumptions)

Determine and Calculate the Summary Measure to be Used

As mentioned earlier, the two most commonly used summary measures are the BCR and the NPV.

Pros and Cons of Using The Benefit–Cost Ratio

The BCR appears to be a simple, easily explained summary measure for presenting the results from a CBA; there will be $X in benefits for every $1 in costs ($X can be either greater than, equal to, or smaller than $1). However, the actual BCR can depend on how costs and benefits are classified. Let us return to the lead-paint removal example, but add the assumption that there are now two methods available for removing the lead paint. Method A costs more than method B, but method A requires less new paint (method A leaves a smoother surface that is easier to paint). A decision maker will recommend funding an intervention using one paint-removal method (program A using method A or program B using method B). The program recommended for implementation will be the one giving the best BCR (i.e., the program with the largest dollar return per $1 of costs). Further, assume that the analyst conducting the CBA of the two programs classified the learning disabilities averted as a negative cost for program A. For program B, the analyst classified learning disabilities averted as a positive benefit. Table 8.2 presents the results of calculating the BCRs for the two programs. The values represent each program relative to a "no program" alternative. Assume that all values have been appropriately discounted over time.

The result appears straightforward: program A is the better choice as it gives the larger BCR. Although program A spends more on paint removal than program B, the savings in new paint appears to make up for those increased costs. However appealing such an explanation may seem, a second look at the data raises an important question. The paint removal in program A costs $1,000,000 more than in program B, yet the new paint in program A is only $500,000 cheaper than in program B. How did the analysis of program A produce a better BCR than that calculated for program B? The answer lies in the way that the benefit "learning disabilities averted" is classified. In the analysis of program A, it is listed as a negative cost, correctly implying a saving or benefit. This classification causes the totals for both costs and benefits for program A to be notably lower than the totals for program B. However, if the analyst had classified "learning disabilities averted" in program A as a benefit (as in program B), the resultant BCR for program A would be 1.07:1 (benefits of $22,000,000, costs of $20,500,000). This reclassification would make program B the preferred program.

This simple example highlights two problems with using BCR as the summary

Table 8.2 Two Proposed Programs to Eliminate Lead-Based Paint: Comparison of Costs, Benefits, and Benefit-Cost Ratios (BCRs)

| | Program Costs and Benefits ($) | | | |
| | Program A | | Program B | |
Item	Costs	Benefits	Costs	Benefits
Removal of old paint		11,000,000	10,000,000	
Temporary housing	4,000,000	4,000,000		
New paint	5,500,000	6,000,000		
Property value increase		9,000,000		9,000,000
Learning disabilities averted	−13,000,000			13,000,000
	7,500,000	9,000,000	20,000,000	22,000,000
BCR	1.2:1		1.1:1	

measure. First, it can be very sensitive to how items are classified. It is not hard to imagine an analyst classifying a saving (benefit) as a negative cost, especially when the intervention contains many inputs and outcomes or when several perspectives are evaluated simultaneously (see above, What Are Costs and Benefits?). The second problem with BCR is that it can be sensitive to size (i.e., the measure is scale-sensitive). The reason that program A has a higher BCR in Table 8.2 is that the totals for both the costs and the benefits are less than half of those calculated for program B. These two problems mean that BCR is not a very good summary measure to compare the results of CBAs from programs of very different sizes (i.e., costs).

For these and other reasons, some analysts consider BCR to be an inferior summary measure of a CBA. Under certain conditions, however, it can be very useful. It can be a very good summary measure when only one program is being considered relative to "no program." If the decision maker is primarily interested in determining if the intervention would have a BCR greater or less than 1:1, then he or she is not concerned about relative scale (i.e., how much larger or smaller). In such a situation, the decision maker is scale-insensitive and will not care if benefits are classified as negative costs (or costs are classified as negative benefits), as long as they are consistently classified in the same manner.

The Pros and Cons of Net Present Value
Using NPV as the summary measure of the results in Table 8.2 would "cure" any problem associated with how the "learning disabilities averted" item was classified. The NPVs (in values appropriately discounted) are as follows:

$$NPV_A = PV \text{ Benefits of } A - PV \text{ Costs of } A = \$9{,}000{,}000 - \$7{,}500{,}000 = \$1{,}500{,}000$$

$$NPV_B = PV \text{ Benefits of } B - PV \text{ Costs of } B = \$22{,}000{,}000 - \$20{,}000{,}000 = \$2{,}000{,}000$$

Assuming that the resources are available to do only one of the two projects, program B should be chosen since it would result in a higher NPV and, thus, a greater gain in social welfare. Also, the result does not depend on the treatment of the value of "learning disabilities averted" (i.e., should it be a negative cost or a positive benefit?) because NPV measures the absolute difference between benefits and costs. The fact that NPV presents the absolute difference between benefits and costs is one of the main reasons that many economists prefer to use NPV as the summary measure of a CBA.

Using NPV to allocate resources can pose problems because the final result (the absolute difference between discounted benefits and costs) provides no direct information about the resource requirements of a project. That is, if a policy maker were told only that the NPV of program B was $2,000,000 and that it was the largest NPV, he or she would have no idea that $20,000,000 worth of resources would be needed to implement the project. What if the policy maker did not have access to such resources? Thus, it is sometimes useful, when presenting an NPV, to also present the discounted benefits and costs. This additional information gives the audience some idea of the scale of the intervention being analyzed.

Other Summary Measures
Other decision criteria are useful in specific situations. Among them are the pay-back period and the internal rate of return. The *pay-back period* is the length of time (usually years in public health interventions) before the benefits equal the costs. For example, stating that a project has a pay-back period of 5 years would mean that for the first 5 years the costs would exceed the benefits, but after year 5 the cumulative benefits would be greater than the cumulative costs. Pay-back period has, however, a number of limitations that prevent it from being as useful a summary measure as NPV. One problem is that it is often not very useful to compare pay-back periods of two very different projects. For example, when considering a vaccination program focused on a local community, does the decision maker really need to know what the payback period is for national vaccination programs? Also, during the course of an intervention, because inputs may have to replenished (e.g., replacement equipment purchased), the cumulative costs may be greater than the cumulative benefits at several different points in time. A single pay-back period calculation can capture only one change, when the cumulative benefits exceed the cumulative costs.

The internal rate of return used to be a very common measure when financial projects were analyzed. The internal rate of return is obtained by altering the discount rate used to calculate the present value of future benefits such that the present value of the future benefits equals the value of the initial investment. If the internal rate of return is equal to or greater than the discount rate appropriate for the perspective of the CBA (e.g., the recommended societal discount rate when considering the societal perspective), then the analyst would state that the present value of the benefits at least equals the value of the resources invested in the intervention. When evaluating an individual project, the NPV and internal rate of return can often give the same accept–reject criterion. However, when evaluating different projects, NPV and internal rate of return can give different results when (*1*) one of the interventions being evaluated has a much larger initial cost than the others and (*2*) each project has a very different time line of costs and benefits. These and other reasons have led to the recommendation, found in many financial textbooks, that most projects should use the NPV method for evaluating investment of resources.[24] For additional information concerning the problems associated with internal rate of return and further discussions on alternative summary measures, the reader should consult standard textbooks on financial management and environmental and natural resource economics.[17,18,24,25]

Incremental Summary Measures
When a CBA of an intervention program(s) is compared to a "no intervention program" option, the summary measure is usually calculated as an average. For example, the NPV would be calculated as follows:

$$Average\ NPV = (PV\ Benefits_A - PV\ Benefits_0) - (PV\ Cost_A - PV\ Cost_0),$$

where *PV* is the present value, *A* is program A, and 0 represents no program.

There may be times, however, when an analyst wishes to know what would be the costs and benefits of either expanding an existing program, adopting a new intervention to replace an existing intervention, or comparing two programs, one of which will definitely be adopted. In such analyses, "no program" is not a realistic option. Thus, the relevant baseline situation is either the existing intervention or the intervention judged as possibly being the least effective. Incremental NPV is a frequently used summary measure of such incremental analyses and is calculated as follows:

$$Incremental\ NPV = (PV\ Benefits_\text{B} - PV\ Benefits_\text{A}) - (PV\ Cost_\text{B} - PV\ Cost_\text{A})$$

Most analysts either would have program B be the new program replacing program A or would assume that program B is more effective than program A.

Evaluate the Results with Sensitivity Analysis

Because most CBAs are based on a mixture of estimates and assumptions, it is absolutely essential that sensitivity analyses be a standard part of a CBA. One of the main goals of a sensitivity analysis of a CBA is to identify which variables exert the greatest influence on the results (i.e., which are the most important). For example, the choice of a discount rate may greatly affect an NPV calculation. When benefits accrue in the distant future, using a low discount rate may make a program appear more worthwhile than when a higher discount rate is used. If a relatively large change in the value of a variable does not change the conclusion, then analysts will state that the conclusion is "robust" to large changes in that variable. For example, in the examination of the economics of vaccinating restaurant workers against hepatitis A, from a restaurant owner's perspective it was found that vaccination was unlikely to result in a positive financial gain.[1] This conclusion was true even if the average cost of vaccinating an employee was just $20. The real-world cost for vaccinating an employee with the recommended two doses would most likely be more than $50 (direct and indirect costs). The authors of the study thus concluded that one of their results (that restaurant owners were unlikely to find routine immunization of their workers to result in a financial gain) was robust over a wide range of probable costs of vaccination.

The values of some variables found to be important in a CBA (i.e., small changes in their values greatly influence the final conclusion) may not be well defined or known. In such situations, an analyst should warn policy makers of the potential problems associated with the uncertainty of the final conclusion because of uncertainty about the value of a variable. At the same time, the analyst could also recommend that a top priority should be further research, designed specifically to obtain a more accurate measurement of the variable in question.

Also, for many CBAs, testing the sensitivity of the outcome by altering the values of one variable at a time (i.e., univariate sensitivity analysis) is often not very informative. This is because CBAs of public health interventions usually consist of mixtures of financial, economic, epidemiological, and even clinical data. The robustness of the overall outcome (i.e., the NPV) may depend more on how the variables interact rather than on the value of a single variable. The only way to dis-cover this fact and which variables interact with each other in a meaningful manner is to conduct multivariate sensitivity analyses. A more complete description of sensitivity analysis is provided in Chapter 7.

Common variables in health care that should be tested with sensitivity analyses are as follows:

1. Patient acceptance of, or compliance with, a program
2. Risk of disease or injury
3. Discount rate
4. Direct costs of the intervention
5. Other costs
6. Value of benefits

Threshold analysis, best- and worst-case-scenario analysis, and Monte Carlo simulations are also useful techniques to evaluate the impact of uncertainty on the conclusions (see Chapter 7).

Prepare the Results for Presentation

Because many analysts will make recommendations based on CBA, it is important to prepare results in a straightforward and useful form for decision makers. The presentation should include the following:

1. Clearly defined questions answered by the analysis
2. Perspective of the study (i.e., who pays and who benefits is clearly identified)
3. Description of the options considered in the analysis
4. Concise listing of the relevant outcomes considered for each option
5. Explanation of valuation of outcomes with particular attention to estimation of intangible costs, benefits, and the differences in timing of when benefits and costs are likely to occur
6. Discussion of the evaluation of results with sensitivity analysis

In essence, the presentation should contain most, if not all, of the elements of a CBA, which were listed earlier.

LIMITATIONS OF COST–BENEFIT ANALYSIS

Like any tool, CBA has limitations. Many health-care interventions, such as therapy for cancer, AIDS research, and treatments for chronic disabling diseases, often do not lend themselves readily to CBA because of difficulties in assessing the monetary value of changes in quality of health. Indeed, just measuring the change in quality of health may prove extremely difficult, and assigning a monetary value to human life will always prove challenging. Some intervention programs, such as programs to protect civil rights or to implement legally mandated requirements, are not designed to achieve results that can be readily expressed in monetary terms. For such programs, because so many variables may be excluded from the analysis, a positive NPV determined by CBA may be neither a necessary nor a sufficient criterion for implementing a program. However, using a CBA to evaluate a program in an emotionally and politically sensitive area can help to make the costs and outcomes explicit, thereby adding clarity to the discussion.

When conducted well and used appropriately, CBA can provide important information for decision making. However, CBA does not make decisions; rather, it is a tool to aid decision making. The use of CBA does not eliminate the need for judgment in public health decision making. Indeed, the use of CBA should force analysts, decision makers, and the public to closely examine the resources required for an intervention, the value of the health outcomes, and the decision-making process. A correctly done CBA will also help to clarify what is and is not known about an intervention and its potential outcomes. It should also highlight important aspects of an intervention that typically are not quantified in a CBA. For example, policy makers may wish to closely examine the distributional effects of an intervention, that is, which segments of society will receive what benefits and which segments will provide the resources so that those benefits can occur. A single NPV will not present answers to such multifaceted concerns.

The usefulness of CBA depends largely on the presentation of uncertainties. Analyses that fail to directly address uncertainties and do not report a range of estimates in sensitivity analyses are limited in their usefulness because they fail to provide comprehensive information for further analysis and interpretation by decision makers.

The CBA cannot be used to determine whether a proposed method for achieving a program's objectives would maximize social benefits. In the lead-paint removal example discussed earlier, we can only say that program B results in a greater increase in social benefits than program A. Without doing further work, we cannot legitimately include in the analysis an additional option (e.g., program C).

Perhaps the greatest problem in CBA is the challenge mentioned earlier of assigning a monetary value to human life or to a change in quality of life. In health, this issue is particularly sensitive since public health programs often have the specific goal of reducing unnecessary morbidity and premature mortality. From an ethical and moral perspective, human life is often considered priceless, so attempting to value it in monetary terms is difficult; or, perhaps more correctly, some segments of society may have difficulty accepting a stated dollar value of human life. As mentioned earlier, investigators routinely try to avoid such controversy by using CEA rather than CBA; but in the end, CEA still forces policy makers to subjectively value human life. That is, the decision makers and society will never avoid the following question: If an intervention costs $X per life saved, is it worthwhile to invest in the program? The advantage of CBA is that it makes certain assumptions, such as the value of life, explicit. Decision makers and society can debate whether or not the assumed value is appropriate. Further, sensitivity analyses can indicate what would happen to the results and conclusions if the value were altered for human life or for changes in quality of life.

AN EXAMPLE OF A COST–BENEFIT ANALYSIS USING THE CONTINGENT VALUATION METHOD

In the following simplified example, assume you wished to conduct a CBA of the use of household water vessels to prevent diarrhea. You decide to estimate consumers' WTP as a measure of the benefits of the program. You use the CVM described earlier and conduct a WTP survey in a village of 100 households. In the description of the intervention, you essentially explain that you wish the villagers to value the water vessel, comparing the bid amount (cost) of the water vessel to the cost of coping with diarrhea in their household. For simplicity, we will not worry about time: both valuation and cost apply to a single time period (of whatever length). From the survey results and other data (e.g., program costs), you produce Table 8.3.

Further, assume that you use the survey data to calculate that the mean WTP is $13 per household, where the mean is weighted by the proportion of households saying "yes" to a given bid amount. The median WTP is $15 per household.

Suppose, as shown in column D, the vessel is sold at a cost of $10 per household. If 80% of the households purchased a vessel, the total cost of the program is $800 (80 households × $10 per vessel), and the total benefits of the program are $1200 (80 households × average WTP of $15). This produces an NPV of $400 ($1200 – $800). Note that each household that purchased a water vessel paid only $10, yet 80% of the village households said they would pay at least $10 (in fact, 65% of households stated they would pay at least $15). Those households that stated they would pay more than $10 actually received excess value, or consumer surplus.

Suppose you now wish to consider increasing the number of households purchasing a water vessel to 95% of the village. To achieve this goal, you lower the price of the vessel to $5. Since the vessel still costs $10 to produce, you give a $5 per vessel subsidy to the manufacturer. The program now costs $950 (95 households × $10 per household). The total benefit is $1300 (95 households × average WTP of $15). The

Table 8.3   Example of Contingent Valuation Method Survey Data

A Bid Amount per Household ($)	B Number of Households Saying "Yes" to Bid Value	C Aggregation of Willingness to Pay for Each Bid Amount (A*B) ($)	D Cumulative Benefits ($)	E Cumulative Program Costs at $10 per Household ($)
0	5	0	0	50
5	15	75	75	200
10	15	150	225	350
15	50	750	975	850
20	10	200	1175	950
25	5	125	1300	1000

NPV of this new program is $350 ($1300 – $950). The incremental NPV of expanding coverage from 80% to 95% is $350 – $400 = –$50. The total NPV is still positive, so the program is still acceptable when coverage is expanded; but what we see is that there is a loss in social benefits resulting from the expansion. The community is worse off, in total, than it was before the expansion. The lesson from this example of an incremental CBA is that achieving full coverage with any prevention program may not maximize the societal economic benefit. Remember that any resources committed to the expansion cannot be used for other purposes that may in fact yield a positive net benefit for the families who would be covered by the expansion.

CONCLUSION

The most comprehensive method of economic analysis is CBA, which attempts to weigh all benefits associated with an intervention against all costs of implementing the intervention. Because the results of CBA are expressed in monetary terms, both health and nonhealth programs can be directly compared.

The greatest area of controversy for CBA is how to value reductions in risks to statistical lives and how to value changes in the quality of life. In CBA, a monetary value is assigned to reducing risks to human life by several methods presented in this chapter. Assigning monetary values to changes in the quality of life is even more difficult; instead, it is usually omitted from CBA and listed as an intangible. However, as the methodology for CBA continues to develop, this method may be used more frequently for prevention-effectiveness studies.

Another apparent difficulty with CBA is that the techniques appear to be precise and objective. If users are not familiar with the underlying assumptions, the results can easily be misinterpreted and misused. The results are only as good as the analysis, assumptions, and valuations and must be skillfully interpreted when used for decision making.

Recommendation 8.1: A comprehensive measure or set of measures (e.g., CVM) designed to fully capture costs and benefits should be used for CBA that take the societal perspective.

Recommendation 8.2: The NPV of benefits, rather than a BCR, should be used as the summary measure in CBA.

Recommendation 8.3: When CBA is used to evaluate more than one competing program or intervention, the incremental or marginal NPVs should be reported. It is acceptable to report average NPVs in CBA of independent programs or interventions.

CHECKLIST FOR COST–BENEFIT ANALYSES

Here, we present a brief checklist of some of the things a user (consumer) should look for when reading a CBA.

1. Have the specific questions to be answered been identified?
2. Have the programs/interventions been clearly identified?
3. Have all reasonable options been clearly stated?
4. Is CBA the appropriate technique for the study?
5. Have all outcomes of the program been identified?
6. Have the assumptions been specified?
7. Is the perspective(s) of the study clearly stated?
8. Have intangible costs and benefits been appropriately included?
9. Are the proper measures of welfare estimated?
10. Have any outcomes been counted more than once?
11. How have the outcomes been valued?
12. Have the appropriate estimation techniques been used?
13. Does the study include inputs and outcomes (costs and benefits) appropriate to the stated perspective(s)?
14. Have calculations for summary measures of all options been appropriately performed?
15. Are the components of the summary measures presented and not just the measures themselves?
16. Have appropriate sensitivity analyses been conducted?
17. Are results presented in a way that clearly outlines to decision makers what options have been evaluated and how robust the CBA is considered to be?

REFERENCES

1. Meltzer MI, Shapiro CN, Mast EE, Arcari C. The economics of vaccinating restaurant foodhandlers against hepatitis A. *Vaccine 2001;* 19:2138–45.
2. Ekwueme DU, Strebel PM, Meltzer MI, et al. Economic evaluation of use of diphtheria, tetanus, and acelluar pertussis vaccine (DTaP) or diphtheria, tetanus and whole-cell pertussis vaccine (DTwP) in the United States. *Arch Pediatr Adolesc Med 2000;* 154:797–803.
3. Dupuit J. On the measurement of utility of public works. *Int Econ Papers 1952;* 2:83–110.
4. United States Federal Inter-Agency River Basin Committee, Subcommittee on Benefits and Costs. *Proposed Practices for Economic Analysis of River Basin Projects.* Washington, DC: U.S. Government Printing Office, 1958.
5. Petty W. *Political Arithmetick, or a Discourse Concerning the Extent and Value of Land, People, Buildings, etc.* London: Robert Caluel, 1699.
6. Rice D. *Estimating the Cost of Illness.* Washington DC: Department of Health, Education and Welfare, Public Health Service, Health Economics Series 6, 1966.
7. Weisbrod B. Costs and benefits of medical research. *J Polit Econ 1971;* 79:527–44.
8. Grosse R. Cost–benefit analysis of health services. *Ann Am Acad Polit Soc Sci 1972;* 89:399–418.
9. Klarman H. Application of cost-benefit analysis to the health services and a special case of technological innovation. *Soc Sci Med 1975;* 4:325–44.
10. Dunlop D. Benefit–cost analysis: a review of its applicability in policy analysis for delivering health services. *Soc Sci Med 1975;* 9:133–51.

11. Pauker S, Kassirer J. Therapeutic decision making: a cost–benefit analysis. *N Engl J Med 1975;* 293:229–38.
12. Harrington W, Portney PR. Valuing the benefits of health and safety regulation. *J Urban Econ 1987;* 22:101–12.
13. Thompson MS. Willingness to pay and accept risks to cure chronic disease. *Am J Public Health 1986;* 76:392–6.
14. Johannesson M. Economic evaluation of hypertension treatment. *Int J Technol Assess Health Care 1992;* 8:506–23.
15. Fisher A, Chestnut LG, Violette DM. The value of reducing risks of death: a note on new evidence. *J Policy Anal Manag 1989;* 8:88–100.
16. Meltzer MI, Cox NJ, Fukuda K. The economic impact of pandemic influenza in the United States: implications for setting priorities for interventions. *Emerg Infect Dis 1999;* 5:659–71.
17. Sassone PG, Schaffer WA. *Cost–Benefit Analysis: A Handbook.* San Diego: Academic, 1978.
18. Randall A. *Resource Economics,* 2d ed. New York: John Wiley and Sons, 1987.
19. Mitchell RC, Carson RT. *Using Surveys to Value Public Goods: The Contingent Valuation Method.* Washington DC: Resources for the Future, 1989.
20. Kopp RJ, Krupnick AJ, Toman M. *Cost–Benefit Analysis and Regulatory Reform: An Assessment of the Science and the Art.* Discussion Paper 97-19. Washington DC: Resources for the Future, 1997.
21. Corso PS, Hammitt JK, Graham JD. Valuing mortality-risk reduction: using visual aids to improve the validity of contingent valuation. *J Risk Uncert* 2001; 23:165–84.
22. Viscusi WK. *Fatal Tradeoffs: Public and Private Responsibilities for Risk.* New York: Oxford University Press, 1992.
23. Viscusi WK. The value of risks to life and health. *J Econ Lit 1993;* 1912–46.
24. Weston JF, Brigham EF. *Essentials of Managerial Finance,* 12th ed. Stamford, CT: Thompson Learning, 2000.
25. Rosen HS. *Public Finance,* 6th ed. Columbus, OH: McGraw-Hill Higher Education, 2001.

BIBLIOGRAPHY

Berwick DM, Weinstein MC. What do patients value? Willingness to pay for ultrasound in normal pregnancy. *Med Care 1985;* 23:881–93.
Binger RR, Hoffman E. *Microeconomics with Calculus.* Boston: Addison Wesley, 1997.
Elbasha EH, Fitzsimmons TD, Meltzer MI. The costs and benefits of a subtype-specific surveillance system to identify *Escherichia coli* O157:H7 outbreaks. *Emerg Infect Dis 2000;* 6:293–7.
Fuchs V, Zeckhauser R. Valuing health: a "priceless" commodity. *Am Econ Rev 1987;* 77:263–8.
Ginsberg GM, Tulchinsky TH. Costs and benefits of a measles inoculation of children in Israel, the West Bank, and Gaza. *J Epidemiol ComOmunity Health 1990;* 44:272–80.
Hammond PB, Coppock R, eds. *Valuing Health Risks, Costs, and Benefits for Environmental Decision Making: Report of a Conference.* Washington DC: National Academy Press, 1990.
Johannesson M, Jonsson B. Economic evaluation in health care: is there a role for cost-benefit analysis? *Health Policy 1991;* 17:1–23.

Johansson PO. *Evaluating Health Risks: An Economic Approach*. Cambridge: Cambridge University Press, 1995.

Phelps C, Mushlin A. On the (near) equivalence of cost–effectiveness and cost-benefit analyses. *Int J Technol Assess Health Care 1991;*7:12–21.

Ponnighaus JM. The cost/benefit of measles immunization: a study from southern Zambia. *Am J Trop Med Hyg 1980;* 83:141–9.

Rice T. *The Economics of Health Reconsidered*. Chicago: Health Administration Press, 1998.

Udvarhelyi IS, Colditz GA, Rai A, Epstein AM. Cost–effectiveness and cost–benefit analyses in the medical literature: are the methods being used correctly? *Ann Intern Med 1992;* 116:238–44.

9

Cost–Effectiveness Analysis

THOMAS L. GIFT
ANNE C. HADDIX
PHAEDRA S. CORSO

Cost–effectiveness analysis (CEA) has become the predominant method for evaluating the costs and effects of alternative health-care strategies. Unlike many clinical decision models, CEAs address questions about population-based health policies and programs. They have has been used to compare strategies designed to address the same health problem (competing interventions) and strategies targeted at different health problems (independent interventions). At the programmatic level, CEAs have been used for planning purposes and at the highest levels of government for setting priorities for resources allocated to health. Their results have been applied by federal, state, and local policy makers in the broad interest of society; by employers, health-plan administrators and managed-care organizations to design health-care packages for employees; and by consumer organizations representing the interests of individuals. CEA is a useful and easily understandable method for evaluating the impact of investment in health on improvements in health status.

This chapter focuses on specific aspects of CEA. It provides guidance on when to use CEA, how to frame study questions, how to construct and analyze models, and how to interpret and present results. The chapter is not intended to stand alone as a guide for performing CEA; rather, it summarizes the techniques described throughout this book, highlighting recommendations specific for CEA. Cost–utility analysis (CUA), a variant of CEA, is also discussed, including the translation of health events into quality-adjusted life years (QALYs).

DEFINITION OF COST–EFFECTIVENESS ANALYSIS AND COST–UTILITY ANALYSIS

Cost–effectiveness analysis is a method used to evaluate the relationship between net investment and health improvement in health-care strategies competing for similar resources. Because CEA is limited to the comparison of strategies designed to improve health, no attempt is made to assign a monetary value to disease averted beyond the cost of care for persons with these conditions and costs of lost productivity from morbidity and mortality. Rather, results are presented in the form of the net cost per health outcome, such as *cost per case prevented* or *cost per life saved*. The decision maker is left to make value judgments about the intrinsic value of the health outcomes.

Unlike cost–benefit analysis (CBA), CEA has not evolved from a single theoretical origin. While CBA was developed primarily within the field of welfare economics, CEA evolved from the disciplines of economics, decision analysis, and operations research. The diversity of disciplines that have contributed to the development of CEA is the basis for the method's strengths as well as its weaknesses.

Cost–effectiveness analyses are designed to produce a cost–effectiveness (CE) ratio, the most commonly used summary measure for comparing health interventions. The numerator of the CE ratio is the cost of the health intervention (including costs of adverse effects of the intervention and other costs induced by the intervention) minus the costs of the health conditions that are prevented as a result of the intervention. The denominator is the improvement in health produced by the intervention. This improvement in health may be measured in natural units, for example, cases of measles prevented, or in terms of the impact on health-related quality of life, for example, QALYs. Ratios may be average, marginal, or incremental measures. These terms are defined later in the chapter.

The CEA is also useful in providing parameter thresholds within which the rank order of strategies is maintained. Threshold analysis assists the decision maker in determining the circumstances under which a specific strategy is the most cost–effective choice. For example, an expensive single-dose antibiotic drug to treat cervical chlamydial infections is more cost-effective than its less expensive multidose competitor when compliance with the multidose therapy is less than about 90%.[1] Based on these findings, a treatment clinic may recommend the less expensive drug for its patients who are likely to be highly compliant and the more expensive drug for noncompliant patients.

CEA differs from CBA in that it does not explicitly include all of the costs and all of the benefits associated with alternative strategies. Most conspicuously absent from CEA are the intangible costs associated with both the intervention and the health outcome. Examples of intangible costs include pain, suffering, social stigma, and lost opportunity. Intangible costs may be incurred by the individual experiencing or at risk for the health problem, family, friends, or the larger community. Methods used to value benefits in CBA generally include the intangible costs. Thus, CBA is a more comprehensive method leading to a clear-cut decision rule. Although proponents of CEA maintain that one of its benefits is that no monetary value is assigned to health, the end user ultimately makes this valuation. For example, if a strategy to prevent cervical cancer costs $25,000 per QALY gained, the decision maker must decide if a QALY is worth at least $25,000. When the health outcome is presented in natural units, such as a case of influenza, the decision maker is faced with an even more difficult task in valuing the outcome; influenza outcomes range from mild self-limited disease to death and affect ages ranging from childhood to the elderly.

CEA is most useful when the goal is to rank prevention strategies by their relative cost–effectiveness. It is an ideal tool for economic analysis of randomized controlled trials (RCTs), which commonly feature a control group and one or more interventions that seek to achieve a common outcome. It is also extremely useful for ranking strategies that address a number of health problems for the purpose of priority setting or resource allocation. For example, a recent project under the auspices of Partnership for Prevention, a nonprofit health-advocacy group, used cost–effectiveness as one of two criteria in prioritizing clinical preventive services. [2,3] More on the uses of CEA for decision making is presented in Chapter 10.

Because outcomes measured in natural units are dependent on the interventions being analyzed, CEA often does not provide a convenient way to compare the cost–effectiveness of interventions for different health conditions. It is difficult, for example, to use CEA to compare an intervention designed to increase seat belt usage with one intended to improve cancer screening. CUA allows comparison across health interventions and has been applied in a diverse array of interventions, including postpartum use of anti-D-γ-globulin,[4] smoking cessation,[5] and phenylketonuria screening.[6] This offers an obvious advantage over CEA, which uses intervention-specific outcome measures but it also imposes limitations. CEA uses outcomes that are directly observable or that can be derived from directly observed outcomes, in most cases. QALYs are not directly observable, except with conditions that deliver only two states: perfect health or death. The greatest limitation for CUA is that a QALY measure has not been defined for many health conditions.

To further illustrate the different potential applications for CUA and CEA, consider the following example. A benefits manager for a health-care provider is weighing two options for annual cholesterol screening for the provider's patients. Screening can be provided to all patients or only to those at special risk. The optimal tool to help determine which approach is most efficient is CEA. If the manager is faced with an allocation decision between cholesterol screening and purchasing blood-glucose meters for use by the provider's diabetic patients, CUA would be a better tool to guide the decision process.

BACKGROUND

The use of CEA in health care began in the mid-1970s in response to a need for systematic analysis of health-care decisions,[7–9] primarily of a clinical nature.[10–12] CBA was considered too burdensome, even if theoretically attractive, and because of controversies over the valuation of health and life, it had fallen from favor. Health practitioners sought a less complex method in which the results were explicitly stated in terms of health outcomes rather than dollars.

The U.S. government began to use CEA in the late 1970s for public health decisions, particularly in vaccine policy.[13] Since then, CEA has become the predominant method for analyzing health-care decisions in both the clinical and public health sectors. Until recently, the quality of the CEA literature was variable. Because no clear standards or guidelines were available, it was difficult to draw comparisons across studies.

During the 1990s, efforts in the United States and other countries led to standards for CEAs, and the quality of the literature has begun to improve. [14–18] As measures for the QALY or DALY impact of health conditions have become more available and reliable, studies using CUA have become more common. Recently, methods have begun to be developed to synthesize information from multiple CEA studies, thus improving their usefulness in policy making. [19] More on this is presented in Chapter 10.

WHEN TO CONDUCT A COST–EFFECTIVENESS ANALYSIS

CEA is most useful when the interventions being compared have one clear and specific outcome. Building on work by Emery and Schneiderman, [20] five scenarios for which CEA is most suited are:

1. Comparing alternative strategies for an identical goal or health problem
2. Identifying which intervention is best for a specific population or setting
3. Prioritizing independent strategies that address different health problems
4. Providing empirical support for the adoption of previously underfunded programs with low cost–effectiveness ratios
5. Identifying practices that are not worth their cost compared to other alternative practices (in some cases, even when the alternative is "do nothing")

When health-related quality of life is the desired health outcome, a CUA may be the most appropriate study design. As noted above, CUA is a specific kind of CEA; it simply uses a standardized measure (DALY or QALY) as the intervention outcome. CUA is appropriate when:[21]

• Quality of life is the important outcome
• Quality of life is an important outcome
• The interventions being evaluated affect both morbidity and mortality
• The interventions being compared have a wide range of different outcomes
• The interventions being compared have both desired and adverse health outcomes
• The interventions being evaluated are being compared with a program that has already been evaluated using CUA

HOW TO CONDUCT A COST–EFFECTIVENESS ANALYSIS

Once CEA has been selected as the method of analysis, there are eight basic steps to conducting one:

1. Frame the problem to be analyzed
2. Identify the baseline and the options to be compared
3. Identify the outcome measures

4. Identify the relevant costs
5. Construct the decision model
6. Analyze and interpret the results
7. Perform sensitivity analysis
8. Prepare presentation of results

Framing the Problem

The first step in CEA, as with any prevention-effectiveness study, is to frame and define the scope of the study. A detailed description of components in framing the study is provided in Chapter 2; the following sections address framing issues specific to CEA.

Study Question
The study question and the scope of the evaluation must be defined. The study question determines which interventions should be included in the study and helps define the scope of the analysis. Some examples of questions that could be answered through CEA include the following:

- Which drug is the most cost–effective for treating persons with chlamydial infection?
- Which tobacco-control program is most cost–effective in the Southeast Asian community?
- Which clinical preventive services recommended by the U.S. Clinical Preventive Services Task Force should be listed as high-priority services?
- Are needle-exchange programs a cost–effective strategy to prevent human immunodeficiency virus (HIV) infections in intravenous drug users, and should such programs be legalized and funded?
- Is surgical treatment of patients with prostate cancer cost–effective when compared to radiation therapy, hormonal therapy, and "watchful waiting"?

Perspective
The perspective of the study determines which costs and outcomes will be included. In questions of public policy, it is usually most appropriate to use a societal perspective because a more narrowly defined perspective may lead to inefficient allocation of public health resources.

This does not mean that all CEAs that bear on public policy should be restricted to the societal perspective only. Often, CEAs are designed to address the needs of different stakeholders. Other perspectives may identify barriers to program implementation. Thus, it may be appropriate to consider more than one perspective. Adopting a particular perspective will often require measuring different costs and consequences or including costs differently in the summary measures.

Time Frame and Analytic Horizon
The *time frame* is the period in which the alternative prevention strategies are being evaluated. Specifically, the time frame of the study should include the period

in which the intervention or treatment is delivered. The time frame should be long enough to ensure that relevant consequences of the intervention are captured. A multiyear time frame may be more appropriate for interventions with extended start-up time, high initial cost, or long treatment period. The *analytic horizon* is the period in which the costs and health outcomes that result from the intervention accrue. The analytic horizon extends for the lifetime of an individual who received the intervention during the time frame of the study.

Choosing Baseline Comparator and Alternative Interventions

Selection of the study baseline and the interventions to be compared is a critcal step in the framing of the CEA. If a CEA does not use an appropriate baseline or evaluate all relevant interventions, it will not be useful to the audience.

The *baseline* is the reference point for the analysis and the one to which the alternative interventions under consideration are compared. Typically, the baseline is "no program," the current practice, or the current standard of care. For example, if the current practice of a sexually transmitted disease clinic is to treat patients who present with signs and symptoms of gonorrhea, then that would be an appropriate baseline intervention; the "no program" option of refusing care to patients with symptoms would not be legally, morally, or ethically appropriate. Inclusion of the baseline comparator, even if it is not going to continue to be used, makes it possible to calculate the incremental costs of the new interventions being evaluated.

Identification of the alternative intervention strategies includes specification of the delivery strategy and the target population. The mode of delivery will affect the costs of the strategy and is closely linked to other parameters in the decision model. For example, an influenza vaccine campaign that provides vaccinations at local supermarkets and other community sites may have a higher adherence rate than one in which the vaccine is available only from health-care facilities. Because of the mode of delivery, the two influenza vaccine options will have different costs.

Target population
When comparing the cost–effectiveness of interventions that address the same health problem, it is important that the populations examined in each of the alternatives are comparable. The population should also include all groups who are affected by the intervention, either directly or indirectly. For example, consider program options designed to increase folic acid intake in women of childbearing years. Low folic acid intake during the first weeks of pregnancy is a risk factor for neural tube defects. Two of the potential strategies for preventing neural tube defects are fortification of cereal grains with folic acid and a public education campaign to encourage women of childbearing years to take folic acid supplements. Although the first strategy is targeted at women of childbearing years, it is delivered to the general population. Therefore, the costs are borne by all consumers of cereal grain products. In addition, increased folic acid intake can mask the signs of vitamin B_{12} deficiency, potentially leading to adverse health outcomes in the elderly population. Thus, the impact of costs in the general population and the adverse health outcomes in the elderly population should be included in the analysis.

When selecting interventions to analyze, all reasonable options should be included, to the extent possible. Interventions must be appropriate for the target population and acceptable to policy makers and society. Measures of effectiveness for the intervention must exist. Finally, CEA must compare options that are directed at achieving comparable health outcomes.

Selecting Health-Outcome Measures

In a CEA, components associated with the health outcome appear in both the numerator and the denominator. The costs of disease averted as a result of the intervention appear in the net-cost calculation, which comprises the numerator. Direct measures of the health outcome (e.g., cases prevented, lives saved, QALYs gained) appear in the denominator of the CE ratio.

The health outcome used in a CEA must be relevant to the study question and should be understandable to the audience. For example, the analyst conducting a CEA of a smoke alarm program to prevent fire-related injuries may select lives saved or injuries prevented rather than the more comprehensive QALY measure because QALYs are an unfamiliar concept to local community health planners. The health outcome must be the same for each intervention in the study. It is not practical to compare cardiac events with cases of lung cancer prevented. A health outcome often used in CEA is life years saved; an alternative is lives saved. However, for health conditions in which morbidity is a significant component, these measures do not capture the full impact of the intervention. Thus, QALYs would be a better choice. When the study is limited to analyzing competing interventions that address the same health condition, outcomes such as cases prevented and cases identified are commonly used.

Intermediate and Final Outcomes

Health outcomes can be categorized as intermediate and final. Final-outcome measures include cases prevented, lives saved, deaths averted, life years gained, and QALYs. Final-outcome measures may be direct measures of an intervention or generated from the intermediate outcomes if the quantitative relationship between the intermediate outcome and final outcome is known. Final-outcome measures should almost always be used for a CE ratio.

Intermediate outcomes are often the only ones that are measurable within the time frame of a study of the effectiveness of an intervention. Examples of intermediate outcomes include cases identified, cases treated, or behaviors changed. Because the time frame for an RCT or a community demonstration project is too short to capture the long-term consequences of the health condition, an intermediate outcome measure is collected. For example, consider a community demonstration project designed to prevent adolescents from beginning to smoke. The adverse health consequences of tobacco use often do not appear for decades after smoking initiation. Thus, the number of new adolescent smokers is the only feasible outcome measure. To examine the cost–effectiveness of the new intervention, the analyst will construct a model of the intervention and link new adolescent smokers with later health outcomes using estimates of risk, cost, and quality-of-life impacts obtained from the literature or other sources.

In rare cases, the relationship between the intermediate and final outcomes may be known but data limitations may make it difficult or impossible to quantify the averted disease costs associated with the final measure. For example, a typical final-outcome measure used in studies of chlamydia and gonorrhea programs is cases of pelvic inflammatory disease averted. Estimates of the medical costs of a case of pelvic inflammatory disease and its sequelae exist for the United States but not for other countries. In situations where precise data are lacking, expert panels can be consulted to assemble reasonable estimates. However, if the scope of an analysis is limited to existing data, the intermediate measure of cases of chlamydia or gonorrhea treated might be used instead of cases of pelvic inflammatory disease prevented. When intermediate-outcome measures are used, the limitations that prevent the use of a final-outcome measure should be discussed in the presentation of the study.

The preference for final outcomes does not mean that the intermediate outcomes are ignored in the study. As noted above, they are often the directly measurable outcomes that will either be collected during the study or found in previously published reports of interventions. In a decision model, intermediate outcomes appear along the path to final outcomes. Their medical costs will be included in the numerator; they just will not appear directly in the denominator.

Adverse Effects of an Intervention

In addition to the health outcomes an intervention is designed to prevent, the intervention itself may cause harmful side effects or adverse health effects. For example, many types of antibiotic therapy are associated with gastrointestinal disorders. This side effect may result in additional treatment costs, which should be factored into the analysis. Minor side effects that do not ultimately change the structure of the decision model can be accounted for in terms of the additional cost they add to the intervention.

If there are serious adverse effects from the intervention, these should appear explicitly in the decision model as an outcome at a terminal node or through changes in the tree structure or the probabilities at the chance nodes. If the adverse effects are severe enough to warrant discontinuing therapy, the probability for treatment compliance should reflect this. Additional outcomes also may be needed to account for the adverse effects. In the example presented earlier, a CEA of strategies to increase folic acid intake for women of childbearing age to prevent neural tube defects evaluated the cost–effectiveness of fortifying all cereal grains. The model included the risk of permanent neurological complications and death due to delayed diagnosis of vitamin B_{12} deficiency in older persons. Because the model used two different sets of health outcomes that were not additive or comparable, all outcomes were converted to QALYs.[22]

Quality-Adjusted Life Years in Cost–Effectiveness Analyses

When QALYs are used in CEAs, the final health outcome measured in natural units is converted to a change in health-related quality of life. Defining and calculating QALYs for specific health conditions was discussed in Chapter 5. This section discusses converting health outcomes in a population or cohort to QALYs in a CEA.

When QALYs are used in a CEA (or CUA), additional information is needed, including the following:

- A list of all possible health outcomes
- Probabilities that the health outcomes will occur
- Average age at onset of health outcomes
- Average duration of health outcomes
- Average life expectancy with and without the health outcomes
- QALY weights for each health outcome

The following example illustrates the use of QALYs as an outcome measure in a CUA that follows a cohort of children. A CUA is conducted for a new vaccine that prevents a serious childhood illness. It examines the cost–effectiveness of the new vaccine in a hypothetical birth cohort. The summary measure is the net cost per QALY gained. Currently, a child has a 25% chance of becoming infected with the disease before age 5. If infected, the disease is fatal in 10% of children. Fifteen percent of infected children have lifelong hearing or vision loss. The remaining 75% of infected children have self-limited disease and make a full recovery. The average age at infection is 2 years. The analysis uses a QALY of 0.8 for a year with hearing or vision loss and assumes a life expectancy of 78 years. The QALYs are discounted at 3% per year.

A simplified decision tree is shown in Figure 9.1. The health outcome at the terminal node is the total lifetime QALYs of a child who proceeded on that branch. A child who does not become infected or who has infection but fully recovers would have 78 QALYs, or 30.91 discounted QALYs. A child who loses hearing or vision at age 2 would have 25.12 discounted QALYs, while a child who dies at age 2 would have 1.97 discounted QALYs. When the tree is averaged out and folded back, a child in the *vaccine* branch, on average, would have 30.91 QALYs. A child in the *no vaccine* branch would have 29.97 QALYs, or an average loss of 0.94 QALYs from the infection. Another way of stating the results is as follows: for every 1000 children in a birth cohort, 250 will become infected, 25 of whom will

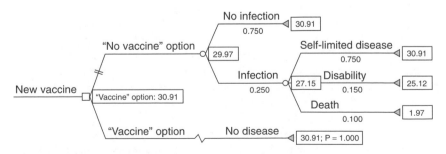

Figure 9.1   A simplified decision tree for calculating quality-adjusted life years in a cost–effectiveness analysis.

die and 38 of whom will experience lifetime vision or hearing loss. This results in a loss of 940 QALYs.

Identifying Intervention and Outcome Costs

Once the relevant intervention strategies and health outcomes have been identified, the next step is to determine the costs of the components in the net-cost equation:[23]

$$Net\ Cost = Cost_{\text{Intervention}} - Cost_{\text{Disease Averted}} - Cost_{\text{Productivity Losses Averted}}$$

Net costs are divided into the total costs for all resources required for the program ($Cost_{\text{Intervention}}$), including the cost of side effects and the costs to participants, the costs of diagnosis and treatment associated with cases of the health problem averted ($Cost_{\text{Disease Averted}}$), and the productivity losses averted as a result of the intervention ($Cost_{\text{Productivity Losses Averted}}$).

The costs of each intervention in the analysis can be ascertained by following the guidelines given in Chapter 4. In CEA, the costs of the disease averted and the productivity losses are assessed using the human capital approach (a form of the cost-of-illness method) detailed in Chapter 4. Whether to include productivity losses will depend on the perspective of the CEA, as described above. Intangible costs, best measured by willingness to pay, as discussed in Chapter 8, are not included in the net-cost calculation.

Productivity Losses in Cost–Utility Analysis

In CUA, the results are usually reported as cost per QALY gained. However, in CUA, if the utility measurement includes the value of lost productivity, productivity losses should not be included in the numerator because this will result in double counting. If the utility measure does not take into account utility lost as the result of a change in productivity due to an illness, productivity losses should be included in the net-cost calculation in the numerator.

Future Unrelated Health-Care Costs

Future unrelated health-care costs are those that would be generated because, as a result of a health care intervention, lives are extended. Continuing the example from above, if an intervention is effective at averting adolescent smoking, the net discounted lifetime health-care costs for the adolescents who do not start smoking, and therefore live longer, may be higher than otherwise.[24] There has been much discussion on whether future unrelated health-care costs should be included in CEAs.[15] Although some researchers argue that it is theoretically correct to include them, practical difficulties exist. Data may not be available on the costs of future disease. Technological changes in health care increase the difficulty in predicting future causes of death. The Panel on Cost–Effectiveness in Health and Medicine recommended that inclusion of future unrelated health-care costs be left to the discretion of the analyst.[15] The analyst should be aware, however, that when these costs are likely to be large, their inclusion could change the rank ordering of the interventions under study. Therefore, it is recommended that sensitivity analyses address the impact of these costs on the results.

Constructing the Decision Model

All of the preceding steps are preparatory. Once they are completed, a decision model can be constructed. This may be the most critical step of the analysis. A decision model can take many forms; one of the most commonly used is a decision tree. The purpose and process of tree construction are described in Chapter 7; software packages designed for decision-tree construction aid in the process (Appendix C). Spreadsheets can also be used, as can mathematical calculation software. Simple decision models can be done by hand.

Regardless of what form of decision model is used, the data requirements are similar and identifying the data needed is the first step in actually constructing the model. A CEA uses a combination of epidemiological and economic data. Unless the interventions being considered have already been carefully evaluated, the first step in data collection is usually a thorough literature review.

The best source for outcome data will, in many cases, be RCTs or other well-designed studies that have undergone peer review and been published in the scientific literature. Other epidemiological data, such as disease prevalence and sequelae rates, may also be available in peer-reviewed publications. Similarly, economic data can sometimes be found in well-designed research studies that have been published. Practically speaking, there are often gaps in the data that must be filled. One way that a gap can be filled is by designing a study to answer the relevant question. However, this is often not feasible because of time and resource constraints and is frequently unnecessary. Such gaps can also be filled by using expert panels to develop the best estimates or by assigning values on the basis of the available evidence. If these methods are used, the variables must be viewed as being uncertain and should be subjected to sensitivity analysis. Those that are critical to the results of the CEA may require additional study. A list of basic types of data needed to construct a CE decision tree is provided in Table 9.1. However, every analysis is different, and some may require additional or different data.

Once the data have been collected, the model itself can be constructed. The process of decision-model construction is a balance between realism and simplification. It is important to account for important events to the extent possible. For example, if a therapy is only 80% effective, accounting for possible treatment failure will improve the value of the decision model, in most instances. However, even the most detailed analysis is still a model and cannot capture all possible chance events. Attempting to include too much detail can quickly lead to excessive complexity and outstrip available data. The model can be simplified to focus on important variables and ones that are of interest.

Figure 9.2 shows a portion of a decision tree constructed for a CEA of azithromycin versus ceftriaxone for treatment of uncomplicated gonorrhea.[25] Numerous adverse gastrointestinal events following treatment with azithromycin were noted in the original publication. These could be modeled as shown in Figure 9.2a. However, the gastrointestinal symptoms were not severe enough to require re-

Table 9.1 Key Data Needed to Construct a Cost–Effectiveness Decision Tree

1. Measurement of the effectiveness of an intervention
   • Efficacy of intervention
   • Compliance, participation, effectiveness in a community setting
   • Sensitivity and specificity of laboratory tests
   • Prevalence of risk factors

2. Risk of side effects

3. Risk of disease or injury with and without the intervention
   • Risk of primary disease or injury averted
   • Risk of sequelae or complications of disease or injury averted

4. Cost of intervention (as appropriate given analytic perspective)
   • Medical and nonmedical costs of intervention
   • Productivity losses associated with disease and participation in intervention
   • Medical and nonmedical costs of adverse effects
   • Productivity losses from adverse effects
   • Medical and nonmedical costs of disease or injury, including costs of sequelae or complications and productivity losses from morbidity and mortality

5. Measurement of health outcomes including life years and QALYs
   • List of all possible health outcomes
   • Risk of health outcome occurring
   • Age at onset of health outcomes
   • Duration of health outcomes
   • Life expectancy with and without health outcomes
   • QALY weight for each health outcome

QALY, quality-adjusted life year.

treatment with a different regimen. A CEA would likely focus primarily on the efficacy of the drug and its cost in comparison to ceftriaxone and use outcomes other than adverse treatment events. Because of that, it would be much simpler (and detract little from the study) to combine all adverse events together as in Figure 9.2b. The probability of each adverse event could be multiplied by its direct medical cost to get a weighted average cost of an adverse event. What would be lost by this approach is the ability to easily perform some forms of sensitivity analysis. If no sensitivity analysis of the frequency of each specific adverse event was contemplated, Figure 9.2b would suffice.

In contrast to using a decision-tree approach for modeling a decision analysis, the analysis could have been set up in a spreadsheet program or with mathematical calculation software. There are many software packages that include CEA as an option, utilizing a decision-tree format. Typically, the first outcome for each terminal node is the cost; the second outcome is the health outcome. The model must, in essence, be computed twice: once to determine the costs of each intervention or program being compared and once to determine the outcomes in each program. The software program can then be used to analyze the dual scales (cost and health outcome) simultaneously in order to compute the expected total cost and the expected value of the health outcome for each strategy. The strategies are ranked in ascending or descending order of cost or effectiveness depending on user preference. Decision-analysis

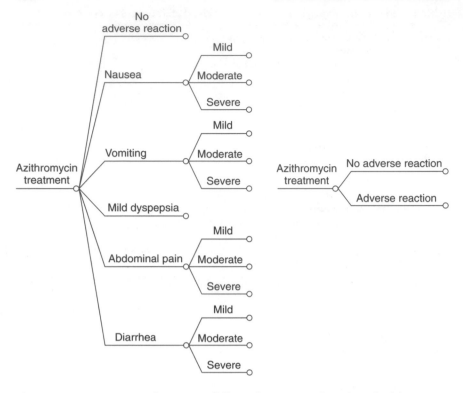

Figure 9.2   Two approaches to modeling adverse reactions in a decision tree comparing gonorrhea treatment options.

software will also compute the average and incremental CE ratios, or the formulas to compute them can be entered into the spreadsheet or computation software.

Analyze and Interpret the Results

Once values have been assigned to both the chance and terminal nodes, the branches are averaged out and folded back to produce expected values for both the costs and the outcomes of the options in the tree. These results are used to calculate both average and incremental CE ratios. When using a spreadsheet, the process is similar, except that the probability, outcome, and cost values are typically listed in different cells and other cells contain formulas to multiply relevant values together to average out and fold back.

Cost-Effectiveness Ratios

Generally, two types of CE ratio are reported for a CEA: average ratio and marginal or incremental. Each provides insight into the efficiency and the affordability of the intervention ratio. The average CE ratio is evaluated against the baseline or reference option and can be calculated by dividing the net cost of a strategy compared to the baseline divided by the total number of health outcomes averted by the intervention, for example, average cost per case prevented or average cost per year of life saved. Net costs in an average CE ratio include intervention costs:

$$Intervention\ Cost = Cost_{Intervention\ A}$$

where $Cost_{Intervention\ A}$ is the cost of the intervention for which the average CE ratio is calculated. This is often expressed in the literature as the *program cost* and shows what amount of funding would be needed to conduct the intervention. As mentioned previously, program costs can also include the costs of side effects associated with the intervention and the costs to participants (depending on the perspective of the analysis).

Other components of the net–cost equation for the numerator of the average CE ratio are the cost of the disease and productivity losses averted as a result of the intervention. The costs averted are as follows:

$$Disease\ and\ Productivity\ Costs\ Averted = (Cost_{Disease\ 0} + Cost_{Productivity\ Losses\ 0}) - (Cost_{Disease\ A} + Cost_{Productivity\ Losses\ A})$$

where $Cost_{Disease\ 0} + Cost_{Productivity\ Losses\ 0}$ are the costs of the disease at the baseline state and $Cost_{Disease\ A} + Cost_{Productivity\ Losses\ A}$ are the costs of the disease that still occur after the intervention is implemented.

The denominator of the average CE ratio is the total number of health outcomes prevented by the intervention

$$Total\ Health\ Outcomes\ Prevented = Outcomes_0 - Outcomes_A$$

where $Outcomes_0$ is the total number of outcomes that occur at the baseline and $Outcomes_A$ is the total number of outcomes that occur after the intervention is implemented.

Based on the above, the formula for the average CE ratio for an intervention is as follows:

$$Average\ CE\ Ratio = \frac{(Intervention\ Cost - Disease\ Cost\ Averted)}{Total\ Health\ Outcomes\ Prevented}$$

When the baseline is "no program," an alternative formula for calculating the average CE ratio that produces the same result can be used.

$$Average\ CE\ ratio = \frac{(Total\ Cost_A - Total\ Cost_0)}{(Total\ Outcomes_0 - TotalOutcomes_A)}$$

where *Total Cost* is

$$Total\ Cost = Cost_{Intervention\ A} + Cost_{Disease\ A} + Cost_{Productivity\ Losses\ A}$$

and *Total Outcomes* is simply

$$Total\ Outcomes = Outcomes_A$$

The two formulas are equivalent. Decision-analysis software, however, usually reports the total cost and total number of outcomes for each intervention and, thus, uses the latter formula. This formula was used to calculate the average CE ratios in Table 9.2.

The average CE ratio provides useful information about the overall affordability of an intervention. In contrast, the marginal CE ratio provides information on the change in cost–effectiveness as a result of expansion or contraction of an intervention and should often be considered in conjunction with an intervention's average CE ratio. Figure 9.3 illustrates this concept. At low vaccination coverage rates (i.e., <70%), the average cost per case prevented is less than 0, indicating that the intervention is cost saving. However, as the percent of people vaccinated increases in this intervention, so too does the cost per case prevented. This suggests that the marginal cost for vaccinating each additional person is relatively high (i.e., the marginal cost per case prevented is much higher than the average cost per case prevented) and should be considered when choosing the optimal level of resource use. Once an efficient (and realistic) level of average cost per case prevented is determined, this amount can be compared to the average CE ratios of other independent interventions that address the same health outcome.

However, prevention-effectiveness studies are also used to examine the efficiency of one strategy relative to another, where the interventions under consideration are mutually exclusive (i.e., are competing for resources). Calculating incremental CE ratios does this. When intervention options are arrayed in order of increasing effectiveness, the incremental CE ratio is the difference in cost of any two adjacent options divided by the differences in number of health outcomes prevented by the two options. The incremental CE ratio is generally reported as the additional cost per additional health outcome prevented and can be interpreted as the incremental cost of producing effectiveness by the intervention compared with the next most effective alternative.[26]

The cost of the intervention in an incremental CE ratio is as follows:

$$\textit{Additional Intervention Cost} = \textit{Cost}_{\text{Intervention B}} - \textit{Cost}_{\text{Intervention A}}$$

where $\textit{Cost}_{\text{Intervention B}}$ is the cost of the intervention for which the incremental CE ratio is calculated and $\textit{Cost}_{\text{Intervention A}}$ is the cost of the next less effective intervention.

Other components of the numerator of the incremental CE ratio are the additional cost of the disease and productivity losses averted as a result of the intervention:

Table 9.2   Incremental Cost–Effectiveness (CE) Ratio for Programs A and B

Mutually Exclusive Intervention	Total Outcomes (Life Years)	Total Costs	Incremental CE Ratio (Cost/Life Year)
Program A	10	$50,000	—
Program B	11	$170,000	$120,000

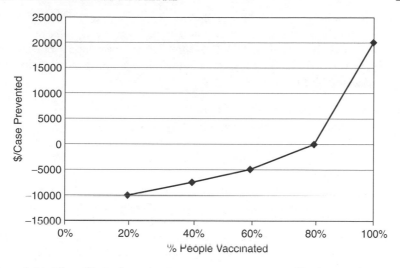

Figure 9.3   The effect of vaccination coverage on cost–effectiveness.

$$Additional\ Disease\ Cost\ Averted = (Cost_{Disease\ A} + Cost_{Productivity\ Losses\ A}) -$$
$$(Cost_{Disease\ B} + Cost_{Productivity\ Losses\ B})$$

where $Cost_{Disease\ A} + Cost_{Productivity\ Losses\ A}$ are the costs of the disease at the adjacent option and $Cost_{Disease\ B} + Cost_{Productivity\ Losses\ B}$ are the costs of the disease
that still occur after the more effective intervention is implemented.

The denominator of the incremental CE ratio is the additional number of
health outcomes prevented by the more effective intervention:

$$Additional\ Health\ Outcomes\ Prevented = Outcomes_A - Outcomes_B$$

where $Outcomes_A$ is the total number of cases that occur after implementation of
the adjacent option and $Outcomes_B$ is the total number of cases that occur after the
more effective intervention is implemented.

Based on the above, the formula for the incremental CE ratio for an intervention
is as follows:

$$Incremental\ CE\ Ratio = \frac{(Additional\ Intervention\ Cost - Additional\ Disease\ Cost\ Averted)}{Additional\ Health\ Outcomes\ Prevented}$$

As with average CE ratios, an alternative formula for calculating the incremental
CE ratio produces the same result:

$$Incremental\ CE\ ratio = \frac{(Total\ Cost_B - Total\ Cost_A)}{(Total\ Outcomes_A - Total\ Outcomes_B)}$$

where *Total Cost* is the sum of the cost of each intervention and the cost of the disease that still occurs after the intervention is implemented and *Total Outcomes* is the total number of outcomes that occur after the intervention is implemented. The incremental CE ratio in Table 9.2 comparing program B to program A was calculated using this formula.

Exclusion of Dominated Alternatives

Because interventions are arrayed in order of increasing effectiveness to calculate incremental CE ratios (and average CE ratios when comparing to a baseline), this calculation requires comparison with the next most effective mutually exclusive alternative under consideration (or the next most effective independent program in the case of average CE ratios). If an intervention is both less effective and more costly than the next most effective alternative, the intervention is considered "strongly dominated" and eliminated from consideration of funding on economic grounds. Table 9.3 illustrates this case. Programs A through C are mutually exclusive programs competing for funding and are first arrayed in increasing order of effectiveness. Since program B is both less effective and more costly than program C, the result is a negative incremental CE ratio for program C.

While a negative CE ratio means an intervention is unambiguously cost-saving and more effective, interpretation of the magnitude is not straightforward. A large increase in effectiveness over the preceding intervention will make the denominator of the CE ratio larger and, therefore, reduce the CE ratio for any given numerator. This reduces the cost per additional unit of outcome when the CE ratio is positive and the apparent savings per additional unit of outcome when the CE ratio is negative. However, in the case of a cost-saving intervention, the smaller CE ratio would point to a more effective intervention; thus, the magnitude of the ratio is less meaningful. Because interpretation of the negative CE ratio is misleading, the program that is less effective and more costly should be eliminated from further funding considerations on economic grounds and is considered strongly dominated. Once the strongly dominated program is eliminated, the incremental CE ratios can be recalculated accordingly, where program C is now compared to program A in Table 9.4.

An intervention can also be dominated when its incremental CE ratio is higher than that of the next most effective intervention. This is known as *extended* or *weak dominance* and is interpreted to mean that effectiveness is produced at a higher marginal cost.[27] In other words, at least two of the alternative interventions would be more cost–effective than the alternative under consideration. For example, sup-

Table 9.3   Analysis of Mutually Exclusive
Programs

Mutually Exclusive Intervention	Total Outcomes (Life Years)	Total Costs	Incremental CE Ratio (Cost/Life Year)
Program A	10	$50,000	—
Program B	11	$170,000	$120,000
Program C	15	$130,000	– $10,000

Table 9.4   Analysis of Mutually Exclusive Programs after Elimination of Strongly Dominated Program (Program B)

Mutually Exclusive Intervention	Total Outcomes (Life Years)	Total Costs	Incremental CE Ratio (Cost/Life Year)
Program A	10	$50,000	—
Program C	15	$130,000	$20,000

pose that a fourth mutually exclusive program, program D, is now under consideration in our hypothetical example (Table 9.5). Because programs are arrayed in order of increasing effectiveness, program D is incrementally compared to program C. Because program C's incremental CE ratio is higher than the next most effective alternative, i.e., program D, this means that there at least two programs (in this case, programs A and D) that would provide a more cost–effective result; therefore, program C should be eliminated because of weak dominance. Once the weakly dominated program is eliminated, the incremental CE ratios can be recalculated accordingly, where program D is now compared to program A (Table 9.6).

Sensitivity Analysis
The final step in analyzing the model is to conduct sensitivity analyses on the variables that have uncertain values or that may change in different population settings. The types of strategy for sensitivity analysis are presented in Chapter 7.

Advantages of using decision-analysis software are that the capacity for sensitivity analysis is built into the programs and graphic displays of results are available. When using spreadsheet models or mathematical computation software, sensitivity analysis can also be performed but it is usually a more cumbersome process, especially when conducting two- or three-way sensitivity analyses. Setting up the equations necessary for threshold analysis in a spreadsheet can also be difficult and time-consuming. Regardless of the platform used for model construction, sensitivity analyses are an extremely important part of the decision analysis because CEA is often conducted under conditions of uncertainty. The researcher must make assumptions about probabilities and costs when data are incomplete.

Sensitivity analyses should be performed on variables in the model for which un-

Table 9.5   Analysis of an Additional Mutually Exclusive Program

Mutually Exclusive Intervention	Total Outcomes (Life Years)	Total Costs	Incremental CE Ratio (Cost/Life Year)
Program A	10	$50,000	—
Program C	15	$130,000	$20,000
Program D	30	$200,000	$4666

Table 9.6   Analysis after Exclusion of Strongly and
Weakly Dominated Programs (Programs B and C)

Mutually Exclusive Intervention	Total Outcomes (Life Years)	Total Costs	Incremental CE Ratio (Cost/Life Year)
Program A	10	$50,000	—
Program D	30	$200,000	$7500

certainty exists. By varying the value of a probability or cost systematically, sensitivity analysis makes it possible to identify the variables that have the greatest impact on the output of the model. This enables the researcher to identify research priorities. If changing the value of a variable about which there is a great deal of uncertainty has a substantial impact on the outcome of the model, a study can be designed to collect data to reduce uncertainty about the value or range of values for that particular variable. However, if substantial changes in the value of an uncertain variable have little impact on the outcome, research resources might be better allocated elsewhere. Some decision-analysis software can do *tornado diagrams*, which are graphical presentations of several one-way sensitivity analyses. Tornado diagrams show the change in the outcome or the cost of the optimal intervention as given variables are varied over their ranges. It is graphically apparent to which variables the outcome or cost value is most sensitive. This can aid in the selection of variables for more elaborate sensitivity analyses. Multiple variables can be varied simultaneously in two- and three-way sensitivity analyses, and their joint impacts can be evaluated. One factor to remember when doing multivariate sensitivity analyses is that the probability of a "best-case" or "worst-case" outcome (where several variables are simultaneously at the high or low end of the ranges used in the analysis) is less than the probability of any one variable being at the high or low end individually. For example, if data exist to use 95% confidence intervals as ranges for sensitivity analysis, the likelihood of both variables simultaneously being at the low end of their range would be much lower than might be apparent, especially if the variables are independent. This does not mean that best- and worst-case results are not relevant but that the selection of ranges for analysis and the presentation of results should be done with care.

Threshold analysis is another form of one-way sensitivity analysis that is sometimes useful in the presentation of results. It shows the value(s) of a given variable for which two or more program options have equal outcomes or costs. Threshold analysis can be used to show under which set of parameter conditions the rank order of interventions remains constant. This is particularly useful in determining under which set of circumstances an intervention is the most cost–effective. For example, universal vaccination may be the most cost–effective strategy when disease incidence is high. However, where the disease incidence is low, a targeted approach may be more cost–effective. Threshold analysis can be used to determine the disease incidence at which it becomes cost effective to switch strategies.

Sensitivity analysis is a critical component of a CEA, and the results and their implications must be included in the presentation of the study.

PRESENTING COST–EFFECTIVENESS ANALYSIS RESULTS

A CEA with an elegant and sophisticated design is of little use if the results are not presented effectively. The CEA is a tool for presenting information in a logical and clear way, to assist in the decision-making process. Presentation is critical. The presentation of a CEA should include the following:

- The study perspective, time frame, and analytic horizon
- The study question
- The assumptions used to build the model
- A description of the interventions
- Evidence of the effectiveness of the interventions
- Identification of all relevant costs
  - Inclusion or exclusion of productivity costs
  - Discount rate
  - Results of incremental analysis
  - Results of sensitivity analysis
  - Discussion of results, addressing all concerns and implications of assumptions

Many reports of CEAs include a graphical representation of the decision tree, although the construction of the tree can also be described in the text. Often, when presenting a tree as a figure in a published article, it is necessary to modify it somewhat to fit space constraints. In any case, sufficient detail should be included to permit a reader to replicate the study and critique the methodology. For readers to gain a better sense of how this type of analysis is presented in the scientific literature, several CE studies are listed in the bibliography.

Recommendation 9.1: The list of intervention strategies in a CEA should include all reasonable options and a baseline comparator.

Recommendation 9.2: Final health-outcome measures should be used in CEAs.

Recommendation 9.3: The numerator in a CUA should include only direct medical and nonmedical costs unless the utility measurement in the denominator does not incorporate productivity losses.

Recommendation 9.4: The QALY measure in the denominator of a CEA should be based on an interval scale and should use preference-based weights. Community preferences for health states are desirable for QALYs used in CEAs that take the societal perspective.

Recommendation 9.5: The numerator of a CEA should include the costs associated with the intervention, adverse health outcomes associated with the intervention, and costs associated with health outcomes that were averted by the intervention. These include medical costs, nonmedical costs, and productivity losses.

Recommendation 9.6: A CEA should report total costs, total effectiveness, incremental or average costs, incremental or average effectiveness, and incremental or average CE ratios. Interventions should be ranked in ascending order of cost and effectiveness. A separate table may be used to report undiscounted health outcomes.

CONCLUSION

A CEA should be used to evaluate interventions that address a single and specific health outcome. Because no attempt is made to assign monetary values to health outcomes, CEA has been widely used in health evaluations. However, care must be taken when using CEA results. The results of CEA are most useful in, and should be limited to, evaluating multiple strategies to prevent a health problem. When analysis across interventions is necessary, CUA is a better choice if adequate quality-of-life measures exist for the health problems being examined.

This chapter has outlined the basic steps in conducting a CEA. Further reading material on the subject of CEA is listed in the bibliography. Two worked examples of CEA in Appendix D provide a supplement to the procedures described in this chapter.

REFERENCES

1. Haddix AC, Hillis SD, Kassler WJ. The cost–effectiveness of azithromycin for *Chlamydia trachomatis* infections in women. *Sex Transm Dis 1995;* 22:174–80.
2. Coffield AB, Maciosek MV, McGinnis JM, et al. Priorities among recommended clinical preventive services. *Am J Prev Med 2001;* 21:1–9.
3. Maciosek MV, Coffield AB, McGinnis JM, et al. Methods for priority setting among clinical preventive services. *Am J Prev Med 2001:* 21:10–9.
4. Torrance GW, Zipursky A. Cost–effectiveness analysis of treatment with anti-D. Cost effectiveness of antepartum prevention of Rh immunization. *Clin Perinatol 1984;* 11(2): 267–81.
5. Williams A. The importance of quality of life in policy decisions. In Walker SR, Rosser RM, eds. *Quality of Life: Assessment and Application.* Lancaster, UK: MTP Press, 1988, pp 279–90.
6. Bush JW, Chen MM, Patrick DL. Health status index in cost–effectiveness: analysis of PKU program. In: Berg R, eds. *Health Status Indexes.* Chicago: Hospital Research and Educational Trust, 1973, pp 172–208.
7. Weinstein MC, Stason WB. Foundations of cost-effectiveness for health and medical practices. *N Engl J Med 1977;* 296:716–21.
8. Cohen DR, Henderson JB. *Health, prevention, and economics.* Oxford: Oxford University Press, 1988.
9. Shepard DS, Thompson MS. First principles of cost–effectiveness analysis in health. *Public Health Rep 1979;* 94:535–43.
10. McNeil BJ, Varady PD, Burrows BA, et al. Measures of clinical efficacy: cost–effectiveness calculations in the diagnosis and treatment of hypertensive renovascular disease. *N Engl J Med 1975;* 293:216–21.

11. Neuhauser D, Lewicki AM. What do we gain from the sixth stool guaiac? *N Engl J Med 1975;* 293:226–8.

12. Weinstein M, Stasson W. Economic considerations in management of mild hypertension. *Ann NY Acad Sci 1976;* 304:424–36.

13. US Congress, Office of Technology Assessment. *A Review of Selected Federal Vaccine and Immunization Policies.* OTA-H-96. Washington DC: Government Printing Office, 1979.

14. Canadian Coordinating Office for Health Technology Assessment. *Guidelines for Economic Evaluation of Pharmaceuticals: Canada,* 2d ed. Ottawa: Canadian Coordinating Office for Health Technology Assessment, 1997.

15. Gold MR, Siegel JE, Russell L, Weinstein MC, eds. *Cost–Effectiveness in Health and Medicine.* New York: Oxford University Press, 1996.

16. National Institute for Clinical Excellence. *Guidance for Manufacturers and Sponsors.* Technology Appraisal Process Series 5. London: National Institute for Clinical Excellence, 2001.

17. Rovira J, Antonanzas F. Economic analysis of health technologies and programmes: a Spanish proposal for methodological standardisation. *Pharmacoeconomics 1995;* 8: 245–52.

18. Drummond MF, Jefferson TO, BMJ Economic Evaluation Working Party. Guidelines for authors and peer reviewers of economic submissions to BMJ. *B Med J 1996;* 313: 275–83.

19. Carande-Kulis VG, Maciosek MV, Briss PA, et al. Methods for systematic reviews of economic evaluations for the *Guide to Community Preventive Services. Am J Prev Med 2000;* 18(Suppl 1):75–91.

20. Emery DD, Schneiderman LJ. Cost–effectiveness analysis in health care. *Hastings Cent Rep 1989,* 8–13.

21. Drummond MF, Stoddard GL, Torrance GW. *Methods for the Economic Evaluation of Health Care Programmes.* Oxford: Oxford University Press, 1987.

22. Kelly AE, Scanlon KS, Mulinare J, et al. Cost–effectiveness of alternative strategies to prevent neural tube defects. In: Gold MR, Siegel JE, Russell LB, Weinstein MC, eds. *Cost–Effectiveness in Health and Medicine.* New York: Oxford University Press, 1996.

23. Teutsch SM. A framework for assessing the effectiveness of disease and injury prevention. *MMWR Morb Mortal Wkly Rep 1992;* 41: i–iv, 1–12.

24. Viscusi WK. The governmental composition of the insurance costs of smoking. *J Law Econ 1999;* 42:575–609.

25. Handsfield HH, Dalu ZA, Martin DH, et al. Multicenter trial of single-dose azithromycin vs. ceftriaxone in the treatment of uncomplicated gonorrhea. *Sex Transm Dis 1994;* 21:107–11.

26. Karlsson G, Johannesson M. The decision rules of cost–effectiveness analysis. *PharmacoEconomics 1996;* 9:113–20.

27. Weinstein MC. Principles of cost–effective resource-allocation in health care organizations. *Int J Technol Assess Health Care 1990;* 6:93–103.

10

Using Economic Evaluations in Decision Making

JOANNA E. SIEGEL
CAROLYN M. CLANCY

The goal of efficiency in the health-care system has broad appeal. Politicians and policy makers periodically have mounted efforts to eliminate or reduce waste. Demands for evidence of the return on investment for health-care services have been prominent for well over a decade, often framed in the context of coverage decisions for health-care services not traditionally reimbursed by insurance policies. Calls for improved cost effectiveness of health-care services are part of the national parlance, reflecting not so much a commitment to the rational allocation of resources as the conviction that improving cost effectiveness, that is, getting value for money, is a widely accepted and legitimate goal. With the increasing emphasis on the quality of medical care, which in part translates into potentially expensive demands for new drugs and technology, redundant safety systems, and greater responsiveness by the health-care system, health-care providers will encounter even greater pressures to improve efficiency, make trade-offs, and develop incentive systems for patients and clinicians to hold down health-care costs.

In large part, clinical preventive and public health policy decisions reflect the pressures confronting the broader health-care system. Preventive services, however, confront an additional set of challenges. Although all medical services are expected to improve quality of life, preventive services are frequently expected to save money as well. Preventive services may pose risks to healthy individuals, so even if expected benefits are great for a large population, individuals may be reluctant to participate in population-wide programs. In addition, because the ultimate beneficiaries of preventive services cannot be identified at the time the services are provided, the quality of and access to services are often difficult to maintain.

Economic evaluations and other prevention-effectiveness studies would appear to be tools of choice for the many involved with health care who directly face budget constraints and complex risk trade-offs. These include public policy makers looking at a besieged Medicare trust fund or at alternative immunization strategies, managed-care administrators and other providers facing steep competitive pressures, clinicians with ever-increasing demands on their time, and patients who must balance their own investments of time and resources in health care. In response to these resource pressures, cost–effectiveness and prevention-effectiveness studies have proliferated in recent years, yet it has been difficult to demonstrate that these studies are widely used by decision makers.

Reasons for reluctance to use these tools are many. Some argue that decision analysis models or cost–effectiveness analyses (CEAs) are too narrow, overlooking many values and other factors influencing real-life decisions and therefore not relevant. Some reject the value of the "transparency" that decision models and CEA bring to decisions, preferring to make decisions on the basis of holistic scenarios. Although economic evaluation is a tool for selecting among competing uses of resources (often situations in which additional expenditures are under consideration), many confuse *cost–effective* with *cost–saving* or *cost–cutting*, perhaps assuming that any policy-level restrictions (organizational, governmental, or otherwise) on the use of health-care resources are undesirable. For these and other reasons, decision makers are often reluctant to admit to using CEA even when they do; in many cases, however, use of economic evaluation is rejected entirely.

This chapter addresses the ideal for the use of CEA and related methods of economic analysis that are integral to prevention effectiveness in policy decisions. It focuses on common critiques of these methods that underlie the reluctance to use them. It describes current and potential efforts to address these critiques, how they may succeed or fail in accomplishing their goals, and implications of these efforts for the practice of prevention effectiveness and other cost–effectiveness studies by analysts. The chapter concludes with recommendations for analysts working to facilitate the use of their research by those in positions to make clinical management, organizational management, and policy decisions. Although much of this chapter focuses on CEA, the general issues apply to other types of economic evaluation and, to a lesser extent, decision analysis.

THE IDEAL: COST–EFFECTIVENESS ANALYSIS TO INFORM POLICY DECISIONS

The ideal for prevention-effectiveness information is that it be a tool to inform decisions, a goal that has been frequently articulated in the literature on technology assessment and CEA. The intention is to differentiate these tools for decision making from the decision-making process itself. Few would accept a mechanistic form of decision making that sought to incorporate all decision elements into an algorithm. The paradigm for using cost–effectiveness information is thus to clarify aspects of a decision through a mathematical analysis with the assumption that this information will be incorporated into a broader decision process.

Prevention effectiveness offers several types of information to the decision maker, including rigorous examination of the evidence for the effectiveness of interventions drawn from clinical trials and observational studies. Meta-analyses and other reviews of the evidence from multiple studies, allowing conclusions about the weight of evidence, are also included (see Chapter 3). Finally, decision, cost–effectiveness, cost–benefit, cost–utility, and similar forms of analysis involve joining studies that describe one link in a chain of events to others to forecast the implications of choices made along the way.

Synthetic prevention-effectiveness tools like decision analysis and economic evaluation are controversial, if for no other reason than that they include the uncertainties in analytic processes and then add more uncertainties, more assumptions. Although even well-accepted components of prevention-effectiveness research (e.g., statistical methods used in clinical trials) contain some controversial elements, many aspects of CEA are much more contested. The ideal task remains to clarify, display, organize, and synthesize information in a form that the decision maker can digest. The analyst can then focus on and debate other aspects of the decision: the ones that are value-dependent, politically sensitive, or require difficult trade-offs among available options.

Prevention-effectiveness information can inform several different types of decision:

- Targeting of interventions (e.g., the varicella vaccine) to the population for which an investment brings the greatest return
- Selecting among strategies (e.g., colonoscopy vs. flexible sigmoidoscopy plus fecal occult blood testing for early detection of colorectal cancer)
- Developing policies for frequency of screening (e.g., the recommendation of biannual vs. triennial pap smears)
- Matching or tailoring interventions to the needs of a specific population, reflecting differences in populations, such as the variation in prevalence of breast cancer by tribe documented among Native-American women[1]
- Prioritizing uses for new funds
- Prioritizing research by modeling the potential downstream outcomes from investments at an early stage or mapping critical gaps in knowledge

These decisions are served by information that reflects the full benefits, harms, and costs of interventions, including costs for following up abnormal results or treating side effects, which are often overlooked in the assessment of preventive interventions. The current task for prevention effectiveness is to address the obstacles to its incorporation into decision making so that it can fulfill its potential to contribute in these ways.

CRITIQUES OF COST–EFFECTIVENESS ANALYSIS AND PROPOSED REMEDIES

Cost–Effectiveness Analysis Methodology is Inconsistent

A very basic critique of CEA has been that the methods used vary across studies, making it difficult to compare the results of one analysis to those from another. Researchers do CEAs differently, and the differences may be arbitrary rather than systematic. The implication is that such studies are not valid (i.e., they do not provide a true picture of the value of interventions) because no one really knows how to do a CEA. On a practical level, it is easy to see that a decision maker will have trouble using a CEA if she or he suspects that the next one that comes along will arrive at a different conclusion purely because another analyst exercises different choices in conducting the analysis.

In fact, there are several issues within this argument. The most basic is a question of whether there is a valid CEA methodology, one which obtains a "true" measure of the cost–effectiveness of an intervention. Some have argued that CEA is a "young" science, still in its formative stages, and ready neither for a systematic articulation of its methods nor use in decision making. In some respects, this is true and in others much less so. The degree of agreement or disagreement on aspects of cost–effectiveness methodology differs from one methodological component to another.[2–4] For example, there is relatively little debate over whether it is correct to use costs rather than charges or to discount costs and quality-adjusted life years (QALYs) at the same rate rather than discounting only one of these, discounting them at different rates, or discounting neither. There is much more debate about appropriate sources for preference weights and other aspects of outcomes measurement and the handling of future costs unrelated to health care.

The variability among analyses reflects not only those areas where it is difficult to define appropriate methods but also cases of poor quality and, until recently, a lack of widely accepted methodological standards. Articles describing the wide variability among analyses in the existing bank of CEAs have identified both instances of poor quality and variability in methods due to analysts' use of multiple defensible methods.[5–8] There are three primary means for addressing the variation in CEA methodology.

Texts

There are now many textbooks describing CEA. To the extent that the variability in CEA can be traced to poor understanding of the methods, texts like these play an important role in improving the practice of CEA, although they do not seek to establish a consistent approach to the same extent as many of the guidelines described in the next section.

The revised *Methods for the Economic Evaluation of Health Care Programmes* is particularly instructive in the practical details of conducting analyses.[9] It addresses cost analysis, CEA, cost–utility analysis (CUA), and cost–benefit analysis (CBA). It also emphasizes the critical analysis of studies, using a general 10-point checklist and numerous examples. Another recently revised text, *Decision Making in Health and Medicine: Integrating Evidence and Values*, instructs on analytic methods used in both decision analysis and CEA.[10] This text provides detail on techniques of outcome valuation, the interpretation and handling of clinical test results, and modeling methods (Markov cohort modeling, Monte Carlo simulations); the section on CEA describes the underlying principles as well as instructions on the calculation of cost–effectiveness ratios.

Guidelines

There have been important efforts to define CEA methods, improve standardization, and reduce variability by establishing guidelines. Although these efforts are consistent with, and in some cases resemble, earlier prescriptions for CEA methods, the newer contributions tend to be more prescriptive and more detailed and many describe areas of controversy more fully, if not always attempting to resolve them.[11–13]

Existing guidelines can be categorized in a number of ways. Drummond[2] and Hjelmgren et al.[14] distinguish methodological guidelines from those required of submissions to inform reimbursement decisions, although these categories clearly overlap. There are also more operational guidelines intended for researchers in managed-care organizations, industry, and international health organizations. The guidelines described here are methodological, intended for use in discussing and improving methods, enhancing the quality of analyses (from a theoretical perspective), and facilitating comparability and consistency.

The Panel on Cost–Effectiveness in Health and Medicine. One of the primary efforts to establish guidelines for the conduct of CEA was undertaken by the Panel on Cost–Effectiveness in Health and Medicine (PCEHM), convened by the U.S. Public Health Service. The panel was initially established to support the conduct and interpretation of CEAs in the area of prevention, but its mandate was broadened when it became clear that the methodological challenges affecting use in prevention applied to the field of CEA more broadly.

The panel's objective was to improve and standardize CEA methodology. It focused on CEAs intending to inform broad resource-allocation decisions, producing a report recommending guidelines for these studies.[15–18] These guidelines, described as a "reference case" set of recommendations, were in some cases drawn from theoretical considerations and in others motivated by practicality, a need for consistency, or other considerations. The reference case analysis is intended to inform resource-allocation decisions, but many of the recommendations apply to CEAs generally, serving as quality standards and helping to make results more comparable.

Canadian Guidelines. In 1997, Canada's Coordinating Office for Health Technology Assessment (CCOHTA) published a second edition of its guidelines on the economic evaluation of pharmaceuticals, which are intended for a variety of uses by governments, manufacturers, and others.[19,20] Although these guidelines focus on pharmaceuticals, their main purpose is to improve the quality and comparability of analyses; the intention is to assist the "doers" of analyses in producing standardized and reliable information for users. The guidelines are detailed and prescriptive, including a separate manual for documenting costs. However, they emphasize that flexibility is needed both in the conduct and in the use of CEAs. Canada does not require the use of these guidelines in drug-regulatory decisions, although they are used in formulary decisions in some provinces.

General Guidelines in Europe. In addition to work at the forefront of submission guidelines (described later), several European countries have developed general guidelines. In Spain, for example, the Ministry of Health commissioned a project for the methodological standardization of economic evaluations of health technologies with the purpose of establishing a higher level of consistency in CEA.[21] These guidelines generally recommend the societal perspective and draw relatively heavily from economic theory in recommending elements to include.[14]

Limitations of Guidelines. Recent guidelines have provided an important contribution to the field of CEA. In the United States, the work of the PCEHM, although the subject of continuing debate, has provided a baseline, one more widely acknowledged than preexisting guidelines in the literature, that has served to focus discussion. In Canada and Australia, where sufficient experience with submission guidelines has accumulated, researchers are beginning to assess their impact.

However, guidelines face some important limitations. First, the jury is still out on the extent to which analysts follow methodological recommendations. Although the PCEHM's work is frequently cited in CEA reports, it is still too early to determine whether those citing it actually follow the guidelines and, if they do, whether improvements in methods or comparability have resulted. A Canadian study of a set of analyses, commissioned by the CCOHTA, was encouraging, concluding that the Canadian guidelines were instrumental in establishing a minimum set of standards, specifically improving uniformity and ensuring a basic level of quality. However, while studies adhered to guidelines fairly consistently in many methodological areas, there was notable divergence in others, particularly perspective and aspects of utility measurement.[20]

Second, adherence to guidelines can only improve the quality and reduce the variability in results to a certain extent. There are both inherent uncertainties and inherent variability in CEA. Sources include the quality of underlying data, the uniqueness of circumstances surrounding the implementation of a studied intervention, and the unavoidable judgments involved in modeling chains of events. Researchers have called for a systematic examination of the reliability of cost–effectiveness methods, for example, by assigning two or more groups to conduct CEAs of the same interventions, to demonstrate the range of results attributable to differences in methods. Although the importance of this source of variability is currently unclear, it remains a concern to researchers and users alike.

Finally, there are concerns about the impact of too much standardization in CEA. Some argue that standardization can lead to a "cookbook" approach to analysis, resulting in analyses that do not reflect the subtleties of real interventions and consequences. Others point to the potential dampening effect of standardization on innovation and advancements in methodology. Also, there are very real concerns that guidelines that are too demanding would make many CEAs too difficult and expensive to conduct. Lessons can be learned from CEAs done at varying levels of detail, if done in a sensible and systematic manner. Thus, very demanding guidelines could essentially prevent the conduct of some valuable studies.

The limitations do not suggest that guidelines are not a good idea. However, guidelines should be flexible and practical and need to evolve over time. Some need to be general and others specific to the different purposes for which CEA can be used. If done well, they will enhance the predictability and credibility of CEA.

Reconciling Cost–Effectiveness Analyses

A different approach to addressing the variability of methods and results in CEA is to reconcile different CEAs on the same topic. This requires analyzing existing studies in detail to determine where methodological differences lie and sometimes adjusting study assumptions and recalculating cost–effectiveness estimates. Brown and Fintor[22] reviewed economic evaluations of mammography and accounted for methodological differences in cost–effectiveness among the studies. Once these differences were accounted for, a much more precise range of cost–effectiveness ratios could be estimated.

The Community Preventive Services Task Force has developed a detailed strategy for synthesizing results from multiple CEAs to inform recommendations on population-based preventive services.[23] To assure basic comparability, this task force established criteria for methodological consistency as a basis for study inclusion. An extensive data-collection instrument is used to extract information from CEAs, and explicit methods are used to adjust results for base year, for categories of costs included or omitted, and for uncertainty. This approach has been applied to vaccination and tobacco interventions.[24,25]

The U.S. Preventive Services Task Force, which reviews evidence and provides recommendations for clinical preventive services, has also described an overall approach to reviewing and synthesizing the cost–effectiveness literature.[26] Cost–effectiveness reviews, which are designed to address specific questions, supplement information on the evidence of effectiveness of services for different age groups, elucidate the advantages of services delivered at different frequencies, or compare the value of different technologies targeted to the same health outcome (e.g., sigmoidoscopy, fecal occult blood testing, and colonoscopy for colorectal cancer screening). The task force has piloted a process and an instrument for abstracting CEAs, based on the work of the Community Preventive Services Task Force and other sources, which includes a system for rating the methodological quality of studies.

Cost–Effectiveness Analysis Is a "Black Box"

Cost–effectiveness analysis is a complex methodology. Although the steps for calculating a cost–effectiveness ratio can be summarized simply, the interpretation of what is or is not included in a given category and the calculation of each step are almost never straightforward. Estimates of effectiveness for an intervention and its alternatives often draw from numerous published studies and are combined in a model that requires compromises, inferences, and extrapolations from existing data. Cost estimates are gathered from administrative or other existing databases, which generally do not provide exactly the estimates required; as a result, they are adjusted to reflect true costs instead of charges, the patient population or setting of interest, and inflation. There are numerous ways of assessing outcome values, and choices must be made concerning the type of measure, source of preferences, methods of scaling responses, and other variables.

It is one thing to do a CEA correctly, that is, in a consistent, generally accepted, valid, and reliable way. It is another to communicate design and other features of the analysis to a reviewer or, especially, a decision maker. The broad initial steps in the analysis (decisions about the perspective of the analysis and the definition of the intervention and alternatives that can profoundly alter its outcome), characteristics of the analysis such as those described above, and results must be presented in a clear, comprehensive, and comprehensible manner if the consumer is to understand and correctly interpret the analysis.

Recommendations for how to report CEA so that it is accessible to its readership appear in the literature and as a component of guidelines (both journal submission guidelines and methodological guidelines). In addition to these comprehensive guidelines, some groups have addressed the reporting of a specific component of CEA. One such example addresses the reporting of utility assessment.[27] Two sets of comprehensive reporting guidelines are described below.

Panel on Cost–Effectiveness in Health and Medicine

The PCEHM report includes recommendations on reporting CEAs.[15,18] The goal of these recommendations is to improve the transparency of analyses, aid the analyst in assuring the completeness of the report, and encourage the presentation of comparable results. The report includes a checklist for authors, which covers the major inputs to a CEA (Table 10.1). Authors are asked to describe the framework of the analysis, including the general design, the target population, program descriptors, and bounds. A Data and Methods section includes a description of sources of data, the approach to combining data on costs, effects, preference weights, and adjustments. The Results section includes model validation, a specified set of reference case results, and sensitivity analyses. (As described earlier, the PCEHM's suggested reference case analysis takes the societal perspective and follows a set of methodological recommendations.) Analysts are asked to present disaggregated results as well as aggregated cost–effectiveness ratios, to provide a better sense of the streams of costs and health outcomes resulting from the intervention and comparators. The Discussion section includes summaries of results designed to help readers interpret the study findings, as well as ethical issues, study limitations, and a discussion of the relevance of results in specific policy contexts. These elements bridge the technical aspects of the analysis and the policy questions.

British Medical Journal *Guidelines*

In 1995, the *British Medical Journal* convened a working group with the goal of improving the quality of submitted and published articles, which published guidelines for CEA and related studies. Although oriented toward the reporting of analyses, these guidelines also serve, to some extent, a methodological role, which is not surprising given that an analysis must be conducted using appropriate methods for these methods to be reported. The emphasis of the guidelines, however, is to communicate to authors and reviewers the components that should be explained in the report, for reviewers and ultimately readers to be able to ascertain the quality of the study and interpret it correctly.

The guidelines prescribe the reporting of study design, data collection, and analysis and interpretation of results, giving the rationale for each recommendation. The guidelines are summarized in a checklist for referees, also intended for use by authors.

The *British Medical Journal* guidelines emphasize transparency in reporting, accomplished through a detailed and systematic description of components of the study and the reporting of disaggregated results in addition to summary ratios. The authors argue that transparency in reporting is essential for the reinterpreta-

Table 10.1 Reporting Checklist, Panel on Cost–Effectiveness in Health and Medicine[15]

1. Framework
   Background of the problem
   General framing and design of the analysis
   Target population for intervention
   Other program descriptors (e.g., care setting, model of delivery, timing of intervention)
   Description of comparator programs
   Boundaries of the analysis
   Time horizon
   Statement of the perspective of the analysis
2. Data and methods
   Description of event pathway
   Identification of outcomes of interest
   Description of model used
   Modeling assumptions
   Diagram of event pathway/model
   Software used
   Complete information on sources of effectiveness data, cost data, and preference weights
   Methods for obtaining estimates of effectiveness, costs, and preferences
   Critique of data quality
   Statement of year of costs
   Statement of method used to adjust costs for inflation
   Statement of type of currency
   Source and methods for obtaining expert judgment
   Statement of discount rates
3. Results
   Results of model validation
   Reference case results (discounted and undiscounted): total costs and effectiveness, incremental costs and effectiveness, and incremental cost–effectiveness ratios
   Results of sensitivity analyses
   Other estimates of uncertainty, if available
   Graphical representation of results
   Aggregate cost and effectiveness information
   Disaggregated results, as relevant
   Secondary analyses using 5% discount rate
   Other secondary analyses, as relevant
4. Discussion
   Summary of reference case results
   Summary of sensitivity of results to assumptions and uncertainties in the analysis
   Discussion of analytic assumptions with important ethical implications
   Limitations of the study
   Relevance of study results for specific policy questions or decisions
   Results of related cost–effectiveness analyses
   Distributive implications of an intervention

tion of cost–effectiveness results necessary for decision makers to apply results to their particular settings. Guidance is also given on the appropriate interpretation of results, including cautions regarding comparisons among studies and admonitions to authors to be "modest" about the generalizability of their results and otherwise conservative in conducting their analyses.

The Information Provided by a Single Cost–Effectiveness Study Is Incomplete, and it is Difficult to Use Multiple Studies Because They Are Hard to Compare

Cost–effectiveness studies provide an estimate of cost per unit of health outcome, essentially the price of an intervention. For price information to be meaningful, a decision maker must be able to compare interventions. This comparison may be implicit, that is, the decision maker may have a general sense of what "price" represents a reasonable expenditure. In CEA, anchoring figures of $50,000 or $100,000 per QALY have been used. These figures are based on the cost effectiveness of interventions in wide use or sometimes on the precedent established when others cite certain CEA cut-off values. They are more or less arbitrary thresholds and have been critiqued for the same reasons any existing price cut-off would be: the cut-off does not reflect inflation, opportunities change over time, or budgets change over time.

An explicit approach to providing comparisons that is gaining in use is the presentation of *league tables*. League tables, named after the tables showing British soccer league standings, list interventions and their cost–effectiveness ratios in rank order. A 1995 league table of life-saving interventions compared health-care, environmental, occupational health, and other interventions based on costs per year of life saved.[28] Chapman and colleagues[29] published a league table drawn from 228 CUAs and containing 647 interventions; a league table containing a subset of clinical preventive services is also available.[30] The cost–effectiveness ratios included in league tables are usually adjusted to improve comparability, at a minimum by correcting for currency differences and inflation. Some authors critique or select the studies they include based on standards such as those of the PCEHM;[31] others do not.[32]

Although the concept of a list of interventions organized by cost–effectiveness is attractive, league tables must be interpreted with caution. The source studies in a league table will generally use different methods and include different outcomes, probabilities, or costs. They may also focus on different populations and use a variety of comparators. It is therefore difficult to devise a league table that is relevant and internally consistent.[33–35] Presumably for this reason, some databases containing CEAs make no attempt to rank interventions. The NHS' extensive Economic Evaluations Database of the U.K. National Health Service (NHS) is an example.[36]

Other approaches have also been used to incorporate data on the cost effectiveness of multiple interventions into information on alternatives and priorities for resource use. The Partnership for Prevention used estimates of clinical preventive burden as well as cost effectiveness to set priorities across the 30 clinical preventive services found to be effective by the U.S. Preventive Services Task Force.[37–39] The project used existing CEAs when possible, selecting those conducted using the PCEHM-recommended methods to enhance comparability and adjusting them in a systematic fashion. When no studies were available, a simplified model was used to estimate cost–effectiveness, again following the PCEHM guidelines. Similarly, the authors used a standardized approach to calculate the clinical preventable burden for each service. The authors presented the quintile ranks for the clinical preventive services on the dimensions of clinical preventable burden and cost–effectiveness, as well as a combined score. Lawrence[40] describes the importance of this type of information, which allows decision makers to reframe the discussion of resource allocation and priority setting at a population level rather than as a negotiation among the many interest groups.

Some researchers have experimented with optimization models to consider combinations of interventions based on cost–effectiveness. Granata and Hillman[41] demonstrated the feasibility of a decision-modeling technique combined with spreadsheet-based optimization to examine the use of several preventive services in scenarios with differing resource constraints. Wang and others[42] compared a model that optimized health outcome under different resource constraints with a model that allocated resources based on cost–effectiveness for services recommended by the United States Preventive Services Task Force. Like many of the league-table projects, these models have been limited by the difficulties of obtaining comparable cost–effectiveness information.

Cost–Effectiveness Analyses Are too General; They Do Not Apply to my Specific Decision

The objection that CEAs are not relevant to a specific decision-making situation is frequently heard in the United States. Both decision makers and analysts take issue with studies that use a perspective that differs from the one used by the decision maker and, as a result, include categories of costs and outcome that do not reflect their interests. Another frequent concern is a target population that does not match the actual population in which an intervention may be implemented, so the analysis is viewed as "theoretical" rather than specific to the decisions at hand.

Those wishing to develop more targeted analyses, usually for managed-care organizations or even government payors, have directed these critiques at the PCEHM and others who have recommended the use of a societal perspective. (It should be noted that the PCEHM does not recommend against perspectives other than the societal but suggest that an analysis from the societal perspective be performed alongside analyses using a different perspective, both to contribute to the bank of CEAs useful for broad resource allocation and to illustrate differences in the perspectives.) Supporters of the societal perspective have argued in turn that it is the societal perspective that captures "true" cost–effectiveness; they suggest that more attention be devoted to developing better processes for using societal CEAs.[43] Because the PCEHM's recommendation to use the societal perspective appears to be frequently ignored, however, it may be useful to develop guidelines that are more relevant to these various organizations. This is particularly true if one believes that more systematic decision making on the part of these individual actors improves the use of CEA and health-care decisions more generally, propositions that merit consideration.

In the absence of well-targeted CEAs, some have suggested that an understanding of the details of economic evaluations be used to interpret and adapt studies to the needs of specific users.[44] Thus, even when cost–effectiveness results are not relevant to a particular situation, the dynamics and processes demonstrated in a cost–effectiveness or decision model may provide valuable insights. For example, a study of an human immunodeficiency virus preventive intervention demonstrated that such interventions are likely to be most effective in low- and medium-risk populations, rather than in very high-risk populations, where the frequency of exposure undermines the effectiveness of the intervention.[45] Similarly, if a cost–effectiveness result turns on a 5% rate of adherence to a counseling intervention, a clinic with a higher rate can interpret the results or revise it using different assumptions.

The problem of lack of relevance to a specific decision-making context is considerably less salient in European and other countries, where national (or provincial) governments have suggested or required the submission of economic information as part of the drug-formulary system and have developed submission guidelines for economic evaluations. Like the more general guidelines described above, these submission guidelines describe, recommend, and may require what is considered "good practice" in CEA. Unlike the general guidelines, the impetus behind these is to improve the ability of CEAs to inform a specific purpose. These bodies usually dictate specifics of how to conduct analyses (types of cost information to include, sources for cost information, discount rate, analytic perspective), balancing concerns for degrees of theoretical correctness with clear imperatives for practicality. The best-established submission guidelines are those for the assessment of pharmaceuticals for inclusion on national health system formularies in Australia and Ontario, Canada.[46,47] The United Kingdom's National Institute for Clinical Excellence (NICE), which provides guidance to the NHS, has developed comprehensive guidelines for submissions to its technology appraisal program.[48]

Although political controversy has prevented U.S. government agencies from formally incorporating cost–effectiveness information into technology coverage or approval processes related to health care, a few private-sector organizations have begun developing submission guidelines similar to other countries' national/provincial government guidelines for their own review processes that include cost–effectiveness information. Regence BlueShield in Washington State and Blue Cross and Blue Shield of Colorado and Nevada require pharmaceutical manufacturers to submit dossiers to their Pharmacy and Therapeutics Committees when requesting new pharmaceutical listings and changes to the formulary status of existing products.[49,50] The dossiers include model-based projections of the impact of new drugs on plan-specific health and economic outcomes, as well as product information, clinical trial information, and other economic studies. In 2000, the Academy for Managed Care Pharmacy (AMCP) released a format for managed-care formulary submissions based on these earlier efforts, intended to standardize the requirements for formulary submissions as well as improve the consistency and quality of drug-review processes across the managed-care industry.[51]

Cost–Effectiveness Analyses Cannot Be Trusted

Often, CEAs are conducted or funded by organizations that have a financial or other interest in their outcome. Because there are many opportunities for methodological discretion in the conduct of a CEA, there are as many opportunities to slant an analysis in a desired direction. Many potential consumers feel that since CEAs are complex and difficult to validate, given the potential for bias, it is better simply to throw them out.

This argument has been made loud and clear. In an editorial in the *Annals of Internal Medicine,* economist Robert Evans[52] described bias as inherent in the structure of pharmacoeconomic studies, where researchers have professional and economic incentives to do CEAs of drugs and pharmaceutical companies have a large economic interest in the outcomes of such research. He decried measures (in this case, ethical guidelines) that would lend these studies a more scientific appearance. A *Journal of the American Medical Association* editorial sounded a similar theme with respect to analyses sponsored by drug companies, the largest and fastest growing area of cost–effectiveness research.[53] The editorial policy of the *New England Journal of Medicine* addresses issues of credibility in CEA more generally but is also largely motivated by the potential for bias in the financial arrangements between drug company sponsors and CEA authors.[54] Citing the discretionary nature of methods used to analyze cost–effectiveness, the journal editors argued that CEAs resemble review articles and imposed restrictions on them.

A primary means of addressing the potential for bias in CEA has been the promulgation of ethical standards, including guidelines for disclosure of financial and other interests. In 1995, the Task Force on Principles for Economic Analysis of Health Care Technology, a group comprised of representatives from the pharmaceutical industry, health-care organizations, and academia, produced a set of recommendations to promote the independence of researchers conducting economic analyses of health-care technology. The task force recommendations emphasize study design and implementation issues, such as the specification of a study protocol prior to initiation and data access, as well as articulating guidelines for financial relationships and disclosure.[55] Formulary submission guidelines frequently contain explicit requirements for disclosure of relationships and other requirements intended to further researcher independence. The CCOHTA guidelines, for example, require CEAs to state the funding and leadership arrangements, listing all key participants and describing administrative arrangements. Investigators are to have independence regarding methodological and publication decisions.

Another means for users to protect themselves from bias in CEA is to develop expertise in evaluating CEAs and detecting bias. Most of the institutions that systematically use CEA rely on health economists to review them. The NHS is a prime example; its NICE employs and contracts with health economists who review evidence of cost–effectiveness and conduct their own CEAs. The NHS Economic Evaluation Database, which contains critical reviews of economic evaluations in the literature commissioned from health economists worldwide, is also designed to inform NHS decisions.[36] In Ontario, Canada, the Drug Quality and Therapeutics Committee, which reviews health economic analyses for the Ministry of Health and Long-Term Care, includes members with expertise in health economics as well as pharmacology and medicine.

In many cases, it is not practical or feasible for organizations to maintain expertise in health economics in-house or through individual contracts. Organizations smaller than a national or provincial government clearly will not have the same level of resources to devote to the review of clinical economics materials as existing review committees. A survey of medical journal editors found a majority using referees without formal training in either health economics or economics to review economic evaluations.[56]

Consumers of CEAs like these are in need of an institution with the capacity and expertise to conduct reviews on a regular basis. Some have called for the establishment of a national institute that would serve as an "authoritative, independent source of reputable research" regarding drugs.[57] In 2000, Blue Cross and Blue Shield initiated a nonprofit research organization, RxIntelligence, designed to serve a similar function. RxIntelligence provides information comparing the costs and effectiveness of pharmaceuticals to its subscribers; the information is provided in a series of reports rather than on demand. If current trends continue, there may well be opportunities for additional services of this type.

The Assumptions Inherent in Cost–Effectiveness Analysis and Many Implications of Its Implementation Are Ethically Problematic, Making It an Ineffective Tool for Real-World Decision Making

There are a number of ethical issues that present challenges for the use of CEA for all health-care services, and most of these are highly relevant to its use in assessing the cost–effectiveness of preventive services. Some of these issues represent fundamental philosophical tensions related to assumptions that are built into cost–effectiveness models. These may be particularly problematic when they are obscured within a CEA. Additional objections derive from the different uses of CEA, while still others are a by-product of health-care delivery in the United States, in which combined public and private financing coupled with frequent movement of individuals across insurers telescopes the time horizon and the scope of relevant analyses.

A fundamental tenet of CEA is that maximizing and aggregating benefits over a population (i.e., maximizing QALYs) demonstrates the policy choice that provides the greatest good for the greatest number. A primary objection to this premise questions the assumption, critical to CEA, that all health benefits can be put on a cardinal scale and summed. Some benefits, it is argued, are incommensurable with others; for example, prevention of a disability is not comparable with prolongation of life. A second problem is that decision makers, or those they represent, may not value equally the benefits accruing to various members of society. Thus, a benefit aggregated over one population subgroup (e.g., the elderly or disabled adults) might be valued more or less than an equivalent benefit to another subgroup. Third, some widely held values may be entirely ignored in CEA. One example is the moral obligation of present generations to ensure the well-being of future ones. This issue is side-stepped in CEA; an analysis may directly compare the value of benefits to a future population with benefits accruing to a (different) current population. Because there is no "step" in CEA requiring a decision with respect to these and many other values, it may not be evident, even to experienced consumers of CEAs, that a decision on these values is in fact implicit within a particular cost–effectiveness ratio.

Although some problematic assumptions are inherent in the cost–effectiveness model, other ethical concerns follow from choices in CEA methods. For example, when analysts use QALYs as the measure of health outcome (as recommended by the PCEHM and other guidelines), they must choose a method for estimating the value of health outcomes. This introduces questions of whose preferences to use. Analysts may find it more practical to ask clinicians about their preferences than patients and have argued that clinicians know more about a given health outcome. However, usually, it is not a physician's QALYs that are being maximized. Whether to use preferences of people who have experienced an illness or disability versus those who have not is also frequently debated. The preferences of these groups have been shown to differ systematically. A related but larger issue is whether the use of QALYs discriminates against persons with disabilities by attaching a lower value to years of life potentially saved by an intervention.

Some of the issues arising in the application of CEA can be illustrated in the context of preventive services. As described earlier, CEA provides information and a framework for assessing the value of specific preventive services. In practical terms, CEA may be more appealing to decision makers for addressing questions of *which* strategy to use for preventing or detecting a condition early, rather than for addressing questions of whether to invest in an intervention. The latter are controversial because they require explicit consideration of difficult issues, such as the value of a possible cure compared with that of preventing a disease or that of a benefit to an identified individual with a visible need versus a benefit spread across a population. It is easier to use CEA to inform decisions such as what sequence of tests should be used to detect colon cancer, what type of smoking-cessation intervention program should be implemented in a particular setting, and other questions where distributional considerations are less prominent.

Even comparisons of which strategy to use, however, are not without controversy. At the most basic level, CEA assumes that the goal of a public health or health care intervention is to maximize health outcomes (years of life, QALYs) on average over the population affected. In reality, this assumption stands in sharp contrast to what stakeholders may perceive as equitable. An important example was documented in a study that asked medical ethicists, prospective jurors, and experts in medical decision making to choose between two screening tests for colon cancer for a low-risk population. One test was more cost-effective but too expensive to be given to everyone; the other could be given to everyone but was less effective. Asked to choose between the more cost–effective test applied to half the population (projected to save 1100 lives) and the alternative that could be given to everyone (projected to save 1000 lives), the majority of participants favored the second test, that is, equity over efficiency.[58] Given these and other results, it is not clear whether a cost–effective strategy that provides services to those at highest risk is acceptable to most people. Moreover, since people often change health plans (by choice or requirement), practical strategies for determining community preferences for these fluid "communities," as recommended by the PCEHM, remain elusive.

The development and evaluation of potential remedies for reconciling the ethical tensions inherent in the use of CEA are essential to its widespread application and represent an area of active research. For example, a recent study suggested that framing effects influence elicitation of public preferences; the authors found that inconsistent approaches to preference assessment may amplify apparent preferences for equity at the expense of efficiency.[59] One proposed solution calls for the assessment of societal value, that is, the strength of public preferences for giving priority to different health-care programs, independently from individual assessment of health-related quality of life, with both measures factoring in decisions.[60] Other strategies include the development of mathematical measures of equity so that the effects of policy decisions can be more readily compared.[61]

DISCUSSION

Cost–effectiveness analysis and related methods of economic evaluation provide one of the few indicators of the relative "price" of an intervention for use in decisions, albeit a price that can be interpreted only given certain assumptions. Whether this information, given these assumptions, is useful with regard to a specific decision is difficult to judge in the abstract. It may often be useful; in other cases, the combination of the underlying assumptions and the characteristics of a particular decision may render it less relevant. What is important is to use CEA with full knowledge of both the assumptions it includes and the considerations it overlooks. Decision makers can then use it when they believe it to be relevant to the decision and, like other types of information, discard it when it is not helpful. Although debates are frequently cast in terms of all-or-nothing use of these methods, few would argue that this piece of information is *never* relevant or even that some other formulation of the information is more generally valuable.

A critical challenge and opportunity for those who wish to apply CEA to decision making is to identify those decisions where the synthesis of information that CEA offers is most useful; that is, in the reverse approach to considering barriers to the use of CEA, the challenge is to identify opportunities for its application while articulating the assumptions and the ethical implications of those assumptions for both individuals and populations. It is also important to remember that CEA is not intended to incorporate all aspects of a decision but, ideally, to quantify the parts that can be quantified. The ethical and political context should be a clear and separate part of the decision, regardless of how the ethical aspects of CEA are handled.

There are specific measures that analysts can take when conducting CEA so that it can be used to its full potential but remain within the limitations of the methodology.

1. Analyses should heed methodological standards, departing from them only with adequate justification and when departures add significantly to the usefulness of the analysis or the development of the field. Particularly in the area of cost–effectiveness, which is regarded as a new field and one in which rigor is lacking, attention to accepted standards of practice is crucial.
2. Analysts need to look for ways to put the results of economic evaluations in a decision context. Elements of the design are critical in this regard, but equally important are thoughtful reviews and discussion of existing evidence and related CEAs. In general, it is important to tailor analyses to the decision maker. This is an important lesson of recent guidelines.
3. In a related sense, analysts should be aware of a range of issues surrounding a decision, including issues of feasibility, legal context, and ethics. These can be raised and addressed in the Discussion section of a CEA, and both the original design and sensitivity analyses can take likely concerns of a decision maker into account to the extent possible and appropriate.
4. The field as a whole needs to look further for ways to guard against bias. In individual cases, consumers should employ reviewers knowledgeable about a cost–effectiveness question to review analyses and should heed minimum disclosure requirements to safeguard against bias.

Some advocates for CEA as a decision-making tool have observed that developing the framework for a specific analysis may be equally or more useful to decision makers than the "answer." That is, the process of clarifying options, risks, and benefits may be more valuable (and much more rapidly accomplished) than the iterative processes used to refine the precision of specific estimates. An example is a CEA focused on primary angioplasty for persons having an acute heart attack, which was conducted by researchers at a large group model health-maintenance organization.[62] The initial framework for the analysis quickly revealed that the cost-effectiveness of this intervention was likely to be quite dependent on the institution performing the procedure because of the superior outcomes obtained in high-volume institutions. Discussion of this result revealed a conflict, namely, that selective contracting for this procedure ran counter to longstanding values of the health-maintenance organization. In this instance, preliminary work helped decision makers to understand the opposing values and focus their attention relatively quickly. When full-fledged analyses are necessary to compare strategies or provide an assessment of the value of an intervention, the task remains one of providing sound, unbiased, and comprehensible analyses as well as facilitated means of presenting and interpreting them.

It is unclear whether improved methods of conducting and presenting CEA will ultimately enhance its use. Undoubtedly, some will argue that it makes no difference; that league tables, efforts to combine analyses, or improved standards will not address the more basic reasons that CEA is not used more often or more consistently. However, it is also clear that the use of CEA has grown tremendously in the past decade, motivated by the demands worldwide for information to assist in making difficult choices that affect populations' health and well-being within tightening resource constraints. A notable feature of this movement has been the focusing of CEA from general, "academic" assessments of interventions to more defined analyses commissioned by identifiable decision-making bodies. The CEA method will always have its flaws. The challenge is to improve the tool and its utility in addressing the dilemmas that now confront health-care systems.

REFERENCES

1. Nutting PA, Calonge BN, Iverson DC, Green LA. The danger of applying uniform clinical policies across populations: the case of breast cancer in American Indians. *Am J Public Health 1994;* 84:1631–6.
2. Drummond MF. Guidelines for pharmacoeconomic studies—the ways forward. *Pharmacoeconomics 1994;* 6:493–7.
3. Luce BR, Simpson K. Methods of cost–effectiveness analysis: areas of consensus and debate. *Clin Ther 1995;* 17:109 20.
4. Drummond M, Brandt A, Luce B, Rovira J. Standardizing methodologies for economic evaluation in healthcare: practice, problems, and potential. *Int J Technol Assess Health Care 1993;* 9:26–36.
5. Udvarhelyi S, Colditz GA, Rai A, Epstein AM. Cost–effectiveness and cost–benefit analyses in the medical literature: are the methods being used correctly? *Ann Intern Med 1992;* 116:238–44.
6. Lee JT, Sanchez LA. Interpretation of "cost-effective" and soundness of economic evaluations in the pharmacy literature. *Am J Hosp Pharm 1991;* 48:2622–7.
7. Mason J, Drummond M. Reporting guidelines for economic studies. *Health Econ 1995;* 4:85–94.
8. Gambhir SS, Schwimmer J. Economic evaluation studies in nuclear medicine: a methodological review of the literature. *Q J Nucl Med 2000;* 44:121–37.
9. Drummond MF, O'Brien BJ, Stoddart GL, Torrance GW. *Methods for the Economic Evaluation of Health Care Programmes,* 2d ed. New York: Oxford University Press, 1997.
10. Hunink MGM, Glasziou P, Siegel JE, et al. *Decision Making in Health and Medicine: Integrating Evidence and Values.* New York: Cambridge University Press, 2001.
11. Shepard DS, Thompson MS. First principles of cost-effectiveness analysis in health. *Public Health Rep 1979;*94:535–43.
12. Weinstein MC, Stason WB. Foundations of cost–effectiveness analysis for health and medical practices. *N Engl J Med 1977;* 296:716–21.
13. Office of Technology Assessment, US Congress. *The Implications of Cost–Effectiveness Analysis of Medical Technology.* Washington DC: US Government Printing Office, 1980.
14. Hjelmgren J, Berggren F, Andersson F. Health economic guidelines—similarities, differences and some implications. *Value Health 2001;* 4:225–50.
15. Gold MR, Siegel JE, Russell L, Weinstein MC, eds. *Cost–Effectiveness in Health and Medicine.* New York: Oxford University Press, 1996.
16. Russell LB, Gold MR, Siegel JE, et al., for the Panel on Cost–Effectiveness in Health and Medicine. The role of cost-effectiveness analysis in health and medicine. *JAMA 1996;* 276:1172–7.
17. Weinstein MC, Siegel JE, Gold MR, et al., for the Panel on Cost–Effectiveness in Health and Medicine. Recommendations of the Panel on Cost–Effectiveness in Health and Medicine. *JAMA 1996;* 276:1253–8.

18. Siegel JE, Weinstein MC, Russell LB, Gold MR, for the Panel on Cost-Effectiveness in Health and Medicine. Recommendations for reporting cost-effectiveness analyses. *JAMA 1996;* 276:1339–41.
19. Canadian Coordinating Office for Health Technology Assessment. *Guidelines for Economic Evaluation of Pharmaceuticals: Canada,* 2d ed. Ottawa: Canadian Coordinating Office for Health Technology Assessment, 1997.
20. Baladi JF, Menon D, Otten N. Use of economic evaluation guidelines: 2 years' experience in Canada. *Health Econ 1998;* 7:221–7.
21. Rovira J, Antonanzas F. Economic analysis of health technologies and programmes: a Spanish proposal for methodological standardisation. *Pharmacoeconomics 1995;* 8:245–52.
22. Brown ML, Fintor L. Cost–effectiveness of breast cancer screening: preliminary results of a systematic review of the literature. *Breast Cancer Res Treat 1993;* 25:113–8.
23. Carande-Kulis VG, Maciosek MV, Briss PA, et al. The Task Force on Community Preventive Services. Methods for systematic reviews of economic evaluations for the *Guide to Community Preventive Services. Am J Prev Med 2000;* 18:75–91.
24. Briss PA, Rodewald LE, Hinman AR, et al. Reviews of evidence regarding interventions to improve vaccination coverage in children, adolescents, and adults. *Am J Prev Med* 2000; 18:97–140.
25. Hopkins DP, Briss PA, Ricard CJ, et al. Reviews of evidence regarding interventions to reduce tobacco use and exposure to environmental tobacco smoke. *Am J Prev Med 2001;* 20:16-66.
26. Saha S, Hoerger TJ, Pignone MP, et al. for the Cost Work Group of the Third US Preventive Services Task Force. The art and science of incorporating cost–effectiveness into evidence-based recommendations for clinical preventive services. *Am J Prev Med 2001;* 20:36–43.
27. Stalmeier PF, Goldstein MK, Holmes AM, et al. What should be reported in a methods section on utility assessment? *Med Decis Making 2001;* 21:200–7.
28. Tengs TO, Adams ME, Pliskin JS, et al. Five hundred life-saving interventions and their cost–effectiveness. *Risk Anal 1995;* 15:369–90.
29. Chapman RH, Stone PW, Sandberg EA, et al. A comprehensive league table of cost–utility ratios and a sub-table of "panel-worthy" studies. *Med Decis Making 2000;* 20:451–67.
30. Stone PW, Teutsch SM, Richard H, et al. Cost–utility analyses of clinical prevention services: published ratios, 1976–1997. *Am J Prev Med 2000;* 19:15–23.
31. Neumann PJ, Stone PW, Chapman RH, et al. The quality of reporting in published cost-utility analyses, 1976-1997. *Ann Intern Med 2000;* 132:964–72.
32. Messonier ML, Corso PS, Teutsch SM, et al. An ounce of prevention . . . what are the returns? *Am J Prev Med 1999;* 16:248–63.
33. Hutubessy RCW, Baltussen RMPM, Evans DB, et al. Stochastic league tables: communicating cost–effectiveness results to decision-makers. *Health Econ 2001;* 10:473–7.
34. Graham JD, Corso PS, Morris JM, et al. Evaluating the cost–effectiveness of clinical and public health measures. *Annu Rev Public Health 1998;* 19:125–52.
35. Drummond MF, Richardson S, O'Brien BJ, Levine M. Users' guide to the medical literature. XIII. How to use an article on economic analysis of clinical practice. A. Are the results of the study valid? *JAMA 1997;* 277:1552–7.
36. National Health Service. *Economic Evaluation Database.* London: NHS, 2001. Available from http://nhscrd.york.ac.uk/welcome.htm.
37. Coffield AB, Maciosek MV, McGinnis JM, et al. Priorities among recommended clinical preventive services. *Am J Prev Med 2001;* 21:1–9.

38. US Preventive Services Task Force. *Guide to Clinical Preventive Services*, 2d ed. Baltimore: Williams and Wilkins, 1996.
39. Maciosek MV, Coffield AB, McGinnis JM, et al. Methods for priority setting among clinical preventive services. *Am J Prev Med 2001;* 21:10–9.
40. Lawrence DM. Priorities among clinical preventive services. *Am J Prev Med 2001;* 21:66–7.
41. Granata AV, Hillman AL. Competing practice guidelines: using cost–effectiveness analysis to make optimal decisions. *Ann Intern Med 1998;* 128:56–63.
42. Wang LY, Haddix AC, Teutsch SM, Caldwell B. The role of resource allocation models in selecting clinical preventive services. *Am J Managed Care 1999;* 5:445–54.
43. Russell LB, Fryback DG, Sonnenberg FA. Is the societal perspective in cost-effectiveness analysis useful for decision makers? *J Qual Improv 1999;* 25:447–54.
44. Teutsch SM, Murray JF. Dissecting cost–effectiveness analysis for preventive interventions: a guide for decision makers. *Am J Managed Care 1999;* 5:301–5.
45. Siegel JE, Weinstein MC, Fineberg HV. Bleach programs for preventing AIDS among IV drug users: modeling the impact of prevalence. *Am J Public Health 1991;* 81:1273–9.
46. Australian Department of Health and Aged Care. *Guidelines for the Pharmaceutical Industry on Preparation of Submissions to the PBAC*, 1999. http://www.health.gov.au:80/pbs/pubs/pharmpac/part1.htm.
47. Ontario Ministry of Health and Long-Term Care. *Ontario Guidelines for Economic Analysis of Pharmaceutical products*. Ontario: Government of Ontario, 2001. Available from www.gov.on.ca/health/english/pub/drugs/drugpro/economic.pdf.
48. National Institute for Clinical Excellence. *Guidance for Manufacturers and Sponsors*. Technology Appraisal Process Series 5. London: National Institute for Clinical Excellence, 2001.
49. Langley PC. Formulary submission guidelines for Blue Cross and Blue Shield of Colorado and Nevada: structure, application and manufacturer responsibilities. *Pharmacoeconomics 1999;* 16:211–24.
50. Mather DB, Sullivan SD, Augenstein D, et al. Incorporating clinical outcomes and economic consequences into drug formulary decisions: a practical approach. *Am J Managed Care 1999;* 5:277–85.
51. Academy of Managed Care Pharmacy. *Format for Formulary Submissions.* Alexandria, VA: Academy of Managed Care Pharmacy, 2000.
52. Evans RG. Manufacturing consensus, marketing truth: guidelines for economic evaluation. *Ann Intern Med 1995;* 123:59 60.
53. Elixhauser A, Halpern M, Schmier J, Luce BR. Health care CBA and CEA from 1991 to 1996: an updated bibliography. *Med Care 1998;* 36:MS1–9.
54. Kassirer JP, Angell M. The journal's policy on cost–effectiveness analyses. *N Engl J Med 1994;* 331:669–70.
55. Task Force on Principles for Economic Analysis of Health Care Technology. Economic analysis of health care technology: a report on principles. *Ann Intern Med 1995;* 122:61–70.
56. Jefferson T, Demicheli V. Are guidelines for peer-reviewing economic evaluations necessary? A survey of current editorial practice. *Health Econ 1995;*4:383–8.
57. Reinhardt UE. How to lower the cost of drugs. *New York Times, 2001*; Jan 3; Sect. A:17.
58. Ubel PA, DeKay ML, Baron J, Asch DA. Cost–effectiveness analysis in a setting of budget constraints. Is it equitable? *N Engl J Med 1996;* 334:1174–7.
59. Ubel PA, Baron J, Asch DA. Preference for equity as a framing effect. *Med Decis Making 2001;* 21:180–9.

60. Ubel PA, Nord E, Gold M, et al. Improving value measurement in cost–effectiveness analysis. *Med Care 2000;* 38:892–901.
61. Williams A. Intergenerational equity: an exploration of the "fair innings" argument. *Health Econ 1997;* 6:117–32.
62. Lieu TA, Gurley RJ, Lundstrom RJ, et al. Projected cost–effectiveness of primary angioplasty for acute myocardial infarction. *J Am Coll Cardiol 1997;* 30:1741–50.

APPENDIX A

Glossary

adequacy When applied to an intervention, the ratio of the expected number of potentially preventable cases to the number of cases that would occur in the absence of an intervention.

adverse event (outcome) Premature death or morbidity.

analytic hierarchy approach A decision-aiding approach in which the attributes of an outcome are ranked in order of importance.

analytic horizon The time period over which the costs and benefits of health outcomes that occur as a result of the intervention are considered.

annuitizing Determining a constant annual value of a capital item for the life of the capital investment.

attributable risk The theoretical reduction in the rate or number of cases of an adverse outcome that can be achieved by elimination of a risk factor.

audience The consumer of the study results. Defined as policy decision makers, program decision makers, or others such as patients, health-care workers, media, other researchers, and the general public.

average cost See **cost**.

average cost–effectiveness See **cost–effectiveness analysis**.

averaging-out-and-folding-back In decision analysis, a series of mathematical computations of probability values multiplied by utility estimates and summed to average the expected value of the branches leading out of each chance node. The results are then folded back from right to left until a value is found for each decision option.

baseline comparator One of the alternative prevention strategies in a decision analysis. May be either the existing-program/strategy alternative or a no-program/strategy alternative, if no program exists at the time of the intervention.

Bayesian methods Techniques of synthesizing data that utilize empiric data and subjective probability. One example is the confidence profile method.

behavioral prevention strategies   Strategies that require that an individual make a personal effort to change lifestyle, such as exercise and dietary improvements.

benefit–cost ratio   A mathematical comparison of the benefits divided by the costs of a project or intervention. When the benefit–cost ratio is greater than 1, benefits exceed costs.

best- and worst-case scenario   A type of sensitivity analysis where the decision-tree model can be used to calculate low- or high-range values that favor one option and recalculated using values that favor another option.

capital costs   The costs of assets with a productive life of more than 1 year required by a program (e.g., equipment, buildings, and land).

case-control study   A study that identifies individuals with a disease or health outcome of interest (cases) and individuals without the disease ot the health outcome of interest (controls) and identifies and compares previous behaviors, risk factors, or characteristics.

case-fatality   See **mortality**.

case series   Studies that focus exclusively on individuals with disease or a specific health event.

cause-specific mortality   See **mortality**.

chance node   In a decision tree, an event that occurs as a consequence of the decision but over which one has no control. Usually drawn as a circle.

clinical prevention strategies   Interventions conveyed by a health-care provider to a patient, often within a clinical setting, such as vaccinations, screening and treatment for diabetic eye disease, and monitoring of tuberculosis treatment.

cohort   Any defined group of persons selected for a special purpose or study.

cohort simulation   In a cohort simulation, a hypothetical cohort of people is cycled through a state-transition model to analyze specific attributes of interest (e.g., duration of survival, quality of life).

cohort study   Longitudinal study where, within a defined population, data on risk factors or health characteristics are collected prior to the occurrence of the health outcome of interest.

concurrently controlled study   A study where the intervention is introduced to one group, and utilizes another similar group as a control, but assignment to these groups is not randomized, also called a quasi-experimental study.

consumer market studies   The determination of the value of nonmarket resources from reference to similar commodities for which a market exists in the context of estimating willingness-to-pay values of health outcomes.

consumer price index (CPI)   Measures relative changes over time in the prices of a specified set of goods and services purchased by households on a regular basis.

consumer surplus   The difference between the value placed on a good or service (i.e., the price a person is willing to pay) and the price that is actually paid.

contingent valuation method The use of surveys of individuals conducted in the context of a hypothetical market situation to elicit consumer valuation of goods and services. Used to estimate the willingness-to-pay values of health outcomes.

cost A measure of what must be given up to acquire or produce something. Economic costs can be differentiated in the following manner:

total cost (TC) Sum of the costs of producing a particular quantity of output.

fixed cost (FC) Costs which do not vary with the quantity of output in the short run (e.g., rent, utilities, and administrative salaries).

variable cost (VC) Costs which vary with the level of output and respond proportionately to change in volume of activity.

average cost (AC) The total cost divided by the total output. Reported as the cost per unit of output.

marginal cost (MC) The additional cost of an intervention to produce one additional unit of output. An intraprogram measure.

incremental cost (IC) When interventions are ranked in ascending order of effectiveness, the additional cost to the next most effective intervention of producing another unit of output. An interprogram measure.

incidence-based See **incidence-based cost**.

prevalence-based See **prevalence-based cost**.

cost analysis The process of estimating the cost of prevention activities, also called **cost identification**.

cost–benefit analysis (CBA) A type of economic analysis in which all costs and benefits are converted into monetary (dollar) values and results are expressed as either the net present value or the dollars of benefits per dollars expended.

cost–effectiveness analysis (CEA) An economic analysis in which all costs are related to a single, common effect. Results are usually stated as additional cost expended per additional health outcome achieved. Results can be categorized in one or all of the following ways:

average cost–effectiveness The total cost of an intervention divided by the health outcomes produced by that intervention.

marginal cost–effectiveness The additional cost incurred by an intervention to produce an additional unit of the health outcome.

incremental cost–effectiveness When strategies are ranked in order of effectiveness, the additional cost incurred by the next most effective strategy to produce an additional unit of the health outcome.

cost identification See **cost analysis**.

cost-of-illness (COI) methodology An approach used to estimate the costs of a health intervention in which two types of cost are collected: the direct medical and nonmedical costs associated with the illness and the indirect costs associated with lost productivity due to morbidity or premature mortality.

cost–utility analysis (CUA)   A type of cost–effectiveness analysis in which benefits are expressed as the number of life years saved adjusted to account for loss of quality from morbidity of the health outcome or side effects from the intervention. The most common outcome measure in CUA is the quality-adjusted life year.

cross-sectional study   A study that collects data on health characteristics and health outcomes at the same time within the study population.

decision analysis   An explicit, quantitative, systematic approach to decision making under conditions of uncertainty.

decision node   In a decision tree, points of choice, usually drawn as a box.

decision-tree model   A graphic representation of how possible choices in a decision analysis relate (stochastically) to the possible outcomes.

delphi process   An iterative consensus process used to determine the "best estimate" of professionals in the field. This process is often used in decision analysis to estimate the probability that an event will occur or to estimate the value of costs and benefits of outcomes when there are insufficient data in the published literature.

demonstration settings   A population- or clinic-based environment in which prevention strategies are field-tested.

direct costs   The measure of the resources expended for prevention activities or health care (compare with **indirect cost**).

   direct medical costs   The measure of the resources for medical care (e.g., the cost of a physician visit).

   direct nonmedical costs   Costs incurred in connection with a health intervention or illness but not expended for medical care itself (e.g., transportation costs associated with a physician visit).

disability   The temporary or long-term reduction in an individual's functional capacity.

discounting   A method for adjusting the value of future costs and benefits to an equivalent value today to account for time preference and opportunity cost, i.e., a dollar today is worth more than a dollar a year from now (even if inflation is not considered).

discount rate   The rate at which future costs and benefits are discounted to account for time preference. See **social discount rate** or **real discount rate**.

distributional effects   The manner in which the costs and benefits of a preventive strategy affect different groups of people in terms of demographics, geographic location, and other descriptive factors.

double counting   When a cost or benefit is captured in more than one measure.

effectiveness   The improvement in health outcome that a prevention strategy can produce in typical community-based settings.

efficacy   The improvement in health outcome that a prevention strategy can produce in expert hands under ideal circumstances.

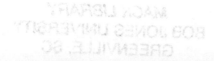

efficiency   A measure of the relationship between inputs and outputs in a prevention strategy. Efficiency goes beyond effectiveness of a prevention strategy by attempting to identify the maximum health output achievable for a set amount of resources.

etiologic fraction   The proportion of cases in the exposed group presumably attributable to the exposure, appropriate only if the exposed group has a higher risk of disease than the unexposed group.

excess fraction   The fractional excess caseload produced by an exposure.

expected utility   The sum of the products of the preference ranking, i.e., utility for an outcome and the probability that the outcome will occur for all of the possible outcomes of a prevention strategy.

expected utility theory   The dominant theory of individual behavior under conditions of uncertainty based on the assumption that, given different alternatives, the alternative with the outcome that has the highest expected utility should be chosen.

expected value   The sum of the products of the value of outcomes and the probability of the outcome occurring for all possible outcomes of a prevention strategy.

extensive margin   Refers to a study that exams the effect of a prevention strategy on different groups of individuals. See also **intensive margin.**

false-negative   A person with a condition who tests negative for that condition. See **sensitivity (test).**

false positive   A person without a condition who tests positive for that condition. See **specificity (test).**

fixed cost (FC)   See **cost.**

health promotion   Disease and injury prevention strategies that depend on behavioral change in individuals.

health-related event (HRE)   Adverse health condition.

health utility   The measure assigned to quality of life.

health utility index (HUI)   A multifaceted measure of utility in which different utility functions (e.g., physical function, role function, social–emotional function, and other coexisting health problems) are weighted and combined to determine an overall preference for a particular outcome.

heuristics   Psychological short-cuts in thinking used to simplify complex decisions.

human capital (HC) approach   A method for estimating the economic impact of disease, which includes the resources used for medical care and the forgone earnings due to morbidity or premature mortality.

incidence   The number of new cases of disease in a defined population initially free of disease, see **incidence rate.**

incidence-based cost   The total lifetime cost of new cases of a disease or injury that occur during a certain period of time.

incidence rate   A measure of the frequency of new cases of disease in a particular population that occurred during a specified period of time.

incremental analysis   A type of comparative analysis used to examine the relationship between the differences in costs and benefits (whether measured in monetary, natural, or quality-adjusted units) between two or more prevention strategies.

incremental cost   The additional cost of producing one more unit of output by an alternative intervention.

incremental cost–effectiveness   See **cost–effectiveness**.

indirect cost   The resources forgone either to participate in an intervention or as the result of a health condition (e.g., earnings forgone because of loss of time from work).

inflation   A sustained rise in the general price level.

injury   An accidental or intentional event that cause physical or mental harm and may lead to disability or death.

intangible benefits   Benefits associated with a good or service for which assigning a specific monetary value is difficult. Intangible benefits are usually quantified using techniques for measuring consumer surplus associated with a good or service.

intangible cost   Cost, such as pain and suffering, for which assigning a monetary value is difficult.

intensive margin   Refers to studies that examine changes in frequency or periodicity of prevention strategy on same group of individuals. See also **extensive margin**.

intermediate measure   The measure most directly associated with the intervention being evaluated, generally reported in terms of the service delivered (e.g., patients tested, number of condoms distributed).

internal rate of return (IRR)   The rate at which the value of future benefits is equal to the value of the initial investiment.

interviewer bias   See **observer bias**.

league tables   Tables used to rank cost–effectiveness and cost–benefit results for various health conditions, usually in ascending order of cost per unit of outcome.

marginal analysis   A type of analysis that examines the additional cost required to produce an additional unit of output by a prevention strategy.

marginal cost   See **cost**.

marginal cost–effectiveness   See **cost–effectiveness**.

Markov cycle   A defined recurring interval in a Markov model during which a person makes a single transition from one state to another. All intervals are of equivalent length and their sum represents the analytic horizon for the model.

Markov model   A type of state-transition model in which transition probabilities depend upon only the current state and not upon the previous state or pathway by which the state was entered.

Markovian assumption   An assumption of a Markov model, which states that knowing only the present state of health of a patient is sufficient to project the entire trajectory of future states. This assumption is a major limitation of Markov models.

meta-analysis   A systematic, quantitative method for combining information from multiple studies to derive the most meaningful answer to a specific question.

Monte Carlo simulation   A type of sensitivity analysis that compares the measure of the central tendency and the variance of results, generated by repeated decision-tree simulations with the expected values of the probabilities and outcome values for the model. Monte Carlo simulation is also used to analyze Markov models.

   first order   Runs a cohort through the model, with the computer making selections randomly at each chance node based on a single value for the probability. A distribution of the accumulated results provides a measure of the central tendency and the variance.

   second order   Runs a cohort through the model a number of times, with the computer making random selections from values in a designated distribution for the probability at the chance node. A distribution of the accumulated results provides a measure of the central tendency and the variance.

morbidity   The absence of health or physical or psychological well-being.

mortality   The number of individuals within a defined population that dies during a specific period, typically expressed as a rate.

   case-fatality   The number of deaths among individuals with the disease, typically expressed as a ratio.

   cause-specific mortality   The number of deaths from a particular disease among individuals at risk for developing or dying from disease.

   premature mortality   (1) Any preventable death (2) Deaths that occur before a specified age, most often age 65, or the average life expectancy of a certain population.

multiattribute utility model   In a cost–utility analysis, the mathematical combination of the utility functions and weights for each of several dimensions into one single function.

net present value (NPV)   The sum that results when the discounted value of the costs of a prevention strategy are deducted from the discounted value of the benefits of the strategy.

normative decision-making models   Models in decision making that provide rules by which decisions "should" be made.

observational study   Epidemiologic study that does not involve any intervention to study participants, but measures health characteristics or risk factors and health outcomes as they naturally occur in a defined population.

observer bias   The influence of the survey interviewer though injection of beliefs or opinions on the reporting of survey participants (also known as interviewer bias).

odds ratio A commonly used measure of association that relies on odds rather than probabilities. The odds of an event happening are the probability of an event happening (p) divided by the probability of the event not happening ($1 - p$).

opportunity cost The value of the resources used in providing a specific set of health-care services valued in terms of forgone alternative uses.

outcome measure The final health consequence (e.g., cases prevented or, quality-adjusted life years) of an intervention.

participant cost Direct and indirect costs borne by the participant in the intervention program. Includes travel and day-care expenses, the purchase of intervention units not accounted for in program costs, and forgone wages due to lost time from work.

payer An individual or organization responsible for payment of health-care costs.

penetrance The extent to which an intervention reaches its intended target.

perspective See **societal perspective**.

policy decision makers Elected officials, agency heads, state and local public health officials, and others responsible for setting public health policy.

population attributable risk The incidence of a disease or condition in a population that is associated with exposure to the risk factor.

premature mortality (1) Any preventable death. (2) Deaths that occur before a specified age, most often age 65, or the average life expectancy of a certain population.

prescriptive decision-making models Models used to guide decision making.

prevalence The number of cases of a given disease or condition in a given population at a designated time.

prevalence-based cost The cost associated with the existing cases of disease or injury that occur during a specified time period.

preventable fraction The proportion of an adverse health outcome that potentially can be eliminated as a result of a prevention strategy.

prevented fraction The proportion of an adverse health outcome that has been eliminated as a result of a prevention strategy.

prevention The promotion and preservation of health, the restoration of health when it is impaired, and the minimization of suffering and distress.

　primary prevention An intervention to reduce risk or exposure to prevent occurence of disease or injury.

　secondary prevention An intervention to detect and treat a disease before it becomes clinically apparent.

　tertiary prevention An intervention implemented after a disease or injury is established to prevent sequelae or to minimize suffering.

prevention effectiveness The systematic assessment of the impact of public health policies, programs, and practices on costs and health outcomes.

preventive medical services   Clinical services provided to patients by a health-care professional to reduce or prevent disease, injury, or disability.

preventive strategies (clinical, behavioral, environmental)   A framework for categorizing programs based on how the prevention technology is delivered, i.e., provider to patient (clinical), individual responsibility (behavioral), or alteration in an individual's surroundings (environmental).

primary prevention   See **prevention**.

process measures   The set of criteria used to evaluate an intervention based on the measurement of either the quantity of inputs used (e.g., number of brochures distributed) or the products produced (e.g., patients tested, by the intervention).

productivity loss   The value of output not produced due to morbidity or premature mortality.

program decision makers   Users of the results of prevention-effectiveness studies who are responsible for decisions about prevention programs.

program evaluation   An assessment of the processes, impacts, and outcomes of intervention programs, with particular attention paid to the purposes and expectations of stakeholders of the program.

publication bias   In the medical literature, studies that show a positive effect are more likely to be published than studies that show no effect.

quality-adjusted life year (QALY)   A frequently used outcome measure in cost–utility analysis that incorporates the quality or desirability of a health state with the duration of survival. Quality of life is integrated with length of life using a multiplicative formula.

quality of life   A multidimensional measure of the physical, emotional, and social effects of disease, treatment, or sequela of injury and disability, usually measured using standardized, validated instruments.

Quality of Well-Being (QWB)   A health utility index widely used for cost–utility analysis.

randomized controlled trial (RCT)   Experimental study where the subjects or communities are randomly assigned to study groups where at least one group receives a therapeutic or other intervention and is compared to best usual care or placebo depending upon the medical condition under investigation.

rank and scale   A method of valuing utilities whereby outcomes are ranked in order of best to worst and then assigned numerical values.

rating scale   A method of valuing utilities based on strength of preference.

ratio   A measure of the frequency of one group of events relative to the frequency of a different group of events.

real discount rate   A discount rate that is free from the effects of inflation.

recall bias   The systematic under- or over-reporting of events by survey respondents.

recipient of services (beneficiary)   Any individual or group who benefits from a prevention strategy; used most often in the context of medical services.

relative hazard   The ratio of the survival time in the group with the risk factor divided by the survival time in the group without the risk factor.

relative risk   The ratio of the incidence rate for a person exposed to a factor to the incidence rate for those not exposed.

required compensation approach   An analytic method that attempts to value the reduction in the risk of a job-related injury by examining the difference in wages for persons in risky occupations versus persons in other occupations.

resource   An input in a prevention intervention without which the intervention would not exist or an input in the treatment of a health outcome.

risk   The likelihood that a person having specified characteristics (e.g., high blood cholesterol, failure to wear seat belts) will acquire a specified disease or injury.

risk ratio   The ratio of the risk among persons with specific risk factors compared to the risk among persons without the risk factors.

safety   An assessment of the level and acceptability of risk of adverse outcomes that occur as a result of a prevention technique in the context of a specific prevention strategy and disease or injury outcome.

scrap value   The resale value of a capital asset at the end of its useful life.

secondary prevention   See **prevention**.

sensitivity analysis   Mathematical calculations that isolate factors involved in a decision analysis or economic analysis to indicate the degree of influence each factor has on the outcome of the entire analysis.

> **one-way sensitivity analysis**   When only one value is changed.

> **multi-way sensitivity analysis**   When several values are changed simultaneously.

sensitivity (test)   The ability of a test to correctly identify those who have the disease. A sensitive test creates few false-negatives.

sequela   An abnormal condition resulting from a disease.

shadow price   An imputed valuation of a commodity or service for which no market price exists. The social opportunity cost of an outcome.

social discount rate   The rate at which society as a whole is willing to trade present costs for future benefits. Used in prevention-effectiveness studies that take the societal perspective; the lower rate indicates that future benefits are also valued highly in the present. See **discount rate**.

societal perspective   The perspective of society as a whole. Economic analyses which take a societal perspective include all benefits of a program regardless of who receives them and all costs regardless of who pays them.

specificity (test)   The ability of a test to identify correctly those who do not have the disease. A specific test creates few false-positives.

stakeholder   An individual or organization with an interest in an intervention or outcome.

standard gamble   In cost–utility analysis, a lottery-based approach to determining the utility of a particular outcome.

state transition model   A model that allocates and reallocates members of the population into health states at defined recurring intervals based upon probabilities of moving from one state to another.

survival   The period from assessment of health characteristics or diagnosis with a disease or condition until death or the end of the observation period.

target audience   See **audience**.

target population   The population for whom the program or policy is intended.

technology   Techniques, devices, drugs, or procedures used to reduce the risk of an adverse health outcome.

terminal node   In a decision tree, the end point of each sequence of events representing a health outcome. Usually represented by a rectangle.

tertiary prevention   See **prevention**.

threshold analysis   A type of sensitivity analysis that identifies the conditions (e.g., the values of variables) that would have to exist for the expected value or expected utility of two interventions to be equivalent. Often used to identify the "switch points" at which cost savings begin or end and to indicate the point at which a different decision should be made.

time frame   The specified period in which the intervention strategies are actually applied.

time series   A study in which multiple observations of historical controls are used for comparison with those after an intervention is implemented.

time trade-off   A method of eliciting utilities from an individual perspective based on the willingness to trade time for health.

total cost (TC)   See **cost**.

transition probability   The probability of moving from one state to another in a state-transition model.

unnecessary morbidity   Any preventable disease, injury, or disability.

utility   In decision analysis, a quantitative measure of the strength of a reference for an outcome.

variable cost (VC)   See **cost**.

wage risk studies   See **required compensation approach**.

welfare economics   The normative aspect of economics. Viewed as an investigation of methods of ordering alternative possible resource allocations. Within the context of prevention effectiveness, it provides the framework for the ranking of prevention strategies by order of net costs and benefits.

willingness to accept (WTA)   A measure of the compensation that must be made to consumers to get them to accept a risk-increasing situation. Implementation of WTA studies is problematic and generally not used.

willingness to pay (WTP)   A method of measuring the value an individual places on reducing the risk of death and illness by estimating the maximum dollar amount an individual would pay in a given risk-reducing situation.

REFERENCES

Some definitions adapted from:

Drummond MF, Stoddart GL, Torrance GW. *Methods for the Economic Evaluation of Health Care Programmes*. Oxford: Oxford University Press, 1987.

Last JM. *A Dictionary of Epidemiology*, 2d ed. New York: Oxford University Press, 1988.

Mausner J, Kramer S. *Epidemiology: An Introductory Text*. Philadelphia: Saunders, 1985.

Pearce DW (ed). *The MIT Dictionary of Modern Economics*, 4th ed. Cambridge, MA: MIT Press, 1994.

Petitti DB. *Meta-analysis, Decision Analysis, and Cost–Effectiveness Analysis: Methods for Quantitative Synthesis in Medicine*. New York: Oxford University Press, 1994.

US Department of Health and Human Services, Centers for Disease Control. *Principles of epidemiology: Self-study course 3030-G*. Atlanta: US DHHS, CDC.

Warner KE, Luce BR. *Cost–Benefit and Cost–Effectiveness Analysis in Health Care: Principles, Practice, and Potential*. Ann Arbor: Health Administration Press, 1982.

APPENDIX B

Recommendations

CHAPTER 2. STUDY DESIGN

2.1: The list of alternative strategies in prevention–effectiveness studies should include all reasonable options and a baseline comparator.

2.2: For decisions that impact public health, prevention–effectiveness studies should take the societal perspective. Additional perspectives may also be studied when relevant to the study question. The perspectives of the analysis should be clearly stated.

2.3: All measurable opportunity costs, representing all groups that are affected by a program or intervention, should be included in the societal perspective.

2.4: The time frame for a prevention–effectiveness study must be long enough to cover the implementation of the program being evaluated.

2.5: The analytic horizon of a prevention–effectiveness study should extend over the time period during which the costs, harms, and benefits of the intervention are incurred.

2.6: Marginal or incremental analysis should always be performed in a prevention-effectiveness study for comparing programs or interventions. Average analyses are acceptable for independent programs or interventions.

2.7: Prevention-effectiveness studies should include all benefits and harms that have a meaningful impact on the results of the analysis.

2.8: Univariate and multivariable sensitivity analyses should be performed and the results reported for a prevention effectiveness study.

2.9: When possible, the distributional and ethical implications of a prevention–effectiveness study should be examined and discussed.

2.10: All assumptions should be explicitly stated, including assumptions about the study structure, probabilities, outcome measures, and costs.

CHAPTER 4. COSTS

4.1:   Incidence-based cost estimates of health outcomes should be used in cost–effectiveness analyses and cost–utility analyses unless the health problem being considered is of sufficiently short duration that prevalence-based estimates are equivalent to incidence-based estimates.

4.2:   Resource costs rather than charges should be obtained when possible.

4.3:   The human-capital approach should be used to estimate productivity losses for cost–effectiveness analyses.

CHAPTER 5. QUALITY OF LIFE

5.1:   Utility assessment for use in QALYs should be preference-based and interval-scaled, on a scale where optimal health has a score of 1 and death has a score of 0. The health state classification system should be generic, that is, not disease-specific. Community preferences are desirable; however, when not available, patient preferences may be used.

CHAPTER 6. TIME EFFECTS

6.1:   Future costs and health outcomes should be discounted to the present value.

6.2:   Future costs and health outcomes should be discounted at the same rate.

6.3:   A 3% real discount rate should be used. A 5% discount rate may also be used for purposes of comparability with older studies or studies from other settings. No adjustments for inflation in the future should be made because this is a real (not a nominal) discount rate. Perform sensitivity analysis on the discount rate over a reasonable range, for example, from 0% to 10%.

CHAPTER 8. COST BENEFIT ANALYSIS

8.1:   A comprehensive measure or set of measures (e.g., contingent valuation methodology) designed to fully capture costs and benefits should be used for cost–benefit analyses that take the societal perspective.

8.2:   The net present value of benefits, rather than a cost–benefit ratio, should be used as the summary measure in a cost–benefit analysis.

8.3:   When a cost–benefit analysis is used to evaluate more than one competing program or intervention, the incremental or marginal net present values should be reported. It is acceptable to report average net present values in cost–benefit analyses of independent programs or interventions.

CHAPTER 9. COST–EFFECTIVENESS ANALYSIS

9.1: The list of intervention strategies in a cost–effectiveness analysis (CEA) should include all reasonable options and a baseline comparator.

9.2: Final health-outcome measures should be used in CEAs.

9.3: The numerator in a cost–utility analysis should include only direct medical and nonmedical costs unless the utility measurement in the denominator does not incorporate productivity losses.

9.4: The quality–adjusted life year (QALY) measure in the denominator of a CEA should be based on an interval scale and should use preference-based weights. Community preferences for health states are desirable for QALYs used in CEAs that take the societal perspective.

9.5: The numerator of a CEA should include the costs associated with the intervention, adverse health outcomes associated with the intervention, and costs associated with health outcomes that were averted by the intervention. These include medical costs, nonmedical costs, and productivity losses.

9.6: A CEA should report total costs, total effectiveness, incremental or average costs, incremental or average effectiveness, and incremental or average cost–effectiveness ratios. Interventions should be ranked in ascending order of cost and effectiveness. A separate table may be used to report undiscounted health outcomes.

APPENDIX C
Software

RICHARD D. RHEINGANS

ANALYTICA, by Lumina Decision Systems, Inc., 59 North Santa Cruz Avenue, Suite Q, Los Gatos, GA 95030; LUMINA; www.lumina.com
Platform: Mac, Windows
Description: Analytica uses influence diagrams to organize and analyze decision analysis problems. Information is entered in a visual environment that facilitates communication of the problem to other users. A variety of graphic and numeric outputs are available. Users can incorporate probabilistic information about individual parameters using a variety of distributions. The program uses "intelligent arrays" to structure problems, making it particularly easy to follow multiple subpopulations or age groups. The program includes features that facilitate the modeling of problems over time. The use of OLE and ODBC protocols allows the user to dynamically link to Excel spreadsheets with input information. Analytica is particularly suited to problems that include both continuous and discrete variables and for developing large models including modules. The user's manual is extensive and available electronically. An interactive tutorial, demo versions, and multiple sample programs are also available online.

CRYSTAL BALL, Decisioneering, Inc., 1515 Arapahoe Street, Suite 1311, Denver, CO 80202; www.decisioneering.com
Platform: Mac, Windows
Description: Crystal Ball is an Excel add-in that allows probabilistic information to be entered for any variable and generation of Monte Carlo analysis. Probabilistic information is entered by selecting from predefined distributions or fitting data to a range of distributions. In a Monte Carlo simulation, input values are selected from each of the distributions and one output value is calculated and stored. A new set of input values is drawn from the distributions and a new output is generated, eventually resulting in a probability distribution for the output values. Crystal Ball is capable of two–dimensional models that separate uncertain parameters (whose actual values are unknown) and variable parameters (which differ within a population).

Model output can be displayed in a number of graphic formats. Several tools are available for sensitivity analysis, including one- and two-way sensitivity analyses and analysis of variance techniques that look at the contribution of each parameter to overall variability in the output parameter. Extensive user manuals and tutorials are available, and a demo version is available for downloading.

DATA, by TreeAge Software, Inc., 1075 Main Street, Williamstown, MA 01267; www.treeage.com
Platform: Mac, Windows
Description: DATA is a stand-alone program that can create models as decision trees or as influence diagrams, using a graphic interface. Input and output data can also be linked to Excel spreadsheets. Certain features in DATA were designed specifically for modeling cost–effectiveness problems, including estimation of multiple outcomes and calculation of cost–effectiveness ratios. Markov models that follow populations over time can also be created (including two-dimensional models). Interactive procedures are available for outcome preferences and risk profiles. Monte Carlo simulations can be added to all models. A wide range of easily accessible graphic outputs is available, including one- and two-way sensitivity analyses. DATA Interactive is a companion program that allows the analyst to create models to be used and manipulated by decision makers on CD-ROMs or at web pages. Demo versions of the program are available at the website. User manuals and documentation pay special attention to the use of DATA for analyzing health-care problems.

DECISION PRO, by: Vanguard Software Corporation, 3111 Trellis Green, Cary, NC 27511; www.vanguardsw.com
Platform: Windows
Description: DECISION PRO is an advanced decision analysis program originally designed for developing and analyzing financial models. Problems are structured as decision trees in graphic interface. Monte Carlo analysis can be incorporated into decision trees. Optimization procedures using linear and non-linear methods can be used for analyzing a wider range of options. Graphic outputs, including three-dimensional graphs, probabilistic distributions, and trend charts are available. Models can be linked to Excel spreadsheets. Using the companion server software, models can be posted on Internet or Intranet sites for use by decision makers. A trial version is available on the company's website.

DPL, by Applied Decision Analysis, 2710 Sand Hill Road, Menlo Park, CA 94025; www.adainc.com
Platform: Windows
Description: DPL allows the analyst to structure problems as decision trees or influence diagrams using a graphic interface. The program was originally designed for business applications but easily can be used for cost–effectiveness analysis. Models can be linked to spreadsheets using the DDE protocol. User-defined distributions, multiple attributes, and utility functions can be added to models. Graphic outputs include sensitivity analyses and cumulative probability distributions. Demo versions of DPL and tutorials are available online.

PRECISION TREE/@RISK, by Palisades Corporation, 31 Decker Road, New-field, NY 14867; www.palisades.com
Platform: Mac, Windows
Description: PRECISION TREE is an Excel add-in that is part of the Decision Tools Suite developed by Palisades. Precision Tree is used to create decision trees and influence diagrams directly in an existing spreadsheet. @RISK is another Excel add-in within the Palisades Decision Tools Suite. It allows for the creation of probabilistic models within spreadsheets (see the description for Crystal Ball as well). @RISK can also be used with Palisade's Precision Tree to generate Monte Carlo analyses for decision trees. A wide range of probabilistic distributions is available for developing models. Other programs within the suite include BestFit, which is used for fitting empirical data to distributions, and RiskView, which provides additional graphic capabilities. A slide show tutorial is available, but no demo version is available.

TREEPLAN, by Decision Support Services, 2105 Buchanan St., #1, San Francisco, CA 94115; www.treeplan.com
Platform: Mac, Windows
Description: TREEPLAN is an Excel add-in that allows the user to construct decision trees within an Excel spreadsheet. Dialog boxes are used for parameter input. Other Excel add-ins from Decision Support Services include SensIt for developing sensitivity analyses and RiskSim for developing Monte Carlo models. The program is simple and inexpensive but includes most of the basic features of more expensive programs. While these programs include fewer options and features compared to other packages, they are much less expensive.

Appendix D

Worked Example: Cost–Effectiveness of Postexposure Prophylaxis Following Sexual Exposure to Human Immunodeficiency Virus

HARRELL W. CHESSON
STEVEN D. PINKERTON

Initiating antiretroviral therapy shortly after exposure to human immunodeficiency Virus (HIV) and continuing therapy for several weeks thereafter can reduce the risk of seroconversion following percutaneous exposure to HIV, such as needle-stick injuries among health-care workers.[1–3] This prevention strategy is known as postexposure prophylaxis (PEP). Although the effectiveness of PEP following sexual exposure to HIV has not been established, some physicians have prescribed PEP for patients who report possible sexual exposure to HIV.[4,5] In addition, PEP prevention programs have been offered on a limited basis in cities such as Boston and San Francisco.[6]

The potential benefits of PEP must be weighed against the cost of this expensive therapy. These costs are not strictly monetary as some patients will have mild to moderate (and sometimes severe) reactions to the multidrug regimen.[2,7–9] Many patients discontinue therapy, possibly due to these side effects or to difficulties following the dosage schedule.[7–9] In addition, the use of HIV-prevention resources to provide PEP precludes the use of these resources for alternative HIV-prevention activities.[5] Information regarding the cost–effectiveness of PEP for potential sexual exposure to HIV could be useful in comparing PEP to other HIV-prevention activities.

FRAMING THE STUDY

Objective of the Analysis

This analysis was conducted to evaluate the cost–effectiveness of a hypothetical program to provide PEP to men who have sex with men (MSM) following accidental exposure to HIV through unprotected receptive anal intercourse. It was based on a recent modeling study which concluded that PEP would be more cost–effective when restricted to partners of persons known to be HIV-infected and to persons reporting unprotected receptive anal intercourse.[5]

Audience for the Study

This study provides a simplified example of a cost–effectiveness analysis. In addition to those wishing to learn more about cost–effectiveness analysis, the intended audience includes decision makers responsible for prioritizing and allocating funding for HIV-prevention activities (e.g., public health program managers at the federal, state, and local levels); governmental agencies and medical societies, which might issue recommendations or guidelines concerning the use of PEP following possible sexual exposure to HIV; physicians considering providing PEP for their at-risk patients; and people with a general interest in HIV prevention.

Perspective of the Analysis

This analysis adopts the societal perspective, meaning that all relevant costs and health outcomes are included regardless of whom they affect. Studies undertaken from this perspective can help to inform resource-allocation decisions at the societal level.

Analytic Method

The results are presented as a cost–effectiveness ratio expressing the cost (in year 2000 dollars) per quality-adjusted life year gained ($/QALY). The QALY measure incorporates the premature mortality and morbidity associated with HIV infection (see Chapter 5). Cost–effectiveness analyses that use a quality-of-life measure are often referred to as *cost–utility analyses*.

Time Frame and Analytic Horizon

This study assesses the lifetime costs and effects of a 1-year PEP intervention. The time frame is therefore 1 year as we estimate the cost of supporting the PEP program and the number of HIV infections averted by the program over the course of 1 year. The analytic horizon includes all of the future benefits (QALYs gained and lifetime medical treatment costs avoided) associated with each case of HIV infection averted by the program within the 1-year time frame.

Target Population for the Intervention

The target population includes all MSM in a hypothetical city who would use PEP following a possible sexual exposure to HIV through receptive anal intercourse.

Defining the Program

The prevention strategy considered in this analysis is the provision of PEP to MSM who report a potential exposure to HIV through unprotected receptive anal intercourse with an HIV-infected man or a man of unknown HIV status. We examined the provision of PEP to a hypothetical cohort of 1000 MSM, all of whom (excluding those who discontinued therapy) were assumed to receive a 4-week course of two antiretroviral drugs, zidovudine and lamivudine.[4] The intervention strategy is compared to a "no-program" option, in which PEP is not offered following possible sexual exposure to HIV.

Scope of the Study

Each instance where PEP was successful at preventing HIV seroconversion was considered to be an HIV case averted; we did not consider the possibility that a man could benefit from PEP today yet acquire HIV later in life due to subsequent sexual exposure.[5,10] This assumption is particularly important as our analysis considers each possible sexual exposure to be an isolated incident. We did not consider the continued use of PEP for those with ongoing behavioral risk for HIV infection. Instead, we assumed PEP would be a "last-resort" intervention to supplement, not replace, individual-level behavioral strategies to prevent HIV, such as condom use. We also did not consider the possibility that PEP might prevent HIV in the future sex partners of men who without PEP would have seroconverted or that some men might alter their future behavior to reduce their HIV risk as a consequence of receiving PEP.

Future Costs and Benefits

Costs and benefits that are projected to occur in the future are discounted to present value using an annual discount rate of 3%.

METHODS

We used standard methods of cost–utility analysis (Chapter 9). Using spreadsheet calculations and DATA 3.5.7 software (TreeAge Software, Williamstown, MA), we constructed a decision tree to model the probability of HIV seroconversion with and without PEP. The intervention was evaluated in terms of cost per QALY gained compared to the option of "no intervention," and the net gain in QALYs was estimated as the QALYs gained by preventing HIV minus the QALYs lost due to side effects of PEP.

Decision Tree

The decision tree (Fig. D.1) was used to estimate the number of HIV cases averted by the program and the number of patients experiencing PEP-associated side ef-

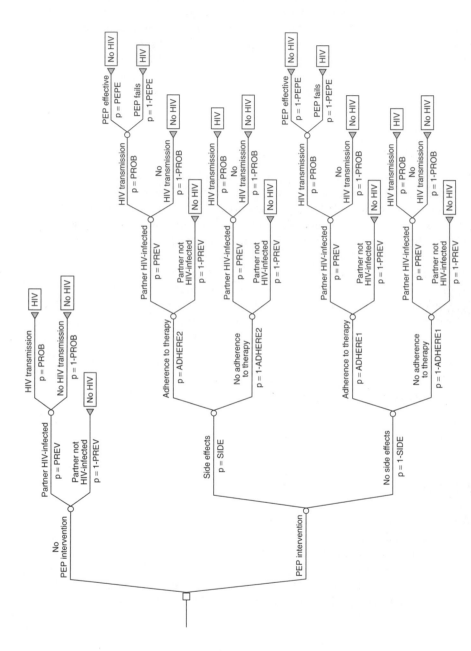

Figure D.1 Decision tree comparing PEP intervention with no PEP intervention.

fects. In our tree, there are two main branches that represent the two options examined here: "no PEP intervention" and "PEP intervention."

Moving from left to right in the "No PEP intervention" branch, there is a chance node that divides the intervention participants into two groups: those whose partner is HIV-infected and those whose partner is not HIV-infected. If the partner is HIV-infected, the subsequent chance node represents the probability of HIV transmission as a result of sexual exposure. This probability is given by PROB, the per-act probability of sexual transmission. There is no risk of HIV infection from sexual exposure if the partner is not HIV-infected.

Moving from left to right in the "PEP intervention" branch, there is a chance node that divides the intervention participants into two groups: those who experience side effects from PEP and those who do not. The next chance node creates two additional groups: those who adhere to therapy and those who do not. Those who experience side effects are assumed to have a lower probability of adherence to therapy (ADHERE2) than those who do not experience side effects (ADHERE1). The next two chance nodes represent the probability that the person's partner is HIV-infected and the probability of HIV transmission as a result of sexual exposure. If transmission does occur, then adherence to PEP may prevent the establishment of HIV infection. This probability that PEP will be effective at preventing seroconversion is defined by the variable PEPE. For intervention participants who adhere to therapy, there is an additional chance node after the event of HIV transmission that represents the possible benefits of PEP.

For simplicity, we assumed that the cost of the therapy (as well as the number of QALYs lost due to the side effects) did not depend on whether or not the person adhered to the therapy. We also assumed that complete adherence to therapy was required to achieve the benefits of PEP; a patient who did not adhere to the therapy would not have any reduction in his probability of acquiring HIV.

Epidemiological and Cost Data

Most of the model inputs (Table D.1) were obtained from the literature, and all costs were adjusted to year 2000 dollars using the "all-items" component of the Consumer Price Index. The per-sex-act probability of HIV transmission (PROB) without the provision of PEP was based on epidemiological studies of the sexual transmission of HIV.[1,11,12] The probability that the person's sex partner is HIV-infected (PREV) was based on a study of HIV prevalence among MSM in urban areas.[13] Reports of medication adherence among health-care workers receiving PEP for occupational exposure to HIV indicate that 50%–87% will complete therapy.[4,7–9] Some patients may discontinue therapy because of side effects such as nausea, fatigue, and headache, as well as difficulty in following the required dosage schedule.[7] We assumed that 79% of patients who do not experience side effects and 59% of patients who do experience side effects would adhere to the full course of therapy (ADHERE1 and ADHERE2). The probability of side effects (SIDE) also was based on studies of health-care workers receiving PEP.[4,7,8] The effectiveness of the full course of PEP at preventing the establishment of HIV infection (PEPE) was based on a case-control study of HIV seroconversion in

Table D.1   Probabilities and Costs Used in Cost–Effectiveness Analysis of
Postexposure Prophylaxis Following Sexual Exposure to Human
Immunodeficiency Virus (HIV)

Parameter	Base-Case Scenario	Best-Case Scenario[a]	Worst-Case Scenario	Source
Per-act probability of HIV infection without PEP (PROB)	0.02	0.03	0.006	4,11,12
Probability partner is HIV-infected (PREV)	0.18	1.0	0.06	13
Probability patient will adhere to full course of therapy in absence of side effects (ADHERE1)[b]	0.79	0.84	0.68	4,7–9
Probability patient will adhere to full course of therapy when side effects occur (ADHERE2)[b]	0.59	0.68	0.50	4,7–9
Effectiveness of full course of PEP at preventing HIV infection (PEPE)	0.79	0.94	0.43	1
Probability of any side effects of PEP (SIDE)	0.50	0.20	0.80	4,7,8
Cost of PEP per person	$679[c]	$439	$1048	5
Discount rate	3%	0%	5%	
Discounted lifetime HIV/AIDS medical-care cost	$214,222	$325,791	$95,533	14
QALYs lost due to side effects of PEP	0.005	0	0.02	Estimate
QALYs saved per averted HIV infection	11.23	13.18	9.34	14

[a] Values in the best-case scenario improve the cost–effectiveness of the post exposure prophylaxis (PEP) intervention; values in the worst-case scenario reduce the cost–effectiveness of the PEP intervention.

[b] Sources cited for probability of adherence suggest that 50%–87% of patients will complete therapy. The distinction between adherence probabilities with and without side effects is assumed by the authors and not directly based on these sources.

[c] Costs were updated to year 2000 dollars using the Consumer Price Index (all urban consumers, all items). QALY, quality-adjusted life year.

health-care workers after percutaneous exposure to HIV-infected blood.[1] The cost of PEP was based on a previous cost–effectiveness study of PEP, which estimated the wholesale drug cost of a 4-week course of zidovudine and lamivudine and the cost of administering PEP (cost of laboratory services and office visits).[5] For simplicity, we did not include costs to the intervention participants (e.g., the cost of transportation to receive PEP). Ideally, all such costs should be included when using the societal perspective.

The discounted lifetime HIV/AIDS medical care cost was based on a cost-of-illness study by Holtgrave and Pinkerton.[14] The cost estimate we applied in our study was based on Holtgrave and Pinkerton's intermediate cost scenario, which assumed that a person would live 16 years after becoming infected with HIV: 2

years while unaware of infection, 1 year while aware of infection and receiving viral load monitoring but no treatment, and 13 years while receiving antiretroviral therapy, prophylaxis and treatment for opportunistic infections, and other medical care as the person progresses to AIDS. These costs were discounted at an annual rate of 3%. For simplicity, we did not include nonmedical HIV/AIDS costs borne by the patient (e.g., the cost of travel to receive treatment), although these costs should be included if possible when using the societal perspective. We did not include productivity losses due to morbidity and mortality as we assumed that these losses were incorporated in the QALY measures discussed below. If these QALY measures were specifically designed not to incorporate such losses in productivity, then the costs associated with these losses could be included as part of the societal cost of HIV/AIDS.

Valuing Outcomes

Holtgrave and Pinkerton[14] used the same disease-progression framework to estimate the number of QALYs saved per HIV infection averted. Their basic approach was to apply quality-of-life weights (ranging from 0 to 1) to each stage of disease progression (e.g., unaware of infection, aware of infection and receiving viral load monitoring but no treatment, etc.). The number of QALYs lost due to HIV infection was then estimated by adding the QALYs lost in each of the 16 years of infection together with the QALYS lost due to premature morbidity, discounted at 3% annually. The quality-of-life weights were drawn from studies in the literature, most of which relied on HIV-infected patients' self-reported quality-of-life estimates.[15-20] These patient-based preferences can be used when community-based preferences (the preferred measure for the base case analysis from the societal perspective) are not available, provided that any potential biases are discussed and addressed. For example, suppose that society's members, on average, would place a smaller quality-of-life weight on each HIV/AIDS state than actual HIV/AIDS patients. If so, then the use of patient-based weights would suggest a smaller number of QALYs lost per HIV infection than would a community-based measure; in turn, this smaller QALY estimate would lessen the apparent cost–effectiveness of all HIV-prevention interventions, including PEP. To address this uncertainty, we applied a range of values to the number of QALYs lost per HIV infection in the sensitivity analysis.

We were unable to find existing estimates of the number of QALYs lost due to side effects of PEP, which most commonly include nausea, fatigue, and headache.[7] We assumed that each person who experiences PEP side effects would suffer a loss of 0.005 QALYs or, equivalently, 1.825 quality-adjusted life days. These 1.825 days could represent 12 days of side effects with a reduction in quality of life of 0.15 per day (e.g., for men who experience side effects and remain on therapy) or 6 days of side effects with a reduction in quality of life of 0.30 per day (e.g., for men who experience side effects and discontinue therapy).

Using the decision tree, we estimated the number of QALYs gained by the intervention by subtracting the number of QALYs lost due to side effects of PEP from the number of QALYs gained by averting new cases of HIV. We calculated the average cost-utility ratio (cost per QALY gained, C) as follows: $C = (I - A) / Q$, where I is the cost of the PEP intervention, A represents direct HIV-related medical-care costs averted by the intervention, and Q represents the QALYs gained by the intervention.

Discounting

Because the analytic horizon includes all of the future benefits (QALYs gained and medical treatment costs averted) associated with each case of HIV infection averted by the program within the 1-year time frame, it is important that these future benefits be discounted appropriately. As discussed above, we applied Holtgrave and Pinkerton's[14] estimates of the QALYs gained and medical costs averted for each HIV infection prevented. Because these published estimates were calculated using 0%, 3%, and 5% discount rates, the discounting was built into our model and we did not have to make additional adjustments for it. After adjusting the treatment cost estimates for inflation to year 2000 dollars, the values we applied for the number of QALYs saved and the averted medical costs per case of HIV prevented were 23.87 and $301,560 (0% discount rate), 11.23 and $214,222 (base case, 3% discount rate), and 7.1 and $172,692 (5% discount rate).

Sensitivity Analysis

After calculating the cost per QALY gained under base-case parameter values, we repeated the analysis, varying other model inputs, such as the probability of HIV seroconversion with and without the provision of PEP, HIV prevalence in the sex partners, the discount rate, and the cost of PEP. First, we varied one input at a time, holding all other model inputs at their base-case values. This method of varying one parameter at a time in a sensitivity analysis is often called a *univariate*, *one-way*, or *one-at-a-time* sensitivity analysis. Second, we performed a multivariate sensitivity analysis, in which we varied two or more inputs at a time, holding other inputs at their base-case values.

Results

At base-case values of all parameters, an estimated 3.6 new HIV cases would occur among a hypothetical cohort of 1000 MSM in the absence of the PEP intervention, resulting in discounted lifetime HIV/AIDS medical-care costs of $771,200 and the loss of 40.4 QALYs (Table D.2). With the PEP intervention, an estimated 1.64 new cases of HIV would occur, resulting in discounted lifetime HIV/AIDS medical-care costs of $350,800 and loss of 18.4 QALYs due to HIV infection and 2.5 QALYs due to side effects of PEP. The incremental cost of the intervention was $258,600, which represents the cost of PEP provided to 1000 men ($679,000) minus the future medical savings ($420,400) from the averted HIV cases. The total number of QALYs gained by the intervention was 19.5 (22 QALYs were gained as a result of preventing new HIV cases, but 2.5 QALYs were lost due to the side ef-

Table D.2 Expected Number of Human Immunodeficiency Virus (HIV) Cases, Average Cost, Quality-Adjusted Life Years (QALYs) Lost, Incremental Change in Cost and QALYs, and Incremental Cost-Effectiveness (CE) Ratio (Cost per QALY Gained) for Postexposure Prophylaxis (PEP) Intervention Compared to No Intervention Under Base Case Parameter Values

Intervention	HIV Cases	Cost (Year 2000 Dollars)[a]			QALYs Lost[b]			Incremental Change		CE Ratio ($ per QALY Gained)[c]
		PEP	HIV	Total	HIV	Side Effects	Total	Cost	QALYs	
No intervention	3.6	0	$771,200	$771,200	40.4	0	40.4	—	—	—
PEP intervention	1.64	$679,000	$350,800	$1,029,800	18.4	2.5	20.9	258,600	19.5	$13,200

[a] Total cost represents cost of providing PEP plus cost of HIV treatment.

[b] Total QALYs lost represent QALYs lost due to PEP side effects and to HIV infection.

[c] Cost-utility ratio compares PEP intervention to no intervention, showing the incremental change in cost divided by the incremental change in effectiveness.

fects of PEP therapy). Dividing the incremental cost of the intervention by the number of QALYs gained yields the cost–utility ratio of $13,200.

In the sensitivity analysis (Table D.3), when we varied one parameter value at a time while holding other parameters at their base-case values, the cost–utility ratio ranged from being cost saving (a negative ratio) to more than $100,000 per QALY gained. Under some scenarios (e.g., when we simultaneously applied the lower bound estimates of PROB and PREV), the intervention resulted in a net loss of QALYs because the QALYs lost due to the side effects outnumbered the slight gain in QALYs from averting HIV infection. In such instances, the intervention is said to be "dominated" by the option "no PEP" since PEP cost more and resulted in a net loss of QALYs. When we assumed an HIV-transmission probability of 0.006 (the approximate per-act risk for insertive anal or vaginal intercourse with an HIV-infected partner[4,5,11,12]), the intervention was much less cost–effective. This finding suggests that providing PEP to men who report engaging in insertive intercourse probably would not be as cost–effective as many other available HIV-prevention interventions, except perhaps in situations when the partner is known or very likely to be HIV-infected.[5]

Table D.3   Sensitivity Analyses: Cost–Utility Ratios when Applying Best-Case and Worst-Case Parameter Values

Parameter Varied	Best-Case Scenario	Worst-Case Scenario
Per-act probability of HIV infection without PEP (PROB)	$1585	$134,483
Probability partner is HIV-infected (PREV)	Cost–saving[a]	$111,205
Probability patient will adhere to full course of therapy in absence of side effects (ADHERE1)	$11,968	$16,429
Probability patient will adhere to full course of therapy when side effects occur (ADHERE2)	$11,023	$15,803
Effectiveness of PEP at preventing HIV infection (PEPE)	$7537	$47,413
Probability of side effects (SIDE)	$9674	$18,310
Cost of PEP per person	$953	$32,124
Discount rate[b]	$1967	$29,749
Discounted lifetime HIV/AIDS medical-care cost	$2031	$25,159
QALYs lost due to side effects of PEP	$11,736	$21,485
QALYs saved per prevented HIV infection	$11,069	$16,339
PROB and PREV	Cost-saving	Dominated by "no PEP"[c]
PREV, ADHERE1, ADHERE2	Cost-saving	$147,886
PREV and PEPE	Cost-saving	$402,267
All of the above parameters	Cost-saving	Dominated by "no PEP"

[a] *Cost-saving* indicates that HIV costs averted were more than the cost of providing PEP. In such instances, PEP dominated the option "no PEP" since PEP saved money and resulted in a net gain of QALYs.

[b] Choice of the discount rate affects the lifetime cost of HIV as well as the number of QALYs saved per HIV case averted. The HIV cost per case is $214,222 at the baseline 3% discount rate, $301,560 when applying a 0% discount rate, and $172,692 when applying a 5% discount rate. The number of QALYs saved per case of HIV averted is 11.23 at the baseline 3% discount rate, 23.87 when applying a 0% discount rate, and 7.1 when applying 5% discount rate.

[c] *Dominated by "no PEP"* indicates that QALYs gained by HIV prevention were outweighed by QALYs lost due to side effects of PEP. In such instances, the option "no PEP" dominated PEP because PEP cost more and resulted in a net loss of QALYs. HIV, human immunodeficiency virus; PEP, postexposure prophylaxis; QALY, quality-adjusted life year.

Sensitivity analysis indicated that the estimated cost–utility ratio was dependent on the choice of discount rate for the future benefits of the intervention (QALYs gained and medical costs averted per case of HIV prevented). The cost–utility ratio was $1967 per QALY gained when the future benefits were not discounted and $29,749 per QALY gained when future benefits were discounted at an annual rate of 5% (Table D.3).

The cost–utility ratio ranged from $11,736 to $21,485 per QALY gained when we varied the number of QALYs lost due to the side effects of PEP from 0 to 0.02. Even larger fluctuations in the cost–utility ratio were obtained when we used a greater range of values for the QALYs lost due to side effects (Fig. D.2). Similarly, the probability that the sex partner is HIV-infected (PREV) is an important variable in the cost–effectiveness analysis (Fig. D.3). The cost–utility ratio is substantially higher when the probability that the partner is infected is 0.1 or lower.

DISCUSSION

This analysis suggests that PEP following possible sexual exposure to HIV through receptive anal intercourse can prevent HIV infection at a cost of $13,200 per QALY gained. However, the estimated cost–utility ratio varied substantially in the sensitivity analyses, suggesting that the cost–effectiveness of PEP might depend on the circumstances of the possible sexual exposure, such as the probability that the partner is HIV-infected. For example, when we assumed that the partner was HIV-infected, the PEP intervention was cost-saving. Thus, PEP can be an efficient use of public health resources when provided to receptive partners of HIV-infected persons, such as in serodiscordant couples.

Limitations

This analysis is subject to several limitations, including uncertainty in parameter values and the demonstrated sensitivity of the results to changes in parameter values. For simplicity, we compared the intervention to the no-intervention option. In reality, there are other HIV-prevention intervention options, such as risk-

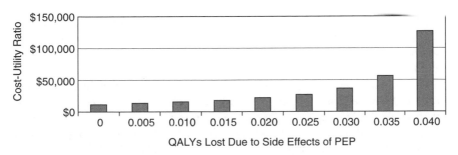

Figure D.2   Estimated cost–utility ratio using a range of values for the number of QALYs lost due to side effects of PEP.

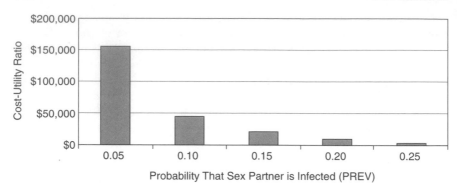

Figure D.3   Estimated cost–utility ratio using a range of values for the probability that sex partner is HIV-infected (PREV).

reduction counseling. The provision of PEP may appear to be less cost–effective compared to risk-reduction counseling, which has been demonstrated to be highly cost–effective in many settings.[21,22] Counseling also could be provided in addition to PEP.[23] If we assume that the effects of counseling would be the same regardless of whether PEP is offered, our analysis could be considered a simplified comparison of "PEP and counseling" to "counseling only."

We did not include costs borne by the intervention participants, such as the cost of travel to receive the PEP therapy. Although these costs should be included in the societal perspective, we note that these omitted costs likely are minor compared to the overall cost of PEP. Further, our results were not particularly sensitive to small changes in the estimated cost per person of PEP therapy.

We also made a number of simplifying assumptions, such as that partially completed PEP would not have any effect on the cost of therapy or on the probability of HIV acquisition. These simplifying assumptions may have resulted in underestimation of the cost–effectiveness of PEP. For example, if partially completed PEP reduces the probability of HIV seroconversion, then our analysis did not account for the potential HIV cases averted in those who discontinued therapy.

The hypothetical intervention would provide PEP to MSM who were the receptive partner in anal intercourse. In reality, it would be difficult to restrict the program in such a manner. For example, men might seek PEP after a possible sexual exposure to HIV in which they were the insertive partner. In such instances, the probability of HIV seroconversion would be lower and the provision of PEP would not be as cost–effective.

Some of our key model inputs may not reflect recent advances in the treatment of HIV/AIDS. For example, although the Holtgrave and Pinkerton[14] estimates of the cost per case of HIV and the number of QALYs lost per case of HIV include the use of combination drug therapy, the scenarios they evaluated do not include recently developed drugs and other improvements in the treatment of HIV/AIDS. Such advances may affect the cost of treatment, the timing of the initiation of antiretroviral therapy, and the expected survival time and quality of life after HIV infection. In addition, although we evaluated the cost–effectiveness of a two-drug PEP therapy, three-drug regimens may be used in some circumstances.[4,5] Our analysis should be viewed as an illustration of cost–effectiveness analysis methodology and not as a definitive determination of the cost–effectiveness of PEP for sexual exposure to HIV.

Finally, as noted earlier, we considered the use of PEP for accidental, episodic sexual exposures and did not examine PEP as a prevention strategy for persons with ongoing risk for sexual acquisition of HIV. Issues concerning the cost–effectiveness, feasibility, and affordability of PEP for accidental sexual exposure to HIV (including the issue of PEP in instances of ongoing risk) are discussed more thoroughly elsewhere.[5,6,23–26]

Public Policy Implications

Although the effectiveness of PEP following sexual exposure to HIV has not been established, cost-effectiveness analyses such as this one can be useful to examine the potential costs and benefits associated with the provision of PEP for sexual exposure to HIV. Of course, the cost-effectiveness of PEP is not the only determinant of its appropriateness as a tool for HIV prevention. Many other important factors, such as the potential for PEP to reduce psychological distress or the possibility that PEP might facilitate the development of drug resistance, also should be considered.[5] An individual's decision of whether or not to seek PEP likely would depend on such factors as risk aversion and willingness to tolerate side effects.

Our results suggest that, in some instances, such as providing PEP to the insertive partner of a person unlikely to have HIV, PEP will not be as cost–effective as other HIV-prevention interventions, such as behavioral risk-reduction programs, many of which have been shown to be cost-saving.[5,27] However, in other situations, such as potential exposure through receptive anal intercourse and exposure involving a partner known to be HIV-infected, the provision of PEP can be a cost-saving strategy in preventing HIV.

REFERENCES

1. Centers for Disease Control and Prevention. Case-control study of HIV seroconversion in health-care workers after percutaneous exposure to HIV-infected blood—France, United Kingdom, and United States, January 1988–August 1994. *MMWR Morb Mortal Wkly Rep 1995;* 44:929–33.
2. Centers for Disease Control and Prevention. Update: provisional Public Health Service recommendations for chemoprophylaxis after occupational exposure to HIV. *MMWR Morb Mortal Wkly Rep 1996;* 45:468–80.
3. Cardo DM, Culver DH, Ciesielski CA, et al. A case-control study of HIV seroconversion in health care workers after percutaneous exposure. Centers for Disease Control and Prevention Needlestick Surveillance Group. *N Engl J Med 1997;* 337:1485–90.
4. Katz MH, Gerberding JL. Postexposure treatment of people exposed to the human immunodeficiency virus through sexual contact or injection-drug use. *N Engl J Med 1997;*336:1097–100.
5. Pinkerton SD, Holtgrave DR, Bloom FR. Cost–effectiveness of post-exposure prophylaxis following sexual exposure to HIV. *AIDS 1998;* 12:1067–78.

6. Merchant RC. Post-exposure prophylaxis affordability: a clearer reality. *AIDS 2001;* 15:541–2.
7. Tokars JI, Marcus R, Culver DH, et al. Surveillance of HIV infection and zidovudine use among health care workers after occupational exposure to HIV-infected blood. The CDC Cooperative Needlestick Surveillance Group. *Ann Intern Med 1993;* 118:913–9.
8. Puro V, Ippolito G, Guzzanti E, et al. Zidovudine prophylaxis after accidental exposure to HIV: the Italian experience. The Italian Study Group on Occupational Risk of HIV Infection. *AIDS 1992;* 6:963–9.
9. Schmitz SH, Scheding S, Voliotis D, et al. Side effects of AZT prophylaxis after occupational exposure to HIV-infected blood. *Ann Hematol 1994;* 69:135–8.
10. Pinkerton SD, Chesson HW, Holtgrave DR, et al. When is an HIV infection prevented and when is it merely delayed? *Evaluation Rev 2000;* 24:251–71.
11. Mastro TD, de Vincenzi I. Probabilities of sexual HIV-1 transmission. *AIDS 1996;* 10 (Suppl A):S75–82.
12. Vittinghoff E, Douglas J, Judson F, et al. Per-contact risk of human immunodeficiency virus transmission between male sexual partners. *Am J Epidemiol 1999;* 150:306–11.
13. Holmberg SD. The estimated prevalence and incidence of HIV in 96 large US metropolitan areas. *Am J Public Health 1996;* 86:642–54.
14. Holtgrave DR, Pinkerton SD. Updates of cost of illness and quality of life estimates for use in economic evaluations of HIV prevention programs. *J Acquir Immune Defic Syndr Hum Retrovirol 1997;* 16:54–62.
15. Tsevat J, Solzan JG, Kuntz KM, et al. Health values of patients infected with human immunodeficiency virus. Relationship to mental health and physical functioning. *Med Care 1996;* 34:44–57.
16. Wu AW, Mathews WC, Brysk LT, et al. Quality of life in a placebo-controlled trial of zidovudine in patients with AIDS and AIDS-related complex. *J Acquir Immune Defic Syndr 1990;* 3:683–90.
17. Revicki DA, Wu AW, Murray MI. Change in clinical status, health status, and health utility outcomes in HIV-infected patients. *Med Care 1995;* 33:AS173–82.
18. Wu AW, Rubin HR, Mathews WC, et al. A health status questionnaire using 30 items from the Medical Outcomes Study. Preliminary validation in persons with early HIV infection. *Med Care 1991;* 29:786–98.
19. Schag CA, Ganz PA, Kahn B, Petersen L. Assessing the needs and quality of life of patients with HIV infection: development of the HIV Overview of Problems-Evaluation System (HOPES). *Qual Life Res 1992;* 1:397–413.
20. Owens DK, Nease RF Jr. Transmission of HIV infection between patient and provider: a quantitative analysis of risk. In: Kaplan EH, Brandeau ML, (eds). *Modeling the AIDS Epidemic: Planning, Policy, and Prediction.* New York: Raven, 1994; 153–77.
21. Holtgrave DR, Qualls NL, Graham JD. Economic evaluation of HIV prevention programs. *Annu Rev Public Health 1996;* 17:467–88.
22. Kamb ML, Fishbein M, Douglas JMJ, et al. Efficacy of risk-reduction counseling to prevent human immunodeficiency virus and sexually transmitted diseases: a randomized controlled trial. Project RESPECT Study Group. *JAMA 1998;* 280:1161–7.
23. Kahn JO, Martin JN, Roland ME, et al. Feasibility of postexposure prophylaxis (PEP) against human immunodeficiency virus infection after sexual or injection drug use exposure: the San Francisco PEP Study. *J Infect Dis 2001;* 183:707–14.
24. Low-Beer S, Weber AE, Bartholomew K, et al. A reality check: the cost of making post-exposure prophylaxis available to gay and bisexual men at high sexual risk. *AIDS 2000;* 14:325–6.

25. Lurie P, Miller S, Hecht F, et al. Postexposure prophylaxis after nonoccupational HIV exposure: clinical, ethical, and policy considerations. *JAMA 1998;* 280:1769–73.
26. Pinkerton SD, Holtgrave DR, Kahn JG. Is post-exposure prophylaxis affordable? *AIDS 2000;* 14:325
27. Pinkerton SD, Johnson-Masotti AP, Holtgrave DR, Farnham PG. Using cost–effectiveness league tables to compare interventions to prevent sexual transmission of HIV. *AIDS 2001;* 15:917–28.

APPENDIX E

Sources for Collecting Cost-of-Illness Data

LAURIE A. FERRELL

Collecting reliable cost-of-illness data is one of the most difficult aspects of conducting an economic analysis. Data are often unavailable, may not be generalizable to another population, or may not reflect true economic costs. This appendix includes sources for collecting costs of illness and injury, including (*1*) literature reviews, (*2*) public-use databases, (*3*) annually published materials, (*4*) miscellaneous journal articles, and (*5*) data collected by the private sector.

LITERATURE REVIEWS

The first step in a cost analysis is a literature review for published studies that assess similar health outcomes. In cases where similar health outcomes have been studied, published studies may provide cost data that can be directly applied to a particular analysis. In other cases, a study of a similar (but not identical) health outcome may provide valuable data that can be extrapolated to fit the study design.

When using data from published studies, however, sensitivity analyses should be conducted to test the effects of changes in cost estimates on the results of the current study.

There are several mechanisms by which to search the literature. Databases such as Medline, The National Health Service Economic Evaluation Database, and the Cochrane Controlled Trial Register can be accessed via the Internet with publicly available search engines. Others, such as The Health Economic Evaluation Database are specialized, include annotated abstracts, and are available on a subscription basis. Other specialized databases are becoming available through academic institutions. The CUA Data Base, available from the Harvard Center for Risk Analysis at the Harvard School of Public Health, is one good example.

MEDLINE

MEDLINE (http://www.nlm.nih.gov/hinfo.html) is produced by the National Library of Medicine (NLM) and contains bibliographic citations from over 3500 medical journals. Topics covered include medicine, nursing, dentistry, veterinary medicine, and preclinical sciences. Over 11 million citations, dating back to 1966, are indexed by over 14,000 medical subject headings (MeSH), including *health-care costs*, *cost–benefit analysis*, and *cost analysis*. Over 80 subheadings, including *economics*, are also used. Most citations entered after 1975 contain abstracts.

National Health Service Economic Evaluation Database

The National Health Service (NHS) Centre for Reviews and Dissemination at the University of York maintains the NHS Economic Evaluations Database (NHS EED). The database contains structured abstracts and bibliographic information on economic evaluations of health interventions. The NHS EED home page is located at http://nhscrd.york.ac.uk/nhsdhp.htm. This site can also be used to search other effectiveness databases, including the Database of Abstracts of Reviews of Effectiveness (DARE) and the Health Technology Assessment (HTA) Database .

Health Economic Evaluations Database

The Health Economic Evaluations Database (HEED) is a subscription database containing more than 25,000 evaluations from peer-reviewed journals and academic and government centers. The database contains articles that have been selected from over 4500 journals and includes cost-minimization, cost–effectiveness, cost–consequences, cost–utility, and cost–benefit analyses. Also included are cost-of-illness and costing studies, methodological articles, and policy applications of economic evaluations. More information is available on the Office of Health Economics (OHE) website at http://www.ohe.org/HEED.htm or by contacting OHE at database@ohe.org.

CUA Data Base

The Harvard Center for Risk Analysis at the Harvard School of Public Health has created the CUA Data Base as a single electronic source for cost–utility analyses (CUAs). The CUA Data Base website includes a reference list of the CUAs of life-saving interventions that have used the quality–adjusted life year (QALY) to measure health benefits, a comprehensive league table of all of the ratios in the database, a modified league table with the ratios from studies that follow the recommendations of the U.S. Public Health Service (USPHS) Panel on Cost–Effectiveness in Health and Medicine (see Chapter 10), and a catalog of preference scores. The database is located at http://www.hsph.harvard.edu/organizations/hcra/cuadatabase/intro.html.

HEALTH CARE UTILIZATION AND COST DATABASES

After completing a literature search, the next step is to gather any data pertaining to the cost and health outcomes under analysis. There are several national data sources administered by federal agencies, such as the National Center for Health Statistics (NCHS), the Centers for Medicare and Medicaid Services (CMS), and the Agency for Healthcare Research and Quality (AHRQ) that provide aggregated data either on the state or national level. There are also commercially available sources of health-care utilization and cost data. One of those, the MEDSTAT Group, sells the widely used MarketScan databases, which are described below. The following list comprises the most frequently used sources of health-care utilization and cost data.

National Center for Health Statistics (NCHS)

The National Center for Health Statistics (NCHS) provides on-line access to a variety of public use databases. The NCHS maintains two major types of data systems: those that contain data collected from interview or examinations and those collected from records. Several of those data systems most useful for estimating cost of illness are described below. NCHS maintains a number of listserves for specific data systems that are designed to keep users up-to-date on new data releases, documentation, and publications. The NCHS Web site is located at http://www.cdc.gov/nchs/

National Health Interview Survey (NHIS)

Implemented since 1957, National Health Interview Survey (NHIS) provides data on self-reported illness. It involves a personal interview performed weekly of a sampling of U. S. households. Prior to 1997, variables included restricted activity days, bed days, work/school lost days, physician visits, hospital episodes, and surgeries. From 1997 on, variables include bed days, work/school loss days, physician and other health-care provider visits, emergency room visits, home care visits, hospital episodes, and surgeries. NHIS data, documentation, and publications are available on-line at http://www.cdc.gov/nchs/nhis.

National Health and Nutrition Examination Survey (NHANES)

The NHANES survey is administered by NCHS to collect information on the health and diet of the U.S. population. Data is collected from personal interviews and health examinations. Data are collected on participant income, health insurance, health-care utilization, and health and health-related behaviors. Further information on NHANES including data, documentation, and publications are available on-line at http://www.cdc.gov/nchs.

National Health Care Survey (NHCS)

The National Health Care Survey (NHCS) is a family of national probability sample surveys that collect data from health-care providers and establishments about characteristics of providers and their patients. Researchers and policy makers use data from the NHCS to profile utilization of health-care services and to study issues such as the epidemiology of health conditions, demand for health resources, patterns of treatment, disposition following receipt of health care, and disparities in health-care utilization. Components of the NHCS and their foci include: the National Hospital Discharge Survey (NHDS, focusing on hospital utilization), the National Ambulatory Medical Care Survey (NAMCS, visits to office based physicians), the National Hospital Ambulatory Medical Care Survey (NHAMCS, visits to hospital outpatient and emergency departments), National Nursing Home Survey (NNHS, nursing home residents and discharges), National Home and Hospice Care Survey (NHHCS, home and hospice care agencies, their residents and discharges), the National Survey of Ambulatory Surgery (hospital and free standing ambulatory surgery centers), and the National Employer Health Insurance Survey (NEHIS, business establishments, government organizations, and self employed individuals). Data are available in publications, on public-use data tapes, data diskettes, CD-ROMs, and downloadable files. Further information on data, publications, and listserves may be found at http://www.cdc.gov/nchs/nhcs.

The Centers for Medicare and Medicaid Services (CMS)

The Centers for Medicare and Medicaid Services sell public-use tapes on Medicare and Medicaid data that provide information on (*1*) utilization, (*2*) enrollment, (*3*) providers, (*4*) cost limits, (*5*) payment rates, and (*6*) cost reports on inpatients, capital, nursing facilities, and outpatients. Two of the most commonly used data sets for health-care utilization and cost studies are the Medicare Provider Analysis and Review (MEDPAR) files, which contain records of hospital inpatient services and the Part B Provider files, which contain claims submitted by a 5% sample of physicians and other outpatient providers of health-care services.

Medicaid data, published annually on a state-by-state basis, provide aggregated information on health-care utilization by and cost for Medicaid recipients. CMS also provides the Medicaid Statistical File, form HCFA-2082, Statistical Report on Medical Care: Eligibles, Recipients, Payments, and Services. This file reports Medicaid costs and utilization data that are submitted annually by states, territories, and the District of Columbia.

A Public Use Files Catalog, which includes both Medicare and Medicaid data, can be downloaded from the CMS Web site at http://www.cms.gov.

Agency for Healthcare Research and Quality (AHRQ)

The Agency for Healthcare Research and Quality (AHRQ), formerly the Agency for Health Care Policy and Research, conducts and funds health services research for the U.S. Department of Health and Human Services. The agency supports two sources of data useful for health-care cost and utilization research: the Medical Expenditure Panel Survey and data from the Healthcare Cost and Utilization Project. The data are available on-line and for purchase. Further information can be obtained at http://www.ahrq.gov.

Medical Expenditure Panel Survey (MEPS)

The MEPS has collected data on health-care use and cost, and health insurance, economic and health status of survey respondents. It is a good source of data for studies of consumer interaction with the health care delivery system. MEPS is comprised of four parts: (*1*) the household, (*2*) nursing home, (*3*) provider, and (*4*) insurance components. Data are available on-line, on diskette, and on CD-ROM. Further information can be found on the AHRQ Web site.

Healthcare Cost and Utilization Project (HCUP)

HCUP is a multi-state information system comprised of several administrative longitudinal databases for the years 1988–1999. The data are obtained from hospital discharge and ambulatory surgery records and contain utilization and cost information classified by diagnosis or procedure code. HCUP data are available for purchase. More information on obtaining the data is located on the AHRQ Web site.

Bureau of Labor Statistics

The Bureau of Labor Statistics (BLS) is the principal fact-finding agency for the federal government in the broad field of labor economics and statistics. This site is particularly useful for obtaining wage and employment information useful in estimating productivity losses. A wide variety of information pertinent to health-care research is located on the BLS Web site at http://stats.bls.gov.

Databases Available from Vendors

Health-care cost databases are also available from private vendors. For example, the MarketScan databases, available from the MEDSTAT Group, are longitudinal databases with patient utilization of inpatient, outpatient, and prescription drug experiences. The database includes the records of millions of privately insured individuals as well as Medicare- and Medicaid-eligible individuals. Health-care utilization records are linked with information on benefit plans, providers, and worker attendance. Interactive software specifically designed to work with the MarketScan databases is also available. Information on the databases and the interactive software is available on the MEDSTAT Group Web site at http://www.medstat.com.

ANNUALLY PUBLISHED MATERIAL

In addition to the data described above, there are several publications that provide nationally aggregated data on an annual basis.

The DRG Handbook: Comparative Clinical and
Financial Benchmarks, 2001

This publication provides a complete charge breakdown and analysis of 53 major diagnosis-related groups (DRGs), and includes a detailed charge analysis providing cost data for ancillary services such as laboratory, radiology, medical supplies, and pharmacy; summary information for all DRGs (includes average length of stay and average total charge per discharge); and comparison group information for all major diagnostic categories (MDCs). The data are further broken down by region and hospital type. *The DRG Handbook* is a good source of cost data only for specific types of studies—those with health outcomes that can be categorized into a DRG. In addition, the handbook assesses Medicare claims only, so one should be cautious in trying to interpolate data for all age groups. *The DRG Handbook* is published annually by HCIA-Sachs and Ernst & Young. HCIA also produces annual publications on hospital inpatient charges, hospital admission rates, and length of stay (LOS). Ordering information on is available on-line at http://www.hcia.com/hcia_library/drgh/default.htm.

Statistical Abstract of the United States

The Statistical Abstract of the United States is published annually by the U.S. Department of Commerce, Economics and Statistics Administration, Bureau of the Census. There are several tables that can provide data for prevention effectiveness studies:

- Medicare Utilization and Charges. Includes percentage of covered charges reimbursed for hospital visits and percentage of covered charges reimbursed for physician visits.
- Consumer Price Indexes of Medical Care Prices. The medical-care commodities include prescription drugs and nonprescription drugs and medical supplies. The medical-care services include professional medical services, (i.e., physician charges, dental services, and eye care), and hospital and related services, (i.e., hospital rooms). See Appendix H.
- Average Cost to Community Hospitals per Patient.
- Average Cost to Community Hospitals per Patient, by State.
- Hospital Discharges and Days of Care, by Sex, Age, and Diagnosis. Diagnoses include diseases of heart, malignant neoplasms, pneumonia (all forms), fractures (all sites), and cerebrovascular diseases.
- Injury, Medical Care, Morbidity, and Mortality Costs, by Sex, Age, and Cause.
- Civilian Labor Force and Participation Rates, by Race, Hispanic Origin, Sex, and Age.
- Employer Costs for Employee Compensation per Hour Worked, by Industry.
- Median Money Income of Year-Round Full-Time Workers with Income, by Sex, Age, Race, and Hispanic Origin.

The Abstract is available in PDF format at no cost or can be ordered from the Government Printing Office (GPO). Information on downloading the PDF files and ordering is available on-line at http://www.census.gov/statab/www/.

Health, United States

Health, United States is published annually by the U. S. Department of Health and Human Services, Centers for Disease Control and Prevention, National Center for

Health Statistics. There are 28 tables that provide economic data over several years. For example,:

- Hospital expenses according to type of ownership and size of hospital.
- Nursing home average monthly charges per resident and percent of residents, according to selected facility and resident characteristics.
- Appendix I. Data Sources. Provides general overview of data sources, methods of data collection, and reliability/validity of data. Also provides contact names for more information on each data set.
- Medicare expenditures according to type of service.

Information on downloading PDF files for the publication is available on-line at http://www.cdc.gov/nchs/hus.htm.

Hospital Statistics

The American Hospital Association (AHA) conducts annual surveys to obtain information on the average cost per hospital day, the average length of a hospital stay, and other hospital statistics. *Hospital Statistics* can be ordered either in hard copy or diskette from the AHA Web site at http://www.aha.org.

INTERNATIONAL RESOURCES

World Bank AIDS Economics

World Bank AIDS Economics is part of the International AIDS Economic Network (IAEN). The IAEN offers data, tools, and analysis for compassionate, cost-effective responses to the global HIV/AIDS epidemic. http://www.worldbank.org/aids-econ/

World Bank Health Nutrition and Population Stats

HNPStats offers country data sheets showing summary indicators for health status, health determinants, and health finance. http://www.devdata.worldbank.org/hnpstats/

WHO Statistical Information System

The purpose of WHOSIS is to describe and provide access to statistical and epidemiological data and information presently available for the World Health Organization. http://www.who.int/whosis/

APPENDIX F

Cost-to-Charge Ratios

Statewide Average Operating Cost-to-Charge Ratios
for Urban and Rural Hospitals (Case-Weighted)
March 2001

State	Urban	Rural
Alabama	0.344	0.410
Alaska	0.417	0.696
Arizona	0.356	0.491
Arkansas	0.466	0.446
California	0.339	0.436
Colorado	0.422	0.577
Connecticut	0.497	0.506
Delaware	0.511	0.450
District of Columbia	0.508	N/A
Florida	0.352	0.369
Georgia	0.459	0.470
Hawaii	0.413	0.554
Idaho	0.545	0.561
Illinois	0.406	0.502
Indiana	0.524	0.533
Iowa	0.486	0.612
Kansas	0.421	0.635
Kentucky	0.479	0.492
Louisiana	0.410	0.488
Maine	0.615	0.543
Maryland	0.759	0.819
Massachusetts	0.512	0.571
Michigan	0.460	0.563
Minnesota	0.494	0.589
Mississippi	0.452	0.447
Missouri	0.405	0.479
Montana	0.537	0.594
Nebraska	0.449	0.610
Nevada	0.306	0.498
New Hampshire	0.549	0.581
New Jersey	0.394	N/A
New Mexico	0.466	0.491
New York	0.528	0.609

(*Continued*)

Statewide Average Operating Cost-to-Charge Ratios
for Urban and Rural Hospitals (Case-Weighted) May
4, 2001 (*continued*)

State	Urban	Rural
North Carolina	0.516	0.464
North Dakota	0.620	0.654
Ohio	0.501	0.570
Oklahoma	0.409	0.494
Oregon	0.613	0.595
Pennsylvania	0.398	0.525
Puerto Rico	0.486	0.583
Rhode Island	0.520	N/A
South Carolina	0.440	0.463
South Dakota	0.529	0.638
Tennessee	0.438	0.453
Texas	0.402	0.494
Utah	0.497	0.586
Vermont	0.572	0.599
Virginia	0.454	0.494
Washington	0.583	0.638
West Virginia	0.568	0.527
Wisconsin	0.525	0.611
Wyoming	0.522	0.717

Source: The Federal Register, Volume 66, No. 87, Friday, May 4, 2001,
pp. 22845–91.

APPENDIX G
Discount and Annuitization Tables

Present Value of $1, Discounted to the nth Year

n	0%	1%	2%	3%	4%	5%	6%	7%	8%	9%	10%
1	1.0000	0.9901	0.9804	0.9709	0.9615	0.9524	0.9434	0.9346	0.9259	09.174	0.9091
2	1.0000	0.9803	0.9612	0.9426	0.9246	0.9070	0.8900	0.8734	0.8573	0.8417	0.8264
3	1.0000	0.9706	0.9423	0.9151	0.8890	0.8638	0.8396	0.8163	0.7938	0.7722	0.7513
4	1.0000	0.9610	0.9238	0.8885	0.8548	0.8227	0.7921	0.7629	0.7350	0.7084	0.6830
5	1.0000	0.9515	0.9037	0.8626	0.8219	0.7835	0.7473	0.7130	0.6806	0.6499	0.6209
6	1.0000	0.9420	0.8880	0.8375	0.7903	0.7462	0.7050	0.6663	0.6302	0.5963	0.5645
7	1.0000	0.9327	0.8706	0.8131	0.7599	0.7107	0.6651	0.6227	0.5835	0.5470	0.5132
8	1.0000	0.9235	0.8535	0.7894	0.7307	0.6768	0.6274	0.5820	0.5403	0.5019	0.4665
9	1.0000	0.9143	0.8368	0.7664	0.7026	0.6446	0.5919	0.5439	0.5002	0.4604	0.4241
10	1.0000	0.9053	0.8203	0.7441	0.6756	0.6139	0.5584	0.5083	0.4632	0.4224	0.3855
11	1.0000	0.8963	0.8043	0.7224	0.6496	0.5817	0.5268	0.4751	0.4289	0.3875	0.3505
12	1.0000	0.8874	0.7885	0.7014	0.6246	0.5568	0.4970	0.4440	0.3971	0.3555	0.3186
13	1.0000	0.8787	0.7730	0.6810	0.6006	0.5303	0.4688	0.4150	0.3677	0.3262	0.2897
14	1.0000	0.8700	0.7579	0.6611	0.5775	0.5051	0.4423	0.3878	0.3405	0.2992	0.2633
15	1.0000	0.8613	0.7430	0.6419	0.5553	0.4810	0.4173	0.3624	0.3152	0.2745	0.2394
16	1.0000	0.8528	0.7284	0.6232	0.5339	0.4581	0.3936	0.3387	0.2919	0.2519	0.2176
17	1.0000	0.8444	0.7142	0.6050	0.5134	0.4363	0.3714	0.3166	0.2703	0.2311	0.1978
18	1.0000	0.8360	0.7002	0.5874	0.4936	0.4155	0.3503	0.2959	0.2502	0.2120	0.1799
19	1.0000	0.8277	0.6864	0.5703	0.4746	0.3957	0.3305	0.2765	0.2317	0.1945	0.1635
20	1.0000	0.8195	0.6730	0.5537	0.4564	0.3769	0.3118	0.2584	0.2145	0.1784	0.1486
21	1.0000	0.8114	0.6598	0.5375	0.4388	0.3589	0.2942	0.2415	0.1987	0.1637	0.1351
22	1.0000	0.8034	0.6468	0.5219	0.4220	0.3418	0.2775	0.2257	0.1839	0.1502	0.1228
23	1.0000	0.7954	0.6342	0.5067	0.4057	0.3256	0.2618	0.2109	0.1703	0.1378	0.1117
24	1.0000	0.7876	0.6217	0.4919	0.3901	0.3101	0.2470	0.1971	0.1577	0.1264	0.1015
25	1.0000	0.7798	0.6095	0.4776	0.3751	0.2953	0.2330	0.1842	0.1460	0.1160	0.0923
26	1.0000	0.7720	0.5976	0.4637	0.3607	0.2812	0.2198	0.1722	0.1352	0.1064	0.0839
27	1.0000	0.7644	0.5859	0.4502	0.3468	0.2678	0.2074	0.1609	0.1252	0.0976	0.0763
28	1.0000	0.7568	0.5744	0.4371	0.3335	0.2551	0.1956	0.1504	0.1159	0.0895	0.0693
29	1.0000	0.7493	0.5631	0.4243	0.3207	0.2429	0.1846	0.1406	0.1073	0.0822	0.0630
30	1.0000	0.7419	0.5521	0.4120	0.3083	0.2314	0.1741	0.1314	0.0994	0.0754	0.0573
31	1.0000	0.7346	0.5412	0.4000	0.2965	0.2204	0.1643	0.1228	0.0920	0.0691	0.0521
32	1.0000	0.7273	0.5306	0.3883	0.2851	0.2099	0.1550	0.1147	0.0852	0.0634	0.0474
33	1.0000	0.7201	0.5202	0.3770	0.2741	0.1999	0.1462	0.1072	0.0789	0.0582	0.0431
34	1.0000	0.7130	0.5100	0.3660	0.2636	0.1904	0.1379	0.1002	0.0730	0.0534	0.0391
35	1.0000	0.7059	0.5000	0.3554	0.2534	0.1813	0.1301	0.0937	0.0676	0.0490	0.0356

(continued)

Present Value of $1, Discounted to the nth Year (*continued*)

n	0%	1%	2%	3%	4%	5%	6%	7%	8%	9%	10%
36	1.0000	0.6989	0.4902	0.3450	0.2437	0.1727	0.1227	0.0875	0.0626	0.0449	0.0323
37	1.0000	0.6000	0.4806	0.3350	0.2343	0.1644	0.1158	0.0818	0.0580	0.0412	0.0294
38	1.0000	0.6852	0.4712	0.3252	0.2253	0.1566	0.1092	0.0765	0.0537	0.0378	0.0267
39	1.0000	0.6784	0.4619	0.3158	0.2166	0.1491	0.1031	0.0715	0.0497	0.0347	0.0243
40	1.0000	0.6717	0.4529	0.3066	0.2083	0.1420	0.0972	0.0668	0.0460	0.0318	0.0221
41	1.0000	0.6650	0.4440	0.2976	0.2003	0.1353	0.0917	0.0624	0.0426	0.0292	0.0201
42	1.0000	0.6584	0.4353	0.2890	0.1926	0.1288	0.0865	0.0583	0.0395	0.0268	0.0183
43	1.0000	0.6519	0.4268	0.2805	0.1852	0.1227	0.0816	0.0545	0.0365	0.0246	0.0166
44	1.0000	0.6454	0.4184	0.2724	0.1780	0.1169	0.0770	0.0509	0.0338	0.0226	0.0151
45	1.0000	0.6391	0.4102	0.2644	0.1712	0.1113	0.0727	0.0476	0.0313	0.0207	0.0137
46	1.0000	0.6327	0.4022	0.2567	0.1646	0.1060	0.0685	0.0445	0.0290	0.0190	0.0125
47	1.0000	0.6265	0.3943	0.2493	0.1583	0.1009	0.0647	0.0416	0.0269	0.0174	0.0113
48	1.0000	0.6203	0.3865	0.2420	0.1522	0.0961	0.0610	0.0389	0.0249	0.0160	0.0103
49	1.0000	0.6141	0.3790	0.2350	0.1463	0.0916	0.0575	0.0363	0.0230	0.0147	0.0094
50	1.0000	0.6080	0.3715	0.2281	0.1407	0.0872	0.0543	0.0339	0.0213	0.0134	0.0085
51	1.0000	0.6020	0.3642	0.2215	0.1353	0.0831	0.0512	0.0317	0.0197	0.0123	0.0077
52	1.0000	0.5961	0.3571	0.2150	0.1301	0.0791	0.0483	0.0297	0.0183	0.0113	0.0070
53	1.0000	0.5902	0.3501	0.2088	0.1251	0.0753	0.0456	0.0277	0.0169	0.0104	0.0064
54	1.0000	0.5843	0.3432	0.2027	0.1203	0.0717	0.0430	0.0259	0.0157	0.0095	0.0058
55	1.0000	0.5785	0.3365	0.1968	0.1157	0.0683	0.0406	0.0242	0.0145	0.0087	0.0053
56	1.0000	0.5728	0.3299	0.1910	0.1112	0.0651	0.0383	0.0226	0.0134	0.0080	0.0048
57	1.0000	0.5671	0.3234	0.1855	0.1069	0.0620	0.0361	0.0211	0.0124	0.0074	0.0044
58	1.0000	0.5615	0.3171	0.1801	0.1028	0.0590	0.0341	0.0198	0.0115	0.0067	0.0040
59	1.0000	0.5560	0.3109	0.1748	0.0989	0.0562	0.0321	0.0185	0.0107	0.0062	0.0036
60	1.0000	0.5504	0.3048	0.1697	0.0951	0.0535	0.0303	0.0173	0.0099	0.0057	0.0033
61	1.0000	0.5450	0.2988	0.1648	0.0914	0.0510	0.0286	0.0161	0.0091	0.0052	0.0030
62	1.0000	0.5396	0.2929	0.1600	0.0879	0.0486	0.0270	0.0151	0.0085	0.0048	0.0027
63	1.0000	0.5343	0.2872	0.1553	0.0845	0.0462	0.0255	0.0141	0.0078	0.0044	0.0025
64	1.0000	0.5290	0.2816	0.1508	0.0813	0.0440	0.0240	0.0132	0.0073	0.0040	0.0022
65	1.0000	0.5237	0.2761	0.1464	0.0781	0.0419	0.0227	0.0123	0.0067	0.0037	0.0020
66	1.0000	0.5185	0.2706	0.1421	0.0751	0.0399	0.0214	0.0115	0.0062	0.0034	0.0019
67	1.0000	0.5134	0.2653	0.1380	0.0722	0.0380	0.0202	0.0107	0.0058	0.0031	0.0017
68	1.0000	0.5083	0.2601	0.1340	0.0695	0.0362	0.0190	0.0100	0.0053	0.0029	0.0015
69	1.0000	0.5033	0.2550	0.1301	0.0668	0.0345	0.0179	0.0094	0.0049	0.0026	0.0014
70	1.0000	0.4983	0.2500	0.1263	0.0642	0.0329	0.0169	0.0088	0.0046	0.0024	0.0013
71	1.0000	0.4934	0.2451	0.1226	0.0617	0.0313	0.0160	0.0082	0.0042	0.0022	0.0012
72	1.0000	0.4885	0.2403	0.1190	0.0594	0.0298	0.0151	0.0077	0.0039	0.0020	0.0010
73	1.0000	0.4837	0.2356	0.1156	0.0571	0.0284	0.0142	0.0072	0.0036	0.0019	0.0010
74	1.0000	0.4789	0.2310	0.1122	0.0549	0.0270	0.0134	0.0067	0.0034	0.0017	0.0009
75	1.0000	0.4741	0.2265	0.1089	0.0528	0.0258	0.0126	0.0063	0.0031	0.0016	0.0008
76	1.0000	0.4694	0.2220	0.1058	0.0508	0.0245	0.0119	0.0058	0.0029	0.0014	0.0007

Annuitization Factor[a]

n	1%	2%	3%	4%	5%	6%	7%	8%	9%	10%
1	0.9901	0.9804	0.9709	0.9615	0.9524	0.9434	0.9346	0.9259	0.9174	0.9091
2	1.9704	1.9416	1.9135	1.8861	1.8594	1.8334	1.8080	1.7833	1.7591	1.7335
3	2.9410	2.8839	2.8286	2.7751	2.7232	2.6730	2.6243	2.5771	2.5313	2.4869
4	3.9020	3.8077	3.7171	3.6299	3.5460	3.4651	3.3872	3.3121	3.2397	3.1699
5	4.8534	4.7135	4.5797	4.4518	4.3295	4.2124	4.1002	3.9927	3.8897	3.7908
6	5.7955	5.6014	5.4172	5.2421	5.0757	4.9173	4.7665	4.6229	4.4859	4.3553
7	6.7282	6.4720	6.2303	6.0021	5.7864	5.5824	5.3893	5.2064	5.0330	4.8684
8	7.6517	7.3255	7.0197	6.7327	6.4632	6.2098	5.9713	5.7466	5.5348	5.3349
9	8.5660	8.1622	7.7861	7.4353	7.1078	6.8017	6.5152	6.2469	5.9952	5.7590
10	9.4713	8.9826	8.5302	8.1109	7.7217	7.3601	7.0236	6.7101	6.4177	6.1446
11	10.3676	9.7868	9.2526	8.7605	8.3064	7.8869	7.4987	7.1390	6.8052	6.4951
12	11.2551	10.5753	9.9540	9.3851	8.8633	8.3838	7.9427	7.5361	7.1607	6.8137
13	12.1337	11.3484	10.6350	9.9856	9.3936	8.8527	8.3577	7.9038	7.4869	7.1034
14	13.0037	12.1062	11.2961	10.5631	9.8986	9.2950	8.7455	8.2442	7.7862	7.3667
15	13.8651	12.8493	11.9379	11.1184	10.3797	9.7122	9.1079	8.5595	8.0607	7.6061
16	14.7179	13.5777	12.5611	11.6523	10.8378	10.1059	9.4466	8.8514	8.3126	7.8237
17	15.5623	14.2919	13.1661	12.1657	11.2741	10.4773	9.7632	9.1216	8.5436	8.0216
18	16.3983	14.9920	13.7535	12.6593	11.6896	10.8276	10.0591	9.3719	8.7556	8.2014
19	17.2260	15.6785	14.3238	13.1339	12.0853	11.1581	10.3356	9.6036	8.9501	8.3649
20	18.0456	16.3514	14.8775	13.5903	12.4622	11.4699	10.5940	9.8181	9.1285	8.5136
21	18.8570	17.0112	15.4150	14.0292	12.8212	11.7641	10.8355	10.0168	9.2922	8.6487
22	19.6604	17.6580	15.9369	14.4511	13.1630	12.0416	11.0612	10.2007	9.4424	8.7715
23	20.4558	18.2922	16.4436	14.8568	13.4886	12.3034	11.2722	10.3711	9.5802	8.8832
24	21.2434	18.9139	16.9355	15.2470	13.7986	12.5504	11.4693	10.5288	9.7066	8.9847
25	22.0232	19.5235	17.4131	15.6221	14.0930	12.7834	11.6536	10.6748	9.8226	9.0770

[a]See chapter 6.

[b]n = Length of capital life.

APPENDIX H
Consumer Price Index

Consumer Price Index for All Items and the Medical-Care Component, 1960–2000

	All Items	Medical Care	Medical-Care Services						Medical-Care Commodities
				Professional Services					
			Total	Total	Physician	Dental	Hospital Room	Hospital Services	
1960	29.6	22.3							
1965	31.5	25.2							
1970	38.8	34.0	32.3	37.0	34.5	39.2	23.6		46.5
1975	53.8	47.5	46.6	50.8	48.1	53.2	38.3		53.3
1980	82.4	74.9	74.8	77.9	76.5	78.9	68.0		75.4
1981	90.9	82.9	82.8	85.9	84.9	86.5	78.1		83.7
1982	96.5	92.5	92.6	93.2	92.9	93.1	90.4		92.3
1983	99.6	100.6	100.7	99.8	100.1	99.4	100.6		100.2
1984	103.9	106.8	106.7	107.0	107.0	107.5	109.0		107.5
1985	107.6	113.5	113.2	113.5	113.3	114.2	115.4		115.2
1986	109.6	122.0	121.9	120.8	121.5	120.6	122.3		122.8
1987	113.6	130.1	130.0	128.8	130.4	128.8	131.1		131.0
1988	118.3	138.6	138.3	137.5	139.8	137.5	143.3		139.9
1989	124.0	149.3	148.9	146.4	150.1	146.1	158.1		150.8
1990	130.7	162.8	162.7	156.1	160.8	155.8	175.4		163.4
1991	136.2	177.0	177.1	165.7	170.5	167.4	191.9		176.8
1992	140.3	190.1	190.5	175.8	181.2	178.7	208.7		188.1
1993	144.5	201.4	202.9	184.7	191.3	188.1	226.4		195.0
1994	148.2	211.0	213.4	192.5	199.8	197.1	239.2		200.7
1995	152.4	220.5	224.2	201.0	208.8	206.8			204.5
1996	156.9	228.2	232.4	208.3	216.4	216.5			210.4
1997	160.5	234.6	239.1	215.4	222.9	226.6		278.4	215.3
1998	163.0	242.1	246.8	222.2	229.5	236.2		287.5	221.8
1999	166.6	250.6	255.1	229.2	236.0	247.2		299.5	230.7
2000	172.2	260.8	266.0	237.7	244.7	258.5		317.3	238.1

Source: Statistical Abstract of the U.S., 2000, Consumer Price Indexes of Medical Care Prices: 1970 to 2000; and 756: Consumer Price Indexes, by major groups: 1960 to 1993; U.S. Bureau of Labor Statistics, *CPI Detailed Report,* January 1995; *Monthly Labor Review* and *Handbook of Labor Statistics,* periodic.

APPENDIX I

Productivity Loss Tables

SCOTT D. GROSSE

Productivity losses, defined as losses in earnings and household production, can often result from illness and disability, as well as premature death. In this appendix, two types of aggregated estimates for productivity losses are presented. First, productivity loss estimates are converted from annual figures to average daily figures and aggregated over age groups to yield estimates of the dollar value of a day of incapacity. Second, the present value of future earnings and household production is calculated by discounting future expected earnings and production for various ages.

EARNINGS ESTIMATES

The largest component of earnings consists of money paid directly to individuals in the form of wage and salary income, overtime pay, bonuses, and self employment earnings. Money earnings estimates used in these tables are from the March 2001 supplement to the *Current Population Survey* (CPS) conducted by the Bureau of the Census.[1]

In addition to money earnings, total employee compensation includes fringe benefits, such as vacation pay, health insurance, retirement benefits, as well as annual and personal leave. To calculate total employee compensation, household-based measures of money earnings must be adjusted for other forms of compensation (i.e., fringe benefits) as reported by employers.

According to the March 2001 *Employer Costs for Employee Compensation* (ECEC) survey conducted by the Bureau of Labor Statistics (BLS), wages and salaries accounted for 72.6% of all compensation for civilian workers.[2] The other 27.4% of compensation, classified as "benefits" by the BLS, included supplemental pay (equal to 2.5% of total compensation) and paid leave (equal to 6.8% of total compensation). Supplemental pay forms part of money earnings and paid leave is relevant for calculating cost per hour worked but not as an adjustment to annual earnings. Excluding paid leave from fringe benefits and including supplemental pay as part of money earnings, fringe benefits constitute 23.9% of money earnings.

Since the ECEC surveys exclude specific worker categories that are likely to receive more fringe benefits (in the case of federal employees) or fewer fringe benefits (in the case of agricultural workers and the self-employed) than the average worker, we adjusted the amount of fringe benefits from 23.9% to 22.4%. Owing to lack of fringe benefit data by age, the same adjustment factor is used for all age and gender groups.

Table I.1 reports earnings for all those with any earnings during the year (adjusted by 22.4% for fringe benefits), along with the percentage of people in each age and gender group who had any earnings. The product of these two sets of numbers represents average earnings for each age and gender group. The choice of age groups for tabulating earnings is constrained by the form in which earnings data are reported. In particular, earnings data are reported for 5-year age groups between ages 25 and 74, for the 10-year age group from 15 to 24, and collectively for all individuals aged 75 and above, as well as for the 18–24 year age group, which allows estimates to be calculated for the 15–17 year age group.

HOUSEHOLD PRODUCTION ESTIMATES

One of the largest components of economic activity is the value of household services performed by household members who do not receive pay for these services. Valuation of household production entails two steps: estimation of annual hours of household services and selection of an appropriate wage rate(s) for valuing the services. The only sources of disaggregated data on allocation of hours to various household tasks are time budget and diary studies. We use estimates derived from the National Human Activity Pattern Survey (NHAPS), conducted during 1992–1994 by the University of Maryland Survey Research Center for the Environmental Protection Agency.[3] This survey collected information on household activities for 9386 subjects of all ages.

Our household production estimates for individuals in each age and gender group are derived from an analysis of the NHAPS data that aggregates household services into three categories: household production, providing care, and personal care.[3] *Household production* is defined to include housework, food cooking and clean-up, outdoor chores, taking care of plants and animals, home and auto maintenance, and obtaining goods and services. *Providing care* is defined as including childcare, child guidance, playing with children, transporting children, and providing care to others (i.e., helping and caring for adults, other personal activities, and personal care travel). Data were provided for the following 10-year age groups: 25–34 to 65–74, along with 12–17 and 18–24 years.

Valuation of weekly hours in household services is taken from the same source.[3] Each detailed activity (e.g., playing with children) was broken down into fractional tasks with a corresponding mean wage in 1999 relevant for that activity. Mean wages were adjusted to include legally mandated benefits (payroll taxes), with three different ratios ranging from 10.3% to 14.1%. Weighted wages were calcu-

Table I.1a   Total for Men and Women, 2000 Data

Age in Years	Proportion with Earnings	Annual Mean Earnings ($)	Annual Mean Earnings in Age Group($)	Proportion in Household	Annual Mean Household Services ($)	Annual Mean Household Services in Age Group ($)	Annual Mean Earnings and Household Services ($)
15–17	0.355	4297	1526	0.996	4624	4606	6132
18–24	0.785	16,692	13,102	0.897	7522	6747	19,849
25–29	0.866	34,758	30,094	0.978	9229	8977	39,071
30–34	0.874	43,013	37,581	0.978	10,498	10,276	47,857
35–39	0.872	47,406	41,339	0.986	12,309	12,149	53,488
40–44	0.866	50,114	43,408	0.986	12,184	12,021	55,428
45–49	0.861	52,792	45,433	0.990	11,976	11,856	57,289
50–54	0.827	52,406	43,321	0.990	11,954	11,834	55,156
55–59	0.728	52,715	38,376	0.990	13,513	13,374	51,751
60–64	0.551	44,926	24,738	0.990	13,613	13,475	38,213
65–69	0.307	33,669	10,335	0.982	14,148	13,888	24,223
70–74	0.178	28,754	5117	0.982	14,191	13,930	19,046
75+	0.072	27,489	1981	0.902	12,950	11,527	13,508

Annual mean earnings for adults with earnings $41,163
Annual mean earnings for all adults $28,542
Annual mean household services $10,805
Annual earnings and household services $39,347
Value of a lost day of work $165
Value of a lost day of primary activity $144
Value of a lost day (unspecified) $108

Value of a lost day of work = average annual earnings of those with earnings/250 days. Value of a lost day of primary activity = annual earnings/250 + annual household services/365. Value of a lost day (unspecified) = (annual earnings + annual household services)/365.

Table I.1b Women, 2000 Data

Age in Years	Proportion with Earnings	Annual Mean Earnings ($)	Annual Mean Earnings in Age Group ($)	Proportion in Households	Annual Mean Household Services ($)	Annual Mean Household Services in Age Group ($)	Annual Mean Earnings and Household Services ($)
15–17	0.324	3647	1182	0.997	4961	4948	6130
18–24	0.767	14,886	11,423	0.915	9806	8968	20,391
25–29	0.806	29,178	23,516	0.992	13,233	13,129	36,645
30–34	0.810	32,403	26,258	0.992	13,233	13,129	39,387
35–39	0.799	34,780	27,801	0.995	15,000	14,920	42,721
40–44	0.808	36,019	29,113	0.995	15,000	14,920	44,033
45–49	0.812	36,446	29,582	0.993	14,958	14,861	44,442
50–54	0.773	37,105	28,692	0.993	14,958	14,861	43,552
55–59	0.656	33,691	22,104	0.993	16,334	16,228	38,332
60–64	0.470	28,778	13,536	0.993	16,334	16,228	29,764
65–69	0.238	20,277	4834	0.981	15,871	15,575	20,409
70–74	0.151	16,070	2428	0.981	15,871	15,575	18,003
75+	0.046	16,344	750	0.873	13,606	11,881	12,631

Annual mean earnings for adults with earnings $29,945
Annual mean earnings for all adults $18,952
Annual mean household services $13,320
Annual earnings and household services $32,272
Value of a lost day of work $120
Value of a lost day of primary activity $112
Value of a lost day (unspecified) $88

Value of a lost day of work = average annual earnings of those with earnings/250 days. Value of a lost day of primary activity = annual earnings/250 + annual household services/365. Value of a lost day (unspecified) = (annual earnings + annual household services)/365.

Table I.1c Men, 2000 Data

Age in Years	Proportion with Earnings	Annual Mean Earnings ($)	Annual Mean Earnings in Age Group ($)	Proportion in Households	Annual Mean Household Services ($)	Annual Mean Household Services in Age Group ($)	Annual Mean Earnings and Household Services ($)
15–17	0.385	5635	2167	0.995	4303	4281	6448
18–24	0.803	18,421	14,784	0.879	5234	4603	19,387
25–29	0.927	39,704	36,795	0.964	7396	7127	43,922
30–34	0.939	52,517	49,338	0.964	7396	7127	56,466
35–39	0.946	58,263	55,115	0.978	9210	9009	64,124
40–44	0.925	62,682	58,001	0.978	9210	9009	67,010
45–49	0.911	67,919	61,906	0.987	9229	9106	71,013
50–54	0.883	66,568	58,737	0.987	9229	9106	67,894
55–59	0.806	69,478	55,386	0.987	11,234	11,084	67,070
60–64	0.643	58,565	37,092	0.987	11,234	11,084	48,766
65–69	0.383	42,911	16,455	0.982	12,395	12,169	28,604
70–74	0.234	39,207	9,157	0.982	12,395	12,169	21,326
75+	0.112	34,430	3,850	0.931	11,351	10,571	14,421

Annual mean earnings for adults with earnings $41,163
Annual mean earnings for adults with earnings $50,649
Annual mean earnings for all adults $39,605
Annual mean household services $8385
Annual earnings and household services $48,040
Value of a lost day of work $203
Value of a lost day of primary activity $182
Value of a lost day (unspecified) $132

Value of a lost day of work = average annual earnings of those with earnings/250 days. Value of a lost day of primary activity = annual earnings/250 + annual household services/365. Value of a lost day (unspecified) = (annual earnings + annual household services)/365.

lated for each detailed category. Weighted hourly costs for the three categories of household services ranged from \$8.16 to \$12.13 in 1999 dollars.

Household surveys by definition exclude individuals not living in households. Approximately one out of 10 individuals between the ages of 18 and 24 and ages 75 and over do not live in households. The Bureau of the Census publishes tabulations of the nonhousehold population by age but not by age and sex. A special Bureau of the Census tabulation of the age and gender distribution of the non household population in 1990 is available.[4] Consequently, average estimates of household production calculated from NHAPS data were multiplied by the percent of each age and gender group in households to determine the average value of household services in each group.

ANNUAL EARNINGS AND DOLLAR VALUE OF A DAY ESTIMATES

Average annual earnings adjusted for fringe benefits and household production estimates are reported in Table I.1 combined for males and females and for each sex separately. Average earnings in an age group is the product of the proportion in each age group with earnings and the mean earnings for all those with any earnings during 2000. Mean earnings are adjusted for fringe benefits by a factor of 1.224, as explained above. Average household production is the product of the proportion in each age group living in households and the mean weekly value of household services times 52 weeks. Total annual earnings is the sum of these two components.

Productivity losses for 1 day lost due to morbidity for an individual of unspecified age are calculated in three ways in Table I.1. First, the expected value of a lost day of work for an adult who is employed is the value of total earnings among all adults with earnings divided by 250, the average number of days of work in a year. This provides an estimate of lost work productivity. Second, the expected value of a lost day of primary activity for an adult is the sum of age-weighted average earnings for all adults (not just those with earnings) divided by 250 and the age-weighted annual value of household services divided by 365. Third, the average value of a lost day in general, including loss of household services, is the sum of market and household production divided by 365, the number of days in a year.

PRESENT VALUE ESTIMATES

The present value of future total earnings (including fringe benefits) and of the combination of future earnings and household production is reported for men and women pooled and separately in Table I.2. Estimates are presented for discount rates ranging from 0% to 10%. The present value of future earnings is reported at each exact age in 5-year intervals, beginning with birth. The exception is that an estimate is provided for age 18 instead of 20, to correspond with the beginning of the age interval used in the CPS earnings estimates. For the final, open interval

Table I.2a Present Value in 2000 of Labor Market Earnings: Total for Men and Women

Exact age in Years	Discount Rate										
	0%	1%	2%	3%	4%	5%	6%	7%	8%	9%	10%
0	2,489,019	1,591,777	1,039,134	691,830	469,281	323,974	227,379	162,057	117,160	85,826	63,641
5	2,387,541	1,635,569	1,101,603	770,455	548,739	397,579	292,714	218,748	165,747	127,199	98,768
10	2,272,545	1,606,995	1,158,824	851,430	636,704	484,145	373,917	292,994	232,675	187,063	152,102
15	2,163,548	1,608,766	1,219,278	941,050	738,928	589,686	477,749	392,524	326,698	275,160	234,286
18	2,102,221	1,609,870	1,255,987	937,409	805,435	660,699	549,952	463,999	396,381	342,496	299,028
25	1,880,332	1,525,497	1,257,218	1,051,528	891,695	765,885	665,627	584,784	518,861	464,526	419,286
30	1,650,572	1,382,126	1,172,408	1,006,585	873,954	766,704	679,071	606,753	546,508	495,869	452,941
35	1,396,281	1,201,999	1,045,470	918,053	813,321	726,440	653,739	592,402	540,247	495,573	457,038
40	1,137,432	1,004,378	894,037	801,724	723,855	657,662	600,984	552,122	509,728	472,723	440,237
45	882,712	797,959	725,877	664,007	610,557	564,075	523,407	487,621	455,963	427,816	402,675
50	631,857	582,870	540,214	502,822	469,838	440,577	414,479	391,087	370,025	350,979	333,689
55	403,762	378,750	356,604	336,874	319,197	303,274	288,862	275,757	263,791	252,821	242,729
60	209,940	198,680	188,623	179,592	171,438	164,042	157,301	151,131	145,460	140,228	135,385
65	89,027	84,194	79,856	75,946	72,407	69,193	66,262	63,580	61,116	58,847	56,749
70	40,732	38,598	36,658	34,891	33,276	31,798	30,442	29,195	28,046	26,985	26,003
75	18,281	17,298	16,377	15,513	14,703	13,942	13,227	12,555	11,923	11,328	10,769

Table I.2b   Present Value in 2000 of Labor Market Earnings: Women

Exact age in Years	Discount Rate										
	0%	1%	2%	3%	4%	5%	6%	7%	8%	9%	10%
0	1,661,703	1,077,625	713,083	481,018	330,433	230,905	163,953	118,153	86,322	63,868	47,806
5	1,592,686	1,086,096	755,349	535,258	386,074	283,140	210,895	159,358	122,023	94,581	74,134
10	1,515,790	1,086,929	794,488	591,421	447,909	344,747	269,367	213,421	171,275	139,077	114,151
15	1,442,738	1,087,862	835,731	653,536	519,695	419,797	344,084	285,850	240,429	204,526	175,787
18	1,399,267	1,086,533	859,191	691,260	565,277	469,339	395,218	337,158	291,071	254,027	223,895
25	1,230,296	1,008,957	839,955	709,179	606,677	525,341	460,035	407,005	363,479	327,385	297,161
30	1,059,045	894,052	763,973	660,243	576,621	508,509	452,481	405,961	366,990	334,064	306,022
35	883,470	766,028	670,574	592,235	527,350	473,144	427,487	388,734	355,600	327,072	302,351
40	709,787	631,072	565,244	509,734	462,562	422,182	387,383	357,200	330,865	307,756	287,370
45	538,865	490,225	448,488	412,416	381,032	353,557	329,366	307,951	288,900	271,871	256,584
50	374,438	347,509	323,905	303,081	284,600	268,108	253,317	239,989	227,927	216,967	206,971
55	222,493	209,446	197,836	187,443	178,089	169,626	161,933	154,910	148,472	142,549	137,081
60	109,335	103,790	98,822	94,347	90,294	86,605	83,233	80,136	77,281	74,639	72,185
65	41,944	39,686	37,659	35,833	34,180	32,678	31,308	30,054	28,901	27,838	26,855
70	19,641	17,713	16,021	14,530	13,212	12,044	11,005	10,079	9251	8508	7840
75	8313	7079	6037	5156	4411	3779	3243	2786	2398	2066	1783

Table I.2c   Present Value in 2000 of Labor Market Earnings: Men

Exact age in Years	Discount Rate										
	0%	1%	2%	3%	4%	5%	6%	7%	8%	9%	10%
0	3,329,188	2,113,597	1,369,892	905,C35	610,104	418,399	291,772	206,675	148,541	108,208	79,814
5	3,195,874	2,133,524	1,453,345	1,009,321	713,946	513,845	375,894	279,185	210,301	160,492	123,962
10	3,042,285	2,135,658	1,529,008	1,115,457	828,487	625,797	480,227	373,986	295,253	236,051	190,922
15	2,897,076	2,138,532	1,609,165	1,233,215	961,736	762,492	613,730	501,152	414,665	347,303	294,152
18	2,818,582	2,142,617	1,659,494	1,308,433	1,049,206	854,756	706,799	592,508	503,031	432,061	375,072
25	2,545,903	2,053,853	1,683,615	1,401,063	1,182,473	1,011,135	875,137	765,584	677,104	604,170	543,631
30	2,258,922	1,885,596	1,591,656	1,361,784	1,178,657	1,031,151	911,012	812,208	730,149	661,366	603,206
35	1,925,424	1,651,288	1,431,311	1,252,945	1,106,884	986,151	885,465	800,785	728,996	667,673	614,913
40	1,581,380	1,391,951	1,235,013	1,104,183	994,206	901,029	821,503	753,154	694,023	642,549	597,478
45	1,243,999	1,121,185	1,016,940	927,785	850,998	784,420	726,339	675,374	630,411	590,540	555,015
50	906,378	833,815	770,757	715,597	667,051	624,079	585,840	551,644	520,923	493,204	468,093
55	600,851	562,890	529,297	499,394	472,629	448,549	426,779	407,010	388,982	372,479	357,316
60	322,855	305,356	289,707	275,640	262,935	251,407	240,900	231,285	222,452	214,307	206,772
65	142,685	135,030	128,131	121,890	116,223	111,061	106,341	102,012	98,028	94,351	90,948
70	68,811	65,456	62,387	59,574	56,990	54,612	52,418	50,390	48,512	46,769	45,148
75	30,298	28,813	27,414	26,097	24,854	23,682	22,576	21,531	20,543	19,609	18,726

Table I.2d Present Value in 2000 of Earnings and Household Production: Total for Men and Women

Exact age in Years	Discount Rate										
	0%	1%	2%	3%	4%	5%	6%	7%	8%	9%	10%
0	3,620,505	2,262,512	1,452,315	955,895	643,931	443,145	310,989	222,171	161,313	118,862	88,759
5	3,472,896	2,282,115	1,539,623	1,064,530	752,961	543,825	400,348	299,891	228,211	176,161	137,750
10	3,305,624	2,284,142	1,619,597	1,176,371	873,664	662,234	511,411	401,678	320,362	259,068	212,134
15	3,080,468	2,252,172	1,686,116	1,290,814	1,008,956	803,955	652,012	537,369	449,408	380,852	326,632
20	3,046,337	2,276,306	1,743,121	1,365,517	1,092,302	890,571	738,760	622,461	531,878	460,228	402,738
25	2,658,233	2,112,937	1,712,638	1,413,488	1,186,092	1,010,423	872,626	762,971	674,525	602,280	542,567
30	2,408,363	1,962,394	1,628,188	1,373,282	1,175,601	1,019,890	895,443	794,630	711,933	643,305	585,737
35	2,015,743	1,699,081	1,451,941	1,256,395	1,099,652	972,469	868,083	781,484	708,917	647,535	595,160
40	1,725,468	1,480,016	1,285,617	1,129,533	1,002,589	898,095	811,111	737,948	675,817	622,584	576,601
45	1,389,917	1,218,836	1,080,036	966,080	871,463	792,070	724,789	667,248	617,616	574,469	536,686
50	1,015,070	914,807	830,426	758,785	697,456	644,540	598,548	558,297	522,843	491,425	463,428
55	768,015	696,931	636,943	585,903	542,131	504,301	471,365	442,487	416,997	394,356	374,125
60	504,568	461,882	425,232	393,577	366,075	342,044	320,925	302,263	285,684	270,877	257,588
65	320,489	295,459	273,509	254,190	237,123	221,990	208,521	196,489	185,703	175,997	167,234
70	212,902	198,822	186,130	174,667	164,296	154,893	146,354	138,583	131,498	125,026	119,104
75	136,008	128,694	121,840	115,414	109,384	103,723	98,405	93,406	88,705	84,281	80,115

Table I.2e Present Value in 2000 of Earnings and Household Production: Women

Exact age in Years	Discount Rate										
	0%	1%	2%	3%	4%	5%	6%	7%	8%	9%	10%
0	3,196,828	1,981,105	1,266,384	832,951	562,376	388,710	274,402	197,395	144,407	107,239	80,711
5	2,943,913	1,934,561	1,308,508	908,974	647,008	470,824	349,496	264,099	202,774	157,922	124,565
10	2,801,778	1,936,044	1,376,309	1,004,350	750,635	573,268	446,397	353,695	284,619	232,217	191,805
15	2,597,880	1,902,227	1,429,359	1,100,233	865,895	695,401	568,800	472,971	399,128	341,275	295,249
20	2,574,779	1,923,245	1,475,883	1,161,009	934,101	766,312	641,139	544,676	469,361	409,581	361,410
25	2,205,534	1,749,095	1,416,817	1,170,195	983,748	840,303	728,112	639,001	567,196	508,555	460,066
30	1,984,973	1,606,271	1,325,751	1,113,934	951,062	823,677	722,455	640,834	574,120	518,908	472,687
35	1,646,709	1,379,405	1,172,870	1,010,893	882,058	778,213	693,463	623,488	565,083	515,841	473,935
40	1,421,724	1,209,279	1,043,140	911,278	805,139	718,570	647,087	587,381	536,981	494,021	457,073
45	1,148,941	998,401	877,820	779,998	699,667	632,936	576,898	529,362	488,657	453,497	422,882
50	838,997	750,417	676,672	614,700	562,157	517,231	478,509	444,884	415,477	389,590	366,660
55	648,902	582,766	527,545	481,049	441,577	407,800	378,670	353,362	331,218	311,711	294,417
60	399,817	367,723	339,926	315,711	294,496	275,809	259,260	244,529	231,354	219,514	208,826
65	299,405	274,628	253,017	234,094	217,461	202,784	189,782	178,221	167,901	158,654	150,338
70	214,978	190,384	169,143	150,743	134,757	120,825	108,649	97,974	88,590	80,315	72,998
75	139,991	119,197	101,653	86,828	74,279	63,640	54,605	46,921	40,376	34,792	30,022

Table I.2f Present Value in 2000 of Earnings and Household Production: Men

Exact age in Years	Discount Rate										
	0%	1%	2%	3%	4%	5%	6%	7%	8%	9%	10%
0	4,412,750	2,737,467	1,743,408	1,138,054	760,167	518,675	360,902	255,673	184,126	134,602	99,752
5	4,032,584	2,652,369	1,787,523	1,232,612	868,389	624,104	456,876	340,170	257,240	197,307	153,311
10	3,838,783	2,655,022	1,880,584	1,362,264	1,007,708	760,078	583,686	455,680	361,153	290,199	236,124
15	3,596,491	2,627,860	1,963,076	1,497,590	1,165,282	923,594	744,660	609,927	506,839	426,765	363,682
20	3,545,550	2,652,366	2,029,451	1,585,983	1,263,991	1,025,782	846,403	709,050	602,211	517,878	450,390
25	3,143,132	2,503,733	2,031,376	1,676,615	1,405,926	1,196,242	1,031,464	900,198	794,275	707,758	636,283
30	2,847,931	2,332,185	1,941,915	1,641,832	1,407,581	1,222,099	1,073,259	952,318	852,891	770,255	700,871
35	2,405,782	2,036,181	1,745,397	1,513,741	1,326,987	1,174,736	1,049,294	944,905	857,219	782,911	719,418
40	2,047,372	1,767,608	1,543,445	1,361,611	1,212,404	1,088,642	984,949	897,256	822,446	758,111	702,369
45	1,649,465	1,457,247	1,299,340	1,168,224	1,058,253	965,143	885,614	817,129	757,705	705,779	660,110
50	1,211,306	1,098,375	1,002,320	919,971	848,843	786,972	732,799	685,072	642,780	605,101	571,363
55	899,687	824,287	759,850	704,359	656,217	614,153	577,152	544,396	515,221	489,088	465,555
60	522,778	487,623	456,668	429,267	404,891	383,099	363,526	345,867	329,868	315,312	302,019
65	338,558	314,282	292,830	273,804	256,869	241,743	228,185	215,989	204,981	195,012	185,954
70	228,260	203,827	182,503	163,844	147,473	133,071	120,369	109,136	99,179	90,330	82,446
75	150,591	129,517	111,560	96,233	83,132	71,916	62,300	54,043	46,943	40,829	35,557

consisting of people aged 75 years and over, the length of the interval is assumed to be the expectation of life at age 75, which in 1998 was 10 years for men and 12 years for women.[5]

The value of average individual worker productivity in future earnings is adjusted for expected future growth in productivity. The conventional assumption is that future growth in labor productivity will occur in line with historically observed rates of increase in labor productivity, empirically measured by changes in employee compensation adjusted for inflation. Between 1970 and 2000, the average rate of growth in employee compensation was just over 1% per year. The usual assumption that long-term growth in labor productivity will continue to be 1% per year is retained in this analysis.

Future productivity is also discounted by the probability of surviving to the age at which the expected production occurs. We use the most recent available life table, an abridged life table for 1998 published by Centers For Disease Control's National Center for Health Statistics that reports survival from birth to each exact age at 5-year intervals.[5] We interpolate to calculate average survival rates from birth for each age interval, except for the last, open-ended interval. For those aged 75 and over, the survival rates to the exact ages of 80 (for males) and 81 (for females) are used. For present value estimates evaluated at birth (discounted lifetime earnings), these average survival rates are directly used to weight future earnings or production. For estimates evaluated at each other exact age, survival rates from the exact age are calculated by dividing the survival rates from birth to age intervals by the survival rate from birth to the exact age.

REFERENCES

1. Bureau of Labor Statistics and Bureau of the Census. Detailed person income (P60 package). *Annual Demographic Survey*, March Suppl, 2001. Available from http://ferret.bls.census.gov/macro/032001/perinc/toc.htm
2. US Department of Labor, Bureau of Labor Statistics. *Employer Costs for Employee Compensation—March 2001*. Washington DC: US Department of Labor, Bureau of Labor Statistics, June 29, 2001. Available from ftp://ftp.bls.gov/pub/special.requests/ocwc/ect/ececrlsc.pdf.
3. Expectancy Data. *The Dollar Value of a Day: 1999 Dollar Valuation*. Shawnee Mission, KS: Expectancy Data, 2001.
4. Expectancy Data. *Healthy Life Expectancy: 1998 Tables*. Shawnee Mission, KS: Expectancy Data, 2000.
5. Anderson RN. United States life tables 1998. *Natl Vital Stat Rep 2001;* 48:18. Available from http://www.cdc.gov/nchs/data/nvsr/nvsr48/nvs48_18.pdf.

Index

Absorbing state, 122
Adjusting earnings to base-year monetary units, 98–99
Administration costs, 63–64
Adverse effects/reactions, modeling, 163, 167, 168
Agency for Healthcare Research and Quality (AHRQ), 235
Analytic horizon, 12, 108, 161, 218
  defined, 17, 108
  vs. time frame, 17–19
Analytic method, 12, 19, 218. See also specific methods
ANALYTICA, 214
Annuitization tables, 243
Annuitizing capital expenditures, 99–101
Asthma Quality of Life Questionnaire, 78
Asymptomatic screening, 42–43
Attributable risk, 3–4, 32
Audience, 11–13, 218
Average cost, 57–58
Averaging out and folding back, 113–114

Base case, analyzing the, 112–113, 121–123
Baseline, 161
Baseline comparator, 12
Base-year monetary units, adjusting earnings to, 98–99
Bayesian methods, 41
Behavioral prevention strategies, 7
Behavioral Risk Factor Surveillance System (BRFSS), 79, 80
Benefit-cost ratio (BCR), 128, 144–145
Benefits. See also specific topics
  direct, indirect, and intangible, 132
  mistakes in assessing and valuing, 144
Best- and worst-case scenarios, 117
Blinded assignment, 37
British Medical Journal guidelines for CEA, 185, 187
Bureau of Labor Statistics (BLS), 236

Canada's Coordinating Office for Health Technology Assessment (CCOHTA) guidelines, 182
Capital costs, 55
Capital expenditures, annuitizing, 99–101
Case fatality, 31
Case series, 40
Case-control studies, 39–40
Cause-specific mortality, 31
Centers for Medicare and Medicaid Services (CMS), 235
Chance node, 109–110
Charges vs. costs, 70–71
Clinical prevention strategies, 7
Clinical trials, 79. See also Randomized controlled trials
Cohort simulation, 121–122
Cohort studies, 39
Comparator, baseline, 12
Complexity, 104
Concurrently controlled studies, 38
Consensus panel, 41–42
Consumer Price Index (CPI), 73, 97, 98, 244
Consumer surplus, 132
Consumer-market studies, 144
Contingent valuation method (CVM), 138–141
  example of, 151–152
  problems with, 141–143
Contingent valuation method (CVM) survey data, 151
Contingent valuation survey, conducting a, 140–141
Cost analysis, framing, 58–61
Cost data, adjustments to, 73
Cost databases, 234–236
Cost inventory, developing a, 61–62
Cost-benefit analysis (CBA), xii–xiii, 5, 19, 127–129
  advantages, 19–20
  defined, 127
  example of, 151–152

Cost-benefit analysis (CBA) (*continued*)
  in health, history of, 129
  limitations, 149–150
  vs. other forms of economic analysis, 130–
    131, 157
  recommendations regarding, 212
  steps in conducting, 132
    assign values to interventions and out-
      comes, 136–144
    define problem, 133–134
    determine and calculate summary mea-
      sure to be used, 144–148
    evaluate results with sensitivity analysis,
      148–149
    health outcomes, 135–136
    identify interventions to be evaluated, 134
    identify outcomes of interventions,
      134–135
    intangible outcomes, 136
    nonhealth outcomes, 136
    outcomes *vs.* costs and benefits, 135
    prepare results for presentation, 149
  when to use, 129–130
Cost-effectiveness analyses (CEAs), multiple
    as difficult to compare, 187–188
    reconciling, 183–184
Cost-effectiveness analysis (CEA), xiii, 5, 20,
    129, 130, 131, 156–158, 175–176,
    193–195
  assumptions inherent in, 191–193
  background, 158–159
  as "black box," 184–185
  cannot be trusted, 190–191
  compared with CBA, 130, 157
  defined, 157
  ethically problems with, 191–193
  guidelines for, 181–183
    limitations of, 183
  how to conduct, 159–160
    analyzing and interpreting results, 168–
      174
    choosing baseline comparator and alterna-
      tive interventions, 161–162
    constructing decision model, 166–168
    framing the problem, 160–161
    identifying intervention and outcome
      costs, 165–166
    selecting health-outcome measures,
      162–165
  implications of its implementation, 191–193
  to inform policy decisions, 179–180
  recommendations regarding, 213
  textbooks on, 181
  as too general, 188–189
  when to conduct, 159

Cost-effectiveness analysis (CEA) method-
    ology, inconsistency of, 180–187
Cost-effectiveness analysis (CEA) results, pre-
    senting, 175–176
Cost-effectiveness (CE) decision tree, 164
  data needed to construct, 166, 167
Cost-effectiveness (CE) ratios, 157
  average and incremental ratios, 168–172
Cost-effectiveness (CE) study, single
  incomplete information provided by, 187
Cost-effectiveness (CE) *vs.* cost-saving/cost-
    cutting, 179
Cost-of-illness (COI) data, sources for collect-
    ing, 232–238
Cost-of-illness (COI) method, 67, 70, 137
Costs, 22, 62, 212. *See also specific topics*
  and benefits, 131–132
    valuation of, 136–137
  future unrelated health-care costs, 165–
    166
  identifying relevant, 12
  of interventions/programs, 58–67, 167
  to others, 62
  quantifying, 62–64
  types of, 53–58
Cost-to-charge ratios, 239–240
Cost-utility analysis (CUA), xiii, 5, 20, 21,
    130–131, 158, 159
Cost-Utility Analysis (CUA) Data Base, 233
Cross-sectional studies, 40
CRYSTAL BALL, 214

DATA, 215
Data sources, 45–47
Decision analysis, 80, 125, 167
  appropriateness, 106
  defined, 103
  as a discipline, 105–106
  elements, 106–107
    develop model to structure problem over
      time, 108–110
    estimating probabilities, 110–111
    evaluating uncertainty, 114–117
    specifying decision problem and its com-
      ponents, 107–108
    valuing consequences, 111–112
  in public health
    examples of, 104
    motivation for, 103–105
Decision models, 4–5. *See also* Models
  estimating model parameters for, 42–45
  public health issues in development of,
    28–29
Decision node, 109
DECISION PRO, 215

Decision tree, 109–112, 219–221
  developing a simple, 109
Decision tree models, limitations of, 118
Declining exponential approximation to life ex-
  pectancy (DEALE) model, 44–45
Delphi method, 42
Disability, 31
Disability-adjusted life years (DALYs), 80
Discount rate, 12, 23, 93–94
  defined, 93
  real, 94
Discount tables, 241–243
Discounting, 224
  defined, 92–93
  nonmonetary benefits, 94–95
Discounting process, 95–97
Disease progression, probability of, 114, 115,
  116, 117
Distributional effects, 12, 24–25
Dollar value of a day estimates, 247–250
Dominance, extended/weak, 172–173
Dominated alternatives, exclusion of, 172–173
DPL, 215
DRG Handbook, The, 236–237

Earnings, adjusted to base-year monetary units,
  98–99
Earnings estimates, 245–250, 257
Economic costs, 53–54
  true, 70–71
Economic evaluations, use of QoL in, 80–81
Economic models, 5
Effectiveness, 34–35
  defined, 34
Efficacy, 34–35
  defined, 34
Employer Costs for Employee Compensation
  (ECEC), 245–246
End stage renal disease (ESRD), 80–83
Environmental prevention strategies, 7
EQ-5D, 83, 85, 88–89
  preference weights for, 89
Europe, guidelines for CEA in, 182
Excess mortality, 44–45
"Exchange rate," 95
Expected value/utility, 106, 111–114
Experimental studies, 37–38. See also Random-
  ized controlled trials
Expert opinion, 41–42
Experts, panel of, 72
Extended dominance, 172

Facilities costs, 63
Federal Register, The, 72
Final outcome (measures), 162–163

Financial costs, 53–54
Fixed costs, 55–56
Fixed effects, 41
Framing a study, 11, 217–219
Framing the question/listing key points,
  11–12, 160–161
Future value (FV), 95–97

Generalizability, 37

Health, United States, 237–238
Health care utilization and cost databases,
  234–236
Health Economic Evaluations Database
  (HEED), 233
Health outcome cost data, sources of, 71–73
Health outcomes, 135–136
  intermediate and final, 162–163
  measurement, 167
  measuring costs of, 67–75
  valuation of, 137–138
Health states, 80
  defined, 118
  delineating a set of mutually exclusive, 119
Healthcare Cost and Utilization Project
  (HCUP), 236
Health-outcome measures, selecting,
  162–165
Healthy Days measure, 79, 80
Healthy People 2010, 79–80
Healthy Utility Index (HUI), 80, 85, 88
Heuristics, 106
HIV/AIDS, 6, 14–16, 24
  cost-effectiveness of postexposure prophy-
  laxis (PEP) following exposure to,
  217–229
Hospital records, charges obtained from, 72
Hospital Statistics, 238
Household production, 250
  defined, 246
Household production estimates, 246, 250
Human-capital (HC) method, 73–74

Incidence, 30
Incidence-based costs, 70
Incremental analysis, 12, 21–22
Indirect costs, 54
Inflation, adjusting for, 97–99
Injuries, 31
Intangible benefits, 132
Intangible costs, 55
Intermediate outcome (measures), 162–163
International resources, 238
Intervention cost, 169. See also specific topics
Intervention strategies, 14–15

Intervention unit, 60–61
Interventions, measures of overall impact of, 32–35
Interviewer bias, 39–40

Labor market earnings. *See* Earnings estimates
Lead time bias, 43
League tables, 187
Life expectancy, estimation of prevention strategy impact on, 44–45
List prices, 71
Literature, data from the, 85–86
Literature reviews, 232–233

Margin, intensive and extensive, 14
Marginal analysis, 12, 21
Marginal cost (MC), 57–58
Marginal cost (MC) effectiveness, 170, 171
MarketScan databases, 236
Markov cycles, 119
Markov models, 118–124
Masked assignment, 37
Material costs, 65
Medical and nonmedical costs, 54
    direct and indirect, 69
Medical Expenditure Panel Survey (MEPS), 236
Medicare reimbursement data, 72
MEDLINE, 233
Meta-analysis, 40–41
Model parameters, estimating, 42–45
Models, 59. *See also* Decision models
    classification of, 109
    development of, 108–110
Monte Carlo analysis, 117
    second-order simulation, 117
Monte Carlo simulation, 122–123
    first order simulation, 122–123
"Moral hazard," 142
Morbidity, 31
Morbidity costs, 74–75
Mortality, 31
    costs of premature, 75
    estimation of prevention strategy impact on, 44–45
Multiple competing objectives, 105
Mutually exclusive health states, delineating a set of, 119
Mutually exclusive programs, analysis of, 172, 173

National Center for Health Statistics (NCHS), 45–46, 85, 234–235
National Health and Nutrition Examination Survey (NHANES), 40, 234

National Health Care Survey (NHCS), 234–235
National Health Interview Survey (NHIS), 40, 80, 234–235
National Health Service (NHS), 190
    Economic Evaluations Database (NHS EED), 233
Net present value (NPV), 128–129, 147–148, 150, 152. *See also* Present value
    calculating, 128
    pros and cons of, 146
Normative theories, 105

Observational studies, 38–40
Observer bias, 39–40
Odds ratio, 33
Operating costs, 55
Opportunity cost, 15
Outbreak investigation data, 72–73
Outcomes, 22–23. *See also specific topics; specific types of outcomes*
    intangible, 136
    nonhealth, 136
    valuing, 223–224
Out-of-pocket expenses, 62
Output, 56

Panel on Cost-Effectiveness in Health and Medicine (PCEHM), 182, 185, 188
Participant costs, 62
    valuing, 66–67
Pay-back period, 146
Penetrance, intervention, 29, 30
Perspective(s), 12, 15–16, 107, 160, 218
    different, 105
    other, 16
Physician visits and charges, 72
Policy decisions, CEA to inform, 179–180
Policy planning, communication of effectiveness data for, 46–47
Population attributable risk, 32. *See also* Attributable risk
Population effects, 30–32
Population surveillance, 79–80
PRECISION TREE/@RISK, 216
Predictive value, 43
Preference measure scores, 84–86
Preferences (for health states of interest), measuring, 81–82
Preferences measurement methods, 82–84
Present value (PV), 95–97, 99. *See also* Net present value
Present value (PV) estimates, 250–257
Prevalence, 30
Prevalence-based costs, 68, 70
Prevented fraction, 3–4, 33

Prevention effectiveness
  defined, xii, 3
  role of, 2
Prevention effectiveness studies
  checklist for evaluating protocol/scope of
    work for, 26
  social, legal, and equity aspects, 6–7
  uses and limitations, 6
Prevention strategies
  conceptual model for development and im-
    plementation of, 2–3
  types of, 7–8
Prevention-effectiveness analysis, building
  blocks of, 107–117
Price indifference/threshold effect, 142–143
Primary prevention, defined, 7
Productivity loss tables, 245–257
Productivity losses, 54–55, 62, 73–75
  in CUA, 165
  defined, 12, 245
Program costs, 61
  fixed, 62–63
  variable, 64–65
Program evaluation research, 4
Program planning, communication of effec-
  tiveness data for, 46–47
Prospective study, 59
Provider cost, 65
Providing care, defined, 246
Public and private data sets, 72
Publication bias, 41

Quality of life (QoL), 32, 77
  measures of, 77–78, 212
    classification of, 78
    disease-specific, 78
Quality of life (QoL) measurement
  applications of, 78–81
  reasons for, 77–78
Quality of Well-Being (QWB), 85
Quality-adjusted life years (QALYs), 80–84,
  86–87, 89, 157
  in CBAs, 130
  in CEAs, 163–165, 192
  in decision analysis, 112
  measuring, for health program evaluation,
    86–89
Quality-adjusted survival, 123
Quasi-experimental studies, 38

Random effects, 41
Randomized controlled trials (RCTs), 34–39,
  41. See also Clinical trials
Rating scale, 83–84
Recall bias, 39

Referral bias, 111
Relative hazard, 33
Relative risk, 33, 46
Reporting, transparency in, 185, 187
Reporting checklist, 186
Required compensation, 143–144
Resources not traded in marketplace, valuing,
  65–66
Retrospective study, 59
Risk
  attributable, 3–4
  relative, 33, 46
Risk factors, 79, 80
  measures of overall impact of, 32–35
Root node, 113

Scrap value, 99–100
Screening strategies, 14
Secondary prevention, defined, 7
Sensitivity analysis, 12, 148–149, 173–174, 224,
  226, 227
  one- vs. multi-way, 115
  questions addressed by, 114–115
Sensitivity vs. specificity, 42–43
SF-36, 77, 78
Social discount rate, 94
Software, 214–216
Staff support costs, 63–64
Standard gamble, 82
State transitions, 119
  specifying, 119
State-transition models, 118–120
  advantages, 123–124
  analyzing the base case, 121–123
  evaluating uncertainty, 123
  identifying probabilities, 119–120
  specifying the decision problem and its com-
    ponents, 118
  valuing consequences, 120–121
Statistical Abstract of the United States, 72,
  237
Study design, 35–42, 58–59
  recommendations regarding, 211
Study perspective, 59
Study question, 13, 160
Study results, comparability of, 25
Summary measures, 12, 24
  calculating, 67, 144–148
  determining which one to use, 144–148
  incremental, 147–148
Supply costs, 65
Surrogate measures, 43–44
Surveys, data from, 85
Synthesis models, 40–41
Systemic changes, 7

Target population, 107–108, 161–162, 218
    defined, 107
Terminal nodes, 110
Tertiary prevention, defined, 8
Threshold analysis, 115–116, 174
Threshold effect, 142–143
Time diaries, 64–65
Time frame, 12, 108, 160–161, 218
    vs. analytic horizon, 17–19
    defined, 17, 108, 160
Time horizon, 17
Time period, factors in selecting, 59–60
Time preference, 23, 212
Time series, 38
Time trade-off, 82–83
Tornado diagrams, 174
Total cost (TC), 56, 169
Total outcomes, 169
Transition probabilities, 119–120
Treat *vs.* no-treat options/strategies, 113, 115, 116
TREEPLAN, 216

Uncertainty, 23–24, 82, 104–105
    evaluating, 114–117, 124
    sources of, 12
Unit cost, 60–61

Utility, 32, 82
    defined, 105–106
    expected, 106
Utility analysis, 111
Utility assessment for health outcomes, 112
Utility scale, 112

Value score, 82
Valuing benefits/outcomes, mistakes in, 143–144
Variable (program) costs, 55–56, 64–65
Volunteer time, 65–66

Weak dominance, 172
Welfare economics, 127
Willingness to accept (WTA), 140
Willingness-to-pay (WTP), 139–141, 142–143
World Bank AIDS Economics, 238
World Bank Health Nutrition and Population Stats (HNPStats), 238
World Health Organization Statistical Information System (WHOSIS), 238

Years of Healthy Life (YHL), 80